DERMATOSCOPY

AND SKIN CANCER

UPDATED EDITION

DERMATOSCOPY AND SKIN CANCER

A HANDBOOK FOR HUNTERS OF SKIN CANCER AND MELANOMA

CLIFF ROSENDAHL

Professor, Faculty of Medicine, The University of Queensland, Australia

AKSANA MAROZAVA

MD, Dermatology Resident at Vitebsk State Medical University, Belarus

Scion

© **Scion Publishing Ltd, 2023**

ISBN 9781914961205

Updated edition published 2023
First edition published 2019

A CIP catalogue record for this book is available from the British Library.

Scion Publishing Limited

The Old Hayloft, Vantage Business Park, Bloxham Road, Banbury OX16 9UX, UK

www.scionpublishing.com

Important Note from the Publisher

The information contained within this book was obtained by Scion Publishing Ltd from sources believed by us to be reliable. However, while every effort has been made to ensure its accuracy, no responsibility for loss or injury whatsoever occasioned to any person acting or refraining from action as a result of information contained herein can be accepted by the authors or publishers.

Readers are reminded that medicine is a constantly evolving science and while the authors and publishers have ensured that all dosages, applications and practices are based on current indications, there may be specific practices which differ between communities. You should always follow the guidelines laid down by the manufacturers of specific products and the relevant authorities in the country in which you are practising.

Although every effort has been made to ensure that all owners of copyright material have been acknowledged in this publication, we would be pleased to acknowledge in subsequent reprints or editions any omissions brought to our attention.

Registered names, trademarks, etc. used in this book, even when not marked as such, are not to be considered unprotected by law.

Cover photograph kindly provided by Brian Mallon, University of Queensland, Australia

Typeset by Evolution Design & Digital Ltd, Kent, UK
Printed in the UK

Last digit is the print number: 10 9 8 7 6 5 4 3 2 1

Contents

CHAPTER 5
The skin examination

CHAPTER 6
'Chaos and Clues' (Chaos, Clues and Exceptions): a decision algorithm for pigmented skin lesions

CHAPTER 7
'Prediction without Pigment': a decision algorithm for non-pigmented skin lesions

Preface

Fifty years ago when I entered my first year of medical studies in 1969, the same year that Neil Armstrong stepped onto the moon, dermatoscopy as we know it was science fiction. Much has changed. Dermatoscopy is now standard of care in the management of skin cancer and melanoma.

My interest in this novel science became focused after a family member, Graham, developed metastatic melanoma. Graham did not blame the GP who dismissed a lesion of concern on his thigh a couple of years earlier, and he made the point to me that GPs were not prepared for this challenge in their training, a challenge that was thrust on them due to a rising incidence of melanoma and an inexplicable shortage of dermatologists in Australia. Graham's GP looked after him well. Right up to the moment of his death, a death which was predictably terrible, aggravated by multi-organ metastases and finally necrotising fasciitis.

My journey since then, commencing with a PhD expertly supervised by David Wilkinson and Peter Soyer and focused on improving skin cancer management in Australia, has been a very steep learning curve. I have been mentored by men of undoubted genius: Harald Kittler and David Weedon, men whose genius was only matched by their generosity. I have been assisted by exceptional colleagues: Ian McColl, Iris Zalaudek, Alan Cameron, Jeff Keir, Greg Canning, Phil Tschandl, Agata Bulinska, Simon Clark and Nisa Akay. I am particularly grateful to Harald Kittler, Stephen Hayes and Jeff Keir for their critical review of the book and to Simon Clark for reviewing and correcting the dermatopathology chapter.

This book would never have been possible without my co-author Aksana Marozava. Aksana worked with me for two years, taught me how to do a skin examination and dispelled any delusions of grandeur by repeatedly discovering significant lesions I had passed over. Her diligence and skill in collating my image collection for the book and preparing all of the graphics has hopefully made this book the masterpiece we wanted to produce.

The hunting metaphor is no accident. Hunting and gathering (Aksana insists that she is a gatherer) are as natural to *Homo sapiens* as is falling in love. The romance and thrill of the hunt elevates what we do to more than the drudgery of repetitive work, and the satisfaction of every success motivates further effort.

Finally, I am indebted to my wife Debbie for putting up with me through this journey and for effectively managing our practice and business affairs so I could focus on hunting, research, teaching and writing.

To conclude, I quote Vice Admiral Horatio Nelson, hunter extraordinaire, speaking at the battle of Copenhagen in 1801:

"It is warm work; and this day may be the last to any of us at a moment. But mark you! I would not be elsewhere for thousands".

Cliff Rosendahl
Brisbane March 2019

Foreword

This new book is an important step forward in the developing art and science of dermatoscopy for skin lesion recognition. The debate as to whether the technique is any good is surely over, but more help as to how to best do it, and (vitally) to best teach it, is most welcome.

Over the last decade or so, Cliff Rosendahl, and more recently Aksana Marozava, have documented some 19,000 excised skin lesions in Cliff's clinic in Capalaba, Brisbane, and fed the data into the SCARD online database which he set up with Tobias Wilson. This book summarises the knowledge gained from the analysis of that histopathological data and the lesion images, plain and dermatoscopic. The sheer scale of the data behind this book gives it an authority that can't be ignored.

The book is built around two algorithms, 'Chaos and Clues' and 'Prediction without Pigment' which, as explained, may not always lead to a diagnosis, but to a safe decision as to whether excision is required. The selected colour images illustrate well the dermatoscopic features and terms set out in the text.

Cliff is fully committed to revised pattern analysis and the use of what he calls objective geometric terminology to describe dermatoscopic structures, building on the 'descriptive' terminology often associated with co-worker Harald Kittler of Vienna. There are no 'arborising' vessels here (if vessels are 'tree like', then what sort of tree?) but branched serpentine (admittedly, 'serpentine', i.e. snake-like, is still a metaphor, but a much more consistent one than tree-like). And it is further explained that the apparent sharp focus of such vessels in BCC is due to the superficial cutaneous vascular plexus being clarified by the translucent BCC stroma, rather than that vessel morphology being unique to BCC.

There is more basic science here than is usual in a book aimed at beginners, but the extra effort put into appreciating the embryology, anatomy and histopathology pays rewards, particularly with regard to dermatoscopic–pathological correlation. Recognising structures like blue clods and polarising-specific white lines is good, but understanding what they mean at the microanatomical level gives insight into the modus operandi of the target of the hunt: malignant tissue.

More recently described signs such as white circles in early invasive SCC and angulated lines and polygons in melanoma *in situ* are detailed. I have witnessed Cliff working in his clinic and I can say that the author has a zero tolerance approach to such lesions, with approximately 80% of the melanomas diagnosed in his clinic being pre-invasive.

Dermatoscopy and Skin Cancer is a more challenging read than some earlier textbooks on this subject, but builds on hard-won, audit-backed knowledge to take us to the next level of advanced pattern analysis. It can be commended to the beginner/improver and indeed expert, who is willing to put in some work to embrace the latest evidence-based approach and terminology, which seems likely to supersede the earlier algorithms based on metaphorical language. This may mean some effort for those of us who learned dermoscopy/dermatoscopy with terms like maple leaf, arborising, comedo-like, ovoid nests, etc., but the new approach makes sense

if for no other reasons than the need for trans-
lation and utility for international research, for
dermatoscopy is now highly globalised.

Dr Stephen Hayes
Independent dermatoscopy educator
Associate Specialist in Dermatology, University Hospital Southampton
UK board member, International Dermoscopy Society

Abbreviations

AK	actinic keratosis
BCC	basal cell carcinoma
DF	dermatofibroma
DOPA	dihydroxyphenylalanine
EFG	elevated, firm and continuously growing
H&E	haematoxylin and eosin
KA	keratoacanthoma
LN	lymph nodes
LPLK	lichen planus-like keratosis
MHC	major histocompatibility complex
Naevus	melanocytic naevus
NMSC	non-melanoma skin cancer
PAM	primary acquired melanosis
pBCC	pigmented basal cell carcinoma
pIEC	pigmented intraepidermal carcinoma
pSCC	pigmented squamous cell carcinoma
RPA	revised pattern analysis
RPE	retinal pigmented epithelial
RR	relative risk
SCARD	skin cancer audit research database
SCC	squamous cell carcinoma
UV	ultraviolet

CHAPTER 1

Introduction to dermatoscopy

 ## 1.1 Why use a dermatoscope?

"Melanoma writes its message on the skin with its own ink and it is there for all to see.
Unfortunately, some see but do not comprehend."
Neville Davis; Modern concepts of melanoma and its management;
Annals of Plastic Surgery, 1978

Since Neville Davis made this statement the advent of dermatoscopy has facilitated earlier diagnosis of melanoma, as well as enhancing diagnostic accuracy for many dermatological conditions both benign and malignant[1]. The handheld dermatoscope is a recent innovation, having first become available in 1987, but there has been a rapid proliferation of research commensurate with the utility and efficacy of this relatively inexpensive instrument. Studies have demonstrated that dermatoscopy improves diagnostic accuracy for pigmented skin malignancies, both melanocytic[2] (naevus and melanoma) and non-melanocytic[3] (basal cell carcinoma (BCC) and squamous cell carcinoma (SCC)), to the extent that it is now standard of care in Australasia for any clinician treating pigmented skin lesions[4]. It has now also been shown that dermatoscopy improves diagnostic accuracy for non-pigmented skin lesions[5] and it is also being increasingly applied to the diagnosis of many inflammatory skin conditions. Not only is dermatoscopy useful for the diagnosis of skin conditions, but it has also been shown to be effective for application in skin cancer surgery, where surgical margins are significantly more likely to be adequate when dermatoscopy is utilised at preoperative

marking[6]. The dermatoscope is an essential tool for dermatologists and, with skin conditions accounting for up to 14.8% of all consultations in general practice[7], there is a compelling argument that it is as applicable for general practitioners (GPs) as the stethoscope (*Figure 1.1*)[8].

1.1.1 The economic impact of dermatoscopy

An American study in 2016 found that the economic costs avoided by diagnosing melanoma 6 months earlier justified over 100 (170 when loss of earnings was considered) benign biopsies[9]. Anything that achieves the same rate of diagnosis and therefore prevention of delayed diagnosis, with greater specificity, will achieve these savings with a smaller investment.

An Australian primary care-based study found that generalist GPs performed 17 benign biopsies for each melanoma treated, whereas GPs subspecialised in skin cancer practice, who also had a high use of dermatoscopy, discovered one melanoma for every 8.5 biopsies[10]. This suggests that with respect to the management of melanoma alone, derma-

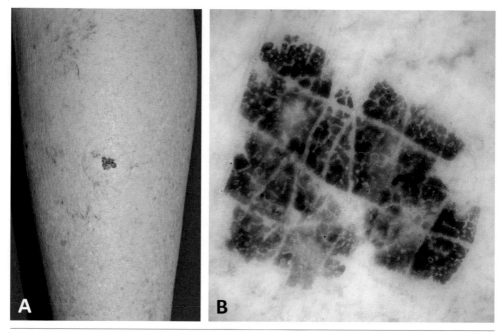

Figure 1.1: *Clinically (A) this irregular pigmented lesion is suspicious for malignancy, but dermatoscopically (B) it has the unequivocal morphology of a seborrhoeic keratosis (see Figure 9.80).*

toscopy could result in economic savings by earlier detection with fewer unnecessary excisions.

It is not unusual in current dermatology and primary care practice for a biopsy to precede many therapeutic surgical procedures for both pigmented and non-pigmented lesions. While suspected melanomas should have an initial excisional biopsy, we have found that with the advent of dermatoscopy and increased diagnostic confidence, a preliminary partial biopsy procedure is not necessary for the majority of suspected non-melanoma skin cancers (NMSC). Unpublished raw data from the skin cancer audit research database (SCARD) gives a snapshot of current practice in Australasia of 848 primary care doctors, either practising in dedicated skin cancer practices or in general practices with a special interest in skin cancer. Of 429,010 specimens of NMSC treated surgically, 316,339 (73.73%) were managed in a 1-step approach, without a preceding biopsy[11]. This suggests that a proportion of primary care doctors are already managing NMSC through a 1-step process in the majority of cases.

There are many advantages of proceeding directly to curative surgical management following a confident dermatoscopic diagnosis. These include the fact that margins are more likely to be more clearly definable without the inflammation that is expected after a partial biopsy. A single procedure is more convenient for the patient and, when the costs of one rather than two surgical episodes and dermatopathological assessments are considered, the economic saving is approximately 50%.

1.2 What is a dermatoscope?

A dermatoscope is essentially a magnifying glass which eliminates surface reflection from the skin by using either a fluid inter-face (non-polarising contact dermatoscopes) or polarising filters (polarising contact or non-contact dermatoscopes) (*Figure 1.2*). This allows pigmented structures to be seen to the level of the deep dermis, up to 1mm into the skin, as well as blood vessels in the dermis when they are not obscured by pigment. A built-in light source allows the device to be used as a compact handheld instrument. Even the early dermatoscopes provided adequate visual information but initial studies were burdened by the need for expensive film photography. The advent of new dermatoscopes with even brighter optics, as well as with the option of polarised light sources, was paralleled by the availability of digital photography. This has facilitated the convenient forwarding of captured images for purposes including research and teledermatoscopy.

Although polarising dermatoscopes can be used without interface fluid, visualisation of structures can be improved with fluid and all the images displayed in this book are taken with fluid immersion, whether the dermatoscope was in polarised mode or not. Initially the interface fluid of choice was oil but that is rarely used now. Alcohol-based fluids (70% ethanol in water, isopropanol in water or alcohol hand gel) are just as effective and have the advantage of having an antiseptic effect as well as of drying very quickly. Ultrasound gel is useful with thicker lesions such as keratoacanthoma (KA) or when examining complex curved surfaces such as the nail unit. Even the use of a sterile alcohol wipe can be effective. Whatever fluid is used should be wiped from the dermatoscope footplate after use for hygienic purposes as well as to protect the footplate from a build-up of residue.

It has been claimed that polarised dermatoscopy provides a superior view of vessel structures – we have found that to be related to footplate pressure rather than to polarisation. Of course, when polarised dermatoscopes are used in non-contact mode vessels will not be compressed. The same can be achieved in contact mode with non-polarised or polarised dermatoscopy if less footplate pressure is applied to the lesion. Sometimes the use of thicker contact fluid such as hand gel or ultrasound gel may facilitate this.

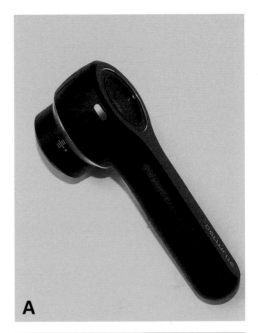

A

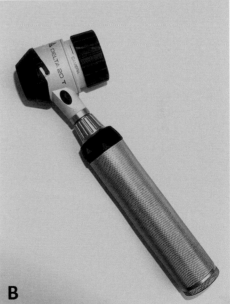

B

Figure 1.2: Dermatoscopes are available from a variety of companies. (A) The DermLite DL4 (3Gen) and (B) the Heine delta 20T (Heine Corporation) both default to polarised mode but can easily be switched to non-polarised mode.

Melanin

The main pigment influencing the colour of fair skin is haem. In people with darker skin

1.3 # Colours in dermatoscopy

The colours seen through a dermatoscope
are shown in *Figure 1.3*.

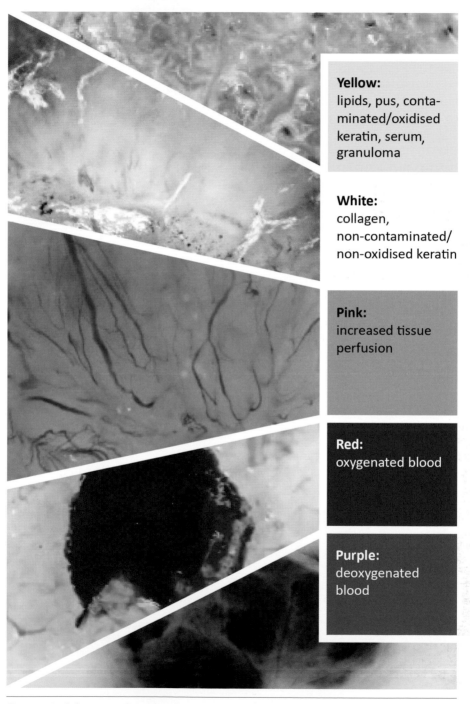

Yellow:
lipids, pus, conta-
minated/oxidised
keratin, serum,
granuloma

White:
collagen,
non-contaminated/
non-oxidised keratin

Pink:
increased tissue
perfusion

Red:
oxygenated blood

Purple:
deoxygenated
blood

Figure 1.3: Colours seen through a dermatoscope and their correlations.

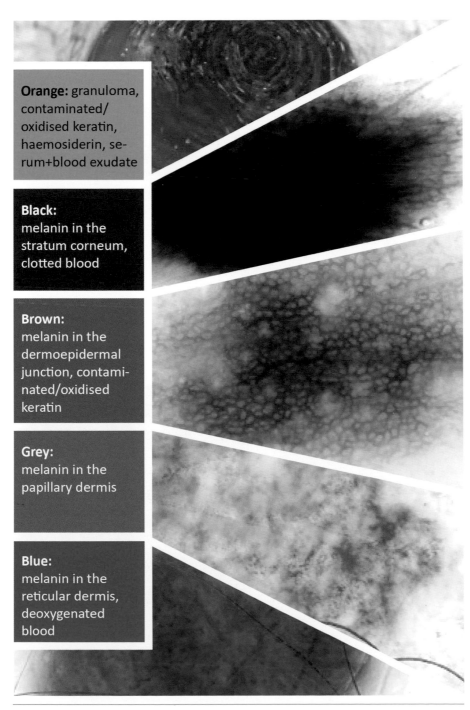

Orange: granuloma, contaminated/oxidised keratin, haemosiderin, serum+blood exudate

Black: melanin in the stratum corneum, clotted blood

Brown: melanin in the dermoepidermal junction, contaminated/oxidised keratin

Grey: melanin in the papillary dermis

Blue: melanin in the reticular dermis, deoxygenated blood

Figure 1.3: continued.

phototypes the melanin concentrated in the epidermis obscures the colour of haem (with the exception of glabrous skin of the palms and soles) and the skin, where pigmented, appears brown.

The colour of melanin in the skin varies according to its depth; the reasons for this, including the Tyndall effect, are explained in *Chapter 2*. Melanin near the surface of the skin appears black at the level of the stratum corneum, brown at the dermoepidermal junction, grey in the superficial dermis and blue in the deeper dermis. This differential colour of melanin at different depths means that the dermatoscopist is actually getting 3-dimensional information, and can often make predictions about the biological behaviour of a tumour from the colours of structures observed through the dermatoscope.

Keratin

Keratin observed through the dermatoscope is white when not pigmented by melanin,

but can vary from yellow through orange to brown if it is pigmented. Pigmented keratin, in horn cysts projecting beneath the dermis in elongated rete ridges in seborrhoeic keratoses, appears blue for the same reasons that melanin in melanocytes in the deep dermis appears blue (see *Figure 1.4*).

Collagen

Collagen laid down in scar tissue or following an immune attack with regression is white.

Blood

The colour of blood varies from red through purple to blue, depending on the degree of oxygenation (red when most oxygenated).

Other

Lipids, sebum, serum and pus, as well as some granulomas, present as dermatoscopic yellow/orange. Exogenous pigment (including tattoo pigment) can present in a variety of colours.

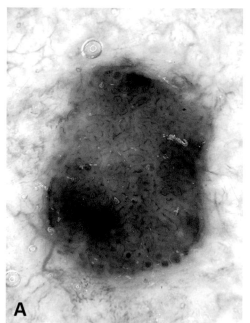
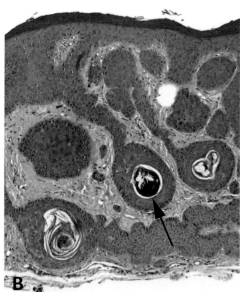

Figure 1.4: *(A) Dermatoscopic and (B) histological images of a seborrhoeic keratosis. A heavily pigmented horn pseudocyst (arrow in B) located in the epidermis but projecting beneath the dermis appears blue on dermatoscopy due to the Tyndall effect.*

1.4 Differences between polarised and non-polarised dermatoscopy

Early studies all used images taken with non-polarised dermatoscopes with fluid immersion used to eliminate the glare caused by reflection of light by the stratum corneum. When dermatoscopes fitted with polarising filters for this purpose were introduced by 3Gen in 2001, it simplified the process of examination because contact fluid was no longer routinely necessary (see *Table 1.1*). However, there are differences in the rendition of colours and structures that must be considered. Non-po-

larised dermatoscopy, being unfiltered, renders colours without modification. This means that the very important colours of grey and blue, which correlate with melanin in the dermis, are more accurately displayed (*Figure 1.5*). This can be crucial in some malignancies in which the only clue to malignancy is the presence of grey colour. Also, the orange clods and bright white dots and clods found in many seborrhoeic keratoses and congenital naevi are only fully revealed with non-polarised dermatoscopy;

Table 1.1: *Important differences between non-polarised and polarised dermatoscopy*

Non-polarised dermatoscopy	Polarised dermatoscopy
• Fluid immersion essential	• Fluid immersion not essential
• Accurate grey–blue rendition	• Impaired grey–blue rendition
• Accurate white clod/dot rendition	• Impaired white clod/dot rendition
• Polarising-specific structures not seen	• Polarising-specific structures seen

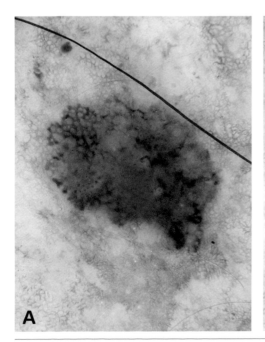
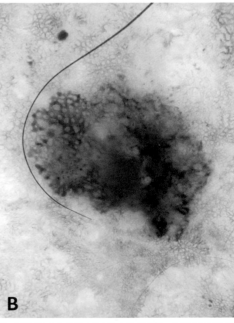

Figure 1.5: *(A) Non-polarised and (B) polarised dermatoscopy of an invasive melanoma. Polarising filters reduce the viewed spectrum of light and therefore grey and blue colours are not as vividly displayed.*

for this reason a non-polarised dermatoscope may be necessary to resolve the diagnosis in these situations, thus preventing unnecessary surgery (*Figure 1.6*).

With increased use of polarised dermatoscopes it became apparent that although these instruments were at times problematic (due to the rendition of certain colours due to selective filtering by polarisation), they did, however, display three types of structures not seen with non-polarised dermatoscopy. It has been shown that dermatoscopes may vary in their rendition of polarising-specific features and that may include not displaying them at all[12].

Polarising-specific white lines

These structures are known to be a valuable clue to the malignancies of BCC and melanoma, as well as the benign conditions dermatofibroma and Spitz naevus. It has been shown that the diagnosis of melanoma can actually depend on this clue (*Figure 1.7*)[13]. Polarising-specific white lines have a distinct

morphology, being straight and oriented perpendicularly to each other. Blue polarising-specific lines with this morphology have the same diagnostic significance (*Figure 1.8*).

Polarising-specific structureless areas

The second polarising-specific feature, polarising-specific structureless areas, are seen frequently over BCC (*Figure 1.9*).

Four-dot clods

The third polarising-specific structure is four bright white dots arranged in a square (4-dot clods), also known as a rosette, which is commonly seen over actinic keratoses (AK, *Figure 1.10*) but also on otherwise normal sun-damaged skin and, not infrequently, on sun-damaged skin on melanomas.

These three polarising-specific clues can be seen in both pigmented and non-pigmented lesions and they may all be altered by rotation of the dermatoscope, consistent with the representation of altered optical qualities of the tissue being examined.

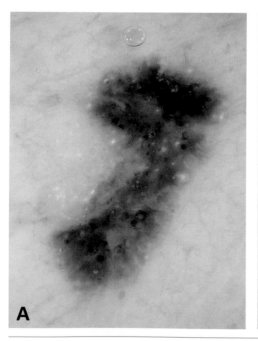 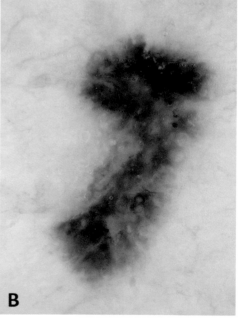

Figure 1.6: *(A) Non-polarised and (B) polarised dermatoscopy of a seborrhoeic keratosis. The non-polarised mode displays the white clods which are not seen with polarised dermatoscopy. Image from* Dermatoscopy: pattern analysis of pigmented and non-pigmented lesions *(Kittler et al., 2016, Facultas).*

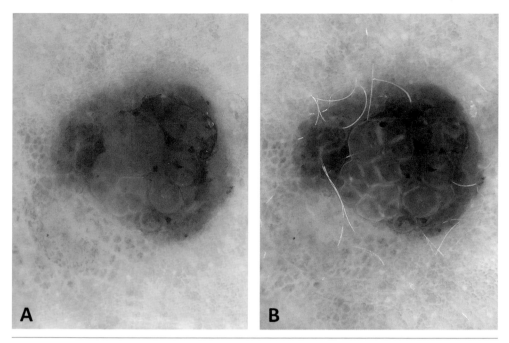

Figure 1.7: *Polarising-specific white lines (B) are the only clue to malignancy in an invasive melanoma arising in a congenital naevus[13], not being seen with non-polarised dermatoscopy (A). Note that terminal hairs are present in the naevus part of the lesion but not in the melanoma. Reproduced from* Dermatol Pract Concept, 2014:4:8312 *with permission from the authors.*

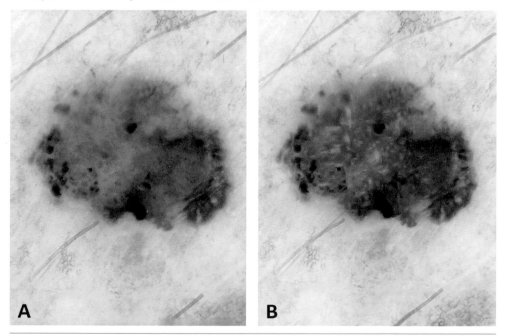

Figure 1.8: *While polarising filters reduce the grey, blue and white in the visible light spectrum they also produce polarising-specific effects. Blue polarising-specific lines in this invasive melanoma (B) have the same significance as white polarising-specific lines. No lines are seen in the non-polarised image (A) but the structureless blue colour is vividly displayed.*

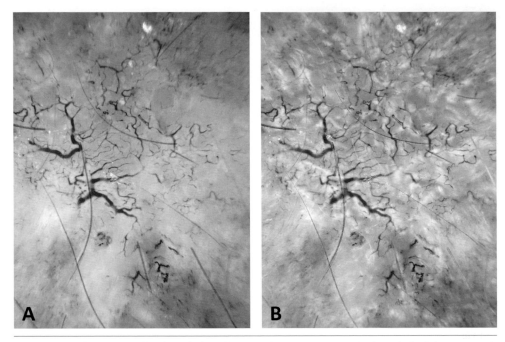

Figure 1.9: *Polarising-specific white clods and structureless areas are seen in the polarised dermatoscopic image of a basal cell carcinoma (B), whereas non-polarised dermatoscopy (A) shows only a large white structureless area.*

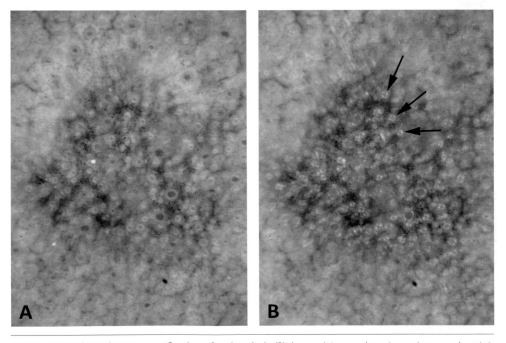

Figure 1.10: *The polarising-specific clue of 4-dot clods (B) (arrows) is seen here in a pigmented actinic keratosis. In the non-polarised view (A) these are seen to correlate with adnexal openings.*

1.5 Uses of dermatoscopy for conditions other than tumours

This book is focused on the use of dermatoscopy in the diagnosis of skin tumours, particularly malignancies, but dermatoscopy can also be applied to the diagnosis of other disorders of the skin, nails and hair.

1.5.1 Dermatoscopy of perilesional skin

The dermatoscopic background to lesions on the skin is variable according to features such as skin type, anatomical location, solar damage and iatrogenic factors including scars and tattoos. Dermatoscopy relies on melanin-pigmented structures, as well as structures containing keratin and collagen, and vascular structures pigmented by haem. Intact perilesional skin forms a uniform struc-

tureless background interrupted by adnexal openings upon which vascular structures may or may not be seen. Where skin is not sun-damaged, traumatised or inflamed, no vascular patterns are expected (*Figure 1.11A*). The context of perilesional skin is important when assessing the significance of lesional pigmented structures. As an example, pigmented circles on the face correlating with hair follicles, which can be a clue to malignancy, are commonly seen on normal facial skin with darker skin phototypes.

Sun-damaged skin is frequently encountered in the context of examination for skin cancer. It differs from normal skin in a variety of ways, including atrophy of the dermis, effacement of the dermoepidermal junction with flattening of the rete ridges, and elastosis

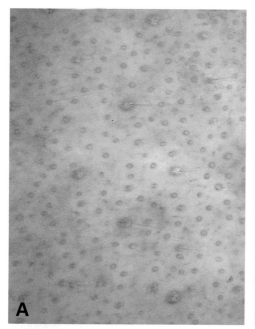
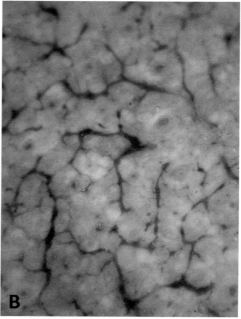

Figure 1.11: (A) Dermatoscopy of normal skin on the cheek of a 38-year-old woman displays a structureless pattern interrupted by adnexal openings. This pattern is more complex on the sun-damaged skin on the face of an 83-year-old man (B), with branched vessels of superficial dermal vascular plexus clearly visible through the atrophic superficial dermis.

in the dermis involving an alteration in the collagen and elastic tissue. Dermal atrophy can increase the visibility of the horizontal dermal vascular plexus and this may appear as a reticular or serpentine-branched vessel pattern on some perilesional skin (*Figure 1.11B*).

The dermatoscopist is encouraged to take note of perilesional skin on all patients because there is an abundance of this to inspect and it achieves the definition of 'baseline' dermatoscopy, which varies between individuals.

1.5.2 Dermatoscopy of inflammatory conditions and dermatoses

Where blood flow is increased by inflammatory conditions such as psoriasis or dermatitis the most superficial vessels, the dermal papillae vessels, normally become apparent as a pattern of dot or coiled vessels. More significant inflammation or epidermal atrophy due to solar damage may cause dermal plexus vessels to become visible as a linear serpentine or reticular pattern, and where this happens the dermal papillary vessels assume less significance although they may still be seen. Apart from vessel pattern, inflammatory conditions and dermatoses may be associated with surface scale (e.g. psoriasis), excoriation, exudation, erosion, traumatic ulceration and exfoliation, all with associated dermatoscopic changes as well as with white structures associated with fibrosis following lichenoid reactions.

It is useful to take time to examine clinically apparent inflammatory dermatoses such as eczema, psoriasis and tinea so as to become familiar with the dermatoscopic appearance of these conditions. Although the diagnosis is often evident, a single lesion of psoriasis can be mistaken for AK or SCC *in situ* and familiarisation with the dermatoscopic features of psoriasis may prevent such an error.

1.5.3 Dermatoscopy of hair

Trichoscopy[14] (hair and scalp dermatoscopy) is relevant to the diagnosis of hair and scalp disorders, but it is not specifically relevant to the diagnosis of skin tumours so is only mentioned here in passing.

1.5.4 Dermatoscopy of skin infestations and infections

Entomodermatoscopy[15] is useful for the diagnosis of skin infections and infestations (such as scabies), but is also not specifically relevant to the diagnosis of skin tumours so is only mentioned here for completeness.

1.5.5 Dermatoscopy of nails

The dermatoscopic appearance of the nail apparatus is very relevant to the diagnosis and management of tumours at that location. Dermatoscopy of the normal nail plate, distal nail matrix (at the level of the lunula), cuticle, proximal nail fold (including nail fold capillaries), lateral nail folds and hyponychium is freely available to every dermatoscopist on any number of patients and familiarity gained by such examination is a prerequisite to recognising pathology. For example, normal nails frequently show a degree of ridging and even mild changes of erythronychia (pink stripe) and so familiarity with what is normal variation is useful in weighing the significance of changes. Similarly, nail plate dystrophy is very common and the dermatoscopist should become familiar with the range of features by examining cases where the involvement of multiple nails supports the diagnosis of benign dystrophy. As with dermatoscopy at any body site it is important to first become familiar with what is either normal, or not suggestive of malignancy.

References

1. Rosendahl C. Dermatoscopy in general practice. *Br J Dermatol*, 2016;175:673.

2. Vestergaard ME, Macaskill P, Holt PE, and Menzies SW. Dermoscopy compared with naked eye examination for the diagnosis of primary melanoma: a meta-analysis of studies performed in a clinical setting. *Br J Dermatol*, 2008;159:669.

3. Rosendahl C, Tschandl P, Cameron A, and Kittler H. Diagnostic accuracy of dermatoscopy for melanocytic and nonmelanocytic pigmented lesions. *J Am Acad Dermatol*, 2011;64:1068.

4. Clinical practice guidelines for the management of melanoma in Australia and New Zealand. Cancer Council Australia and Australian Cancer Network, Sydney and New Zealand Guidelines Group, Wellington, 2008;xxii.

5. Sinz C, Tschandl P, Rosendahl C, *et al*. Accuracy of dermatoscopy for the diagnosis of nonpigmented cancers of the skin. *J Am Acad Dermatol*, 2017;77:1100.

6. Caresana G, and Giardini R. Dermoscopy-guided surgery in basal cell carcinoma. *J Eur Acad Dermatol Venereol*, 2010;24:1395.

7. Britt H, Miller GC, Charles J, *et al*. General practice activity in Australia 2009–2010. General Practice Series no. 27 cat.no. GEP 27. Canberra: AIHW. Available from: www.aihw. gov.au/publication-detail/?id=6442472433 [accessed 18 Mar 2011].

8. Rosendahl C, Cameron A, McColl I, and Wilkinson D. Dermatoscopy in routine practice – "Chaos and Clues." *Aust Fam Physician*, 2012;41:482.

9. Aires DJ, Wick J, Shaath TS, *et al*. Economic costs avoided by diagnosing melanoma six months earlier justify >100 benign biopsies. *J Drugs Dermatol*, 2016;15:527.

10. Rosendahl C, Williams G, Eley D, *et al*. The impact of subspecialization and dermatoscopy use on accuracy of melanoma diagnosis among primary care doctors in Australia. *J Am Acad Dermatol*, 2012;67:846.

11. SCARD Skin Cancer Audit Research Database. https://scard.co/ [accessed 2 Feb 2018].

12. Whybrew C, Pietkiewicz P, Kohut I, Chia JC, Akay BN, Rosendahl C. Not all polarized-light dermatoscopes may display diagnostically critical polarizing-specific features. *Dermatol Pract Concept*, 2022; in press.

13. Cohen YK, Elpern DJ, Wolpowitz D, and Rosendahl C. Glowing in the dark: case report of a clue-poor melanoma unmasked by polarized dermatoscopy. *Dermatol Pract Concept*, 2014;4:83.

14. Romero JAM, and Grimalt R. Trichoscopy: essentials for the dermatologist. *World J Dermatol*, 2015;4(2):63.

15. Tschandl P, Argenziano G, Bakos R, *et al*. Dermoscopy and entomology (entomodermoscopy). *J Dtsch Dermatol Ges*, 2009;7:589.

CHAPTER 2

Skin – the organ

2.1 Skin as an organ

Skin was the first organ to evolve in multi-cellular organisms and, weighing approximately 4kg over a surface area of 2m^2, it is the largest organ in the human body[1]. Because skin covers the external surface it is vulnerable to injury from many sources, including incident radiation, and so unsurprisingly it is the most common site of malignancy. For the same reason those malignancies are more accessible to direct visual inspection, making the development of tools to assist such inspection highly relevant. Knowledge of the microanatomy and physiology of skin is fundamental to an understanding of dermatoscopic correlation in relation to pigmented, collagen and keratin structures, as well as with respect to vascular structures and patterns.

The significance of certain patterns and clues vary according to anatomical site and this is particularly relevant on the head and neck, in the nail apparatus and on volar skin.

Finally, skin type as defined in the Fitzpatrick phototype classification, influences both patterns of disease prevalence and the interpretation of dermatoscopic clues.

2.2 Embryology of skin

After fertilisation of the ova by a spermatozoon, a single pluripotent cell, the zygote, carries the genetic blueprint for a unique integrated individual which commences life as a developing embryo. This genetic material will launch a cascade of events where each stage in the sequence leads to subsequent ones throughout the development, growth, maturation, reproduction and decline of that individual, until terminated by death. The resulting progression will include the differentiation of multiple cell types and their organisation into organs, including the first organ to evolve in multicellular organisms, the skin[1].

Immune system

Development of the embryo includes the differentiation and integration of the components of an immune system. Invertebrates develop an innate immune system which responds to an immune attack in a generic manner, but vertebrates also develop an adaptive immune system which allows them to tailor an immune response to specific antigens[2]. Both responses are employed in the vertebrate's response to tumours, including skin tumours. Sexual reproduction is relevant because it provides a virtually infinite number of potential combinations of genetic material relevant to the innate and adaptive immune systems, for forces of natural selection to sort and select or reject. This gives the species the greatest chance of surviving in a hostile and changing environment.

Formation of the skin precursors: the ectoderm, neural crest and mesoderm

After fertilisation and formation of the zygote, the process of cell division forms a hollow ball or 'blastula' and then it undergoes 'gastrulation' (*Figure 2.1*)[1]. A pouch forms at one end of the blastula and bulges into its centre so that a 3-layered structure or 'gastrula' is formed. The outer layer of cells is the ectoderm and the inner layer of cells formed by the pouch is the endoderm. The pouch will eventually form the gut, with the opening of the pouch, the blastopore, being its excretory orifice. The mesoderm will develop between the ectoderm and endoderm in the space labelled blastocoele in the image on the far right of *Figure 2.1*.

During the fourth week of embryo development, the single cell thick ectoderm and underlying mesoderm begin to proliferate and differentiate. The neural crest develops from the ectoderm as do specialised structures formed from skin elements, including sebaceous glands, sweat glands, apocrine glands, mammary glands, fingernails and toenails. The teeth and hair follicles formed from both the ectoderm and the mesoderm also begin to appear during this period.

Melanocytes

The neural crest develops from the ectoderm and melanocytes are derived from neural crest cells produced at the dorsal neural tube, from where they migrate to the basal layer of the epidermis to populate all parts of the skin[3]. Also, growing nerves projecting throughout the body as a stem/progenitor niche, contain Schwann cell precursors, from which some skin melanocytes also originate[4,5].

The migration of melanocytes proceeds in a cephalad-to-caudal and axial-to-peripheral sequence. By week 8 melanocytes are present both in the dermis and in the basal layer of the epidermis, as well as in the hair bulbs, choroid, inner ear and pia arachnoid[6]. This melanocyte migration may lead to 'rests' of naevus precursor melanocytes within the dermis, explaining the appearance of congenital naevi later in life as well as possibly explaining the occurrence of primary dermal (nodular) melanomas. This distribution of melanocytes also accounts for melanocytosis and the risk of developing melanoma in the eye (e.g. choroid). It also explains melanoma developing in the leptomeninges that is seen in some patients with naevus of Ota, as well as the occurrence of neurocutaneous melanocytosis in patients with large and/or multiple congenital melanocytic naevi[6]. Dermal melanocytes first appear in the head and neck region, and they begin to produce pigment at a gestational age of approximately 10 weeks. However, by the time of birth, active dermal melanocytes have disappeared, with the exception of three anatomical sites – the head and neck, the dorsal aspects of the distal extremities, and the pre-sacral area. Of note, the three locations of persistent dermal melanocytes

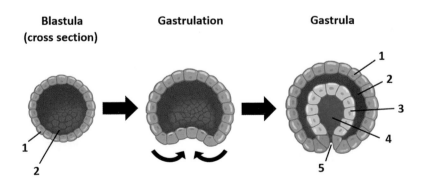

Blastula (cross section) **Gastrulation** **Gastrula**

Figure 2.1: Early stages of embryo development. 1 – ectoderm; 2 – blastocoele; 3 – endoderm; 4 – archenteron; 5 – blastopore.

correspond to the most common locations for dermal melanocytosis and blue naevi[6]. This fits with Ackerman's assertion that blue naevi are congenital[7].

Association between keratinocytes and melanocytes

The cells which derive directly from the ectoderm are called keratinocytes in recognition of their keratin-producing function. These include cells of the basal layer of the epidermis (basal cells) and squamous cells. The other major cell type located at the dermoepidermal junction, in a ratio of approximately 1:10–30 to basal cells, is the melanocyte. As described, some melanocytes migrate to that location from the neural crest via the dermis, while others derive from Schwann cell precursors.

Another cell type in the epidermis is the mobile Langerhans cell; like the melanocyte it is dendritic, but unlike the melanocyte it is of mesodermal origin derived from bone marrow and, rather than using its dendrites to transfer melanosomes to keratinocytes, it uses them to present antigens to cells of the immune system.

Merkel cells

Merkel cells are also believed to migrate from the neural crest to the epidermis.

Fibroblasts

The other major cell in the skin is the fibroblast, of mesodermal derivation, and located in the dermis where it is responsible for collagen synthesis.

Why melanomas are not carcinomas

By convention, malignant tumours are named according to the cell of origin. Those of epithelial origin (ectoderm or endoderm), being naturally continuously proliferative, are 'carcinomas'. Melanocytes, not being naturally continuously proliferative, are not epithelial and therefore melanomas are not carcinomas.

2.3 The microanatomy of skin

The skin develops as a complex organ comprising a thin outer epidermis surmounted by a barrier layer, the stratum corneum, and a thicker inner (papillary and reticular) dermis. In most parts of the body a layer of subcutaneous fat, the subcutis, is located deep to the dermis (see *Table 2.1* and *Figure 2.2*). The thickness of the epidermis varies from 0.04mm on the eyelids to 1.5mm on the soles of the feet[8] and this variation is predominantly due to variation in the thickness of the stratum corneum. In fact, if the stratum corneum is excluded the thickness of the epidermis is fairly constant at 0.1mm (it is about half that on the eyelids). This is 100μm and represents the thickness of approximately 7 full-sized keratinocytes. The thickness of the dermis varies from 0.3mm on the eyelid to 3.0mm on the back, possibly an evolutionary response to the selective force produced by the fact that predators may preferentially attack from behind.

A dermatoscope employs either fluid immersion or polarising filters for the specific purpose of rendering the stratum corneum invisible, so it is not surprising that surface keratin is generally better visualised clinically than dermatoscopically. Light from a dermatoscope is expected to pass through the stratum corneum and be reflected and/or scattered back from pigmented and keratin structures in the epidermis and pigmented structures, collagen fibrils and vascular structures in the dermis.

Tumours of the skin can be derived from any of the cells that are present in normal skin or they can be metastatic, from other organs in the body.

2.3.1 Epidermis

The epidermis is essentially a binary system of cells comprising keratinocytes and melanocytes, separated from the dermis by a basement membrane and from the external

Table 2.1: *Skin microanatomy definitions*

Epidermis: the outermost layer of the skin. Lacking blood and lymphatic vessels, nutrition and excretion are achieved by diffusion across the basement membrane which separates it from the vascular layer of the dermis.

- **Stratum corneum**: the outermost layer of the epidermis, consisting of non-viable cells with a high concentration of keratin and functioning as a barrier. Highly specialised structures derived from the stratum corneum include hair shafts and digital nails.
- **Stratum lucidum**: a clear layer separating the stratum corneum from the stratum granulosum.
- **Stratum granulosum**: a dark thin layer representing viable squamous cells (see *Figure 2.3*) with a high concentration of keratin.
- **Stratum spinosum**: the thickest layer of squamous cells named due to prominent desmosomes appearing as spines.
- **Stratum basale**: a single layer of basal cells (see below) lined up on the basement membrane (see below).
- **Keratinocyte**: the most populous cell type in the epidermis, derived from the embryonic ectodermal layer. The keratinocytes in the stratum basale are termed 'basal cells' and those located above the stratum basale are termed 'squamous cells'.
- **Melanocyte**: a cell type derived from the embryonic neural crest. Melanocytes migrate to the stratum basale of the skin via the peripheral nerves and are interspersed between basal cells in a ratio of about 1:10–30.
- **Basement membrane**: a physical membrane which separates the non-vascular epidermis from the vascular dermis.

Dermis: the layer of skin beneath the basement membrane mainly comprising water and collagen and containing blood vessels, lymphatics, nerves and adnexal structures (see below).

- **Papillary dermis**: a layer of fine, vertically orientated, collagen fibrils located immediately beneath the basement membrane.
- **Reticular dermis**: a layer of coarse, horizontally oriented collagen fibrils, which lies between the papillary dermis and the subcutis.
- **Fibroblast**: the most populous cell in the dermis and the producer of collagen.
- **Collagen**: the structural protein which contributes approximately 80% of the dry weight of the skin.
- **Adnexal structures**: eccrine (sweat glands), sebaceous and apocrine glands as well as hair follicles – all being located within the dermis, with eccrine ducts and hair follicles also traversing the epidermis.

Subcutis: located beneath the dermis, primarily composed of fat.

---

environment by a compact layer of non-viable cells, the stratum corneum (*Figure 2.3*).

Keratinocytes

Keratinocytes ('*kerato*' – Greek for '*horn*') derive from a layer of basal cells at the base of the epidermis, called the stratum basale (*Figure 2.3*). As new basal cells are formed they displace cells formed earlier, causing these cells to effectively move away from the basal layer towards the stratum corneum. Keratino-cytes are joined to each other by interlocking cytoplasmic processes, desmosomes, and by an intercellular cement of glycoproteins and lipoproteins[9]. Because the desmosomes resemble spines or prickles, this layer of cells is called the stratum spinosum (*Figures 2.3 and 2.4*). As keratinocytes migrate upwards from the basal layer they differentiate into keratin-producing cells known as squamous cells ('*squamous*' – Latin for '*scale-like*'), which extend to the level of the stratum corneum.

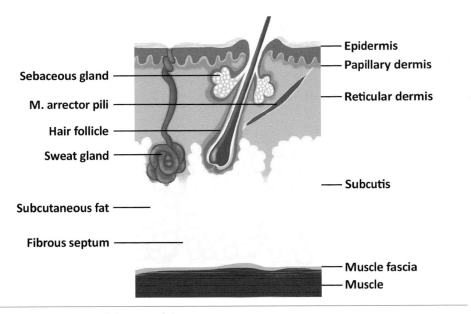

Epidermis
Papillary dermis
Reticular dermis

Sebaceous gland
M. arrector pili
Hair follicle
Sweat gland

Subcutis

Subcutaneous fat

Fibrous septum

Muscle fascia
Muscle

Figure 2.2: Cross-sectional diagram of skin.

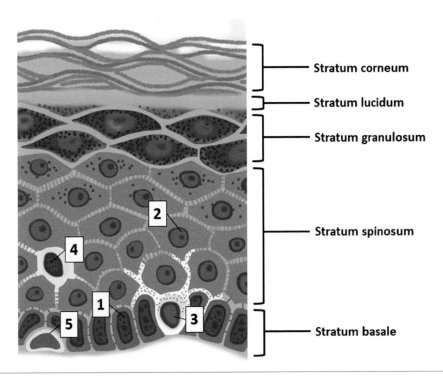

Stratum corneum
Stratum lucidum
Stratum granulosum
Stratum spinosum
Stratum basale

Figure 2.3: Diagrammatic representation of the principal layers and cells of the epidermis. Key: 1 – basal cell (keratinocyte); 2 – squamous cell (keratinocyte); 3 – melanocyte; 4 – Langerhans cell; 5 – Merkel cell.

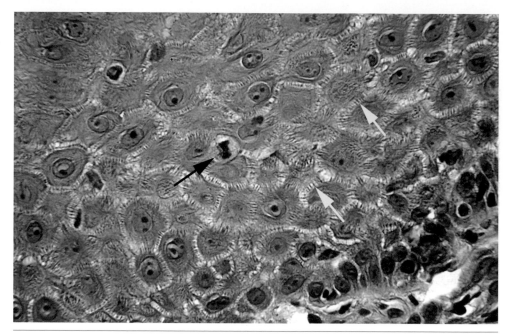

Figure 2.4: *A high-power view of a section from the stratum spinosum of the epidermis in a squamous cell carcinoma illustrating desmosomes (yellow arrows), which are seen as short linear projections between keratinocytes. A prominent mitotic figure is seen centrally (black arrow).*

The time from a basal cell being formed at the stratum basale until natural proliferation of basal cells displaces it to the level of the stratum corneum, is approximately 40–56 days in normal skin[10]. This may be accelerated in conditions such as psoriasis (7 days) and keratinocyte neoplasia.

The outermost layer of viable epidermis comprises 2–3 layers of cells containing keratohyalin granules. The keratohyalin granules make this layer of cells appear as a thin, hyperchromatic (densely coloured) layer and it is called the stratum granulosum (*Figures 2.3* and *2.5*). This layer is used as the level from which to measure the Breslow thickness of malignant skin tumours, this being defined as the distance from the stratum granulosum to the deepest malignant cell.

The stratum corneum is the final organic barrier between the individual and the external environment. It is slightly permeable to water but relatively impermeable to ions such as sodium and potassium and to substances such as glucose and urea.

Normally the cells of the stratum corneum have shed their nuclei and such stratum corneum is described as orthokeratotic ('ortho' meaning 'normal', as in orthodox) with so-called basket-weave morphology (*Figure 2.6*). This is the expected morphology on all skin surfaces except on the palms and soles, where the keratin is densely packed (compact orthokeratosis). Compact orthokeratosis can also occur in pathological skin conditions such as lichen simplex chronicus.

In pathological conditions associated with rapid proliferation of keratinocytes, such as psoriasis and squamous cell neoplasia, the stratum corneum can become thicker (hyperkeratosis) and may have cornified squamous cells that have retained their nuclei (parakeratosis) (*Figure 2.7*).

Keratin, produced by the keratinocytes in the epidermis, is a fibrous structural protein which assembles into filaments to form a semipermeable barrier as the outermost layer of skin. Keratin also forms into specialised structures including hair and nails. As

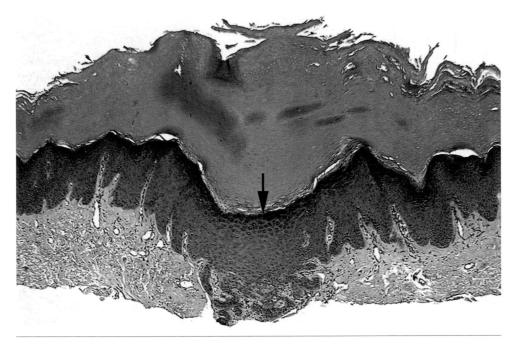

Figure 2.5: *The stratum granulosum is seen as a hyperchromatic (dark) layer (arrow) separating the stratum spinosum from the (hypertrophic) stratum corneum.*

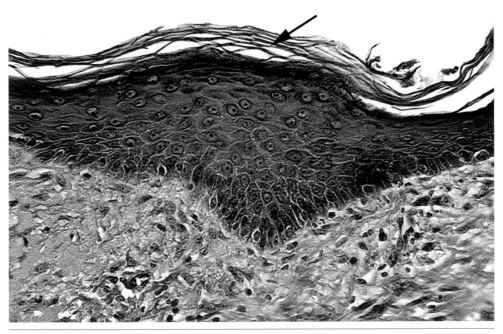

Figure 2.6: *Photomicrograph of skin showing an orthokeratotic stratum corneum in the normal basket-weave pattern (arrow).*

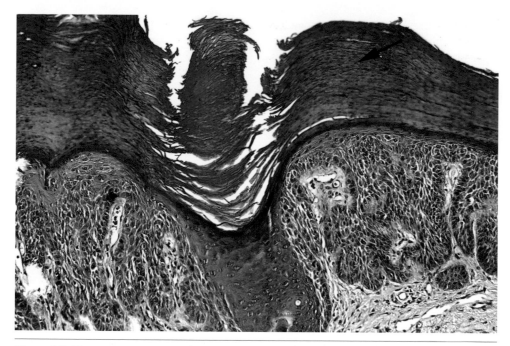

Figure 2.7: *The stratum corneum seen in this section of an actinic keratosis is thickened (hyperkeratotic). Centrally, overlying relatively normal epidermis it is dense but orthokeratotic (compact orthokeratosis), but on each side of this, where it overlies neoplastic squamous cells, the retained nuclei can be seen as fine dots (compact parakeratosis) (arrow).*

well as sometimes being dermatoscopically visible on the surface of the skin as scale (white through yellow to brown, and structureless), keratin can be seen within benign or malignant lesions as white dots and clods (commonly seen in seborrhoeic keratoses and congenital naevi) and in neoplastic lesions as surface scale, white structureless areas and white circles. Surface scale and compacted keratin are best observed clinically. The dermatoscopic clues of white structureless areas and white circles are particularly useful in the diagnosis of AK, SCC and KA. These structures correlate, respectively, with masses of highly keratinised keratinocytes (white structureless areas in SCC/KA), or invasion of hair follicles, also by highly keratinised neoplastic keratinocytes (white circles in AK and SCC/KA)[11].

Melanocytes

The other major cell type in the epidermis, apart from the keratinocyte, is the melano-cyte. As discussed in *Section 2.2* on embryology, melanocytes are thought to be derived from the neural crest and to migrate through the dermis, possibly via nerve cells, and from Schwann cell precursors in nerve fibres, ending up in the basal layer of the epidermis in a ratio to basal cells of approximately 1:10–30. While epithelial cells at all sites where they occur, including skin, are naturally proliferative, melanocytes are not. Melanocyte numbers in skin appear to increase slightly in response to UV radiation, although this certainly does not amount to proliferation. The fact that mitotic figures are not seen in melanocytes in normal skin makes it likely that the increase involves the activation of existing melanocyte precursors rather than an increase in melanocyte numbers. While continual natural proliferation of keratinocytes makes the development of dysplasia of epithelial cells (e.g. in cervix or skin) understandable, with successive mutations leading through sequential stages of neoplasia to frank malignancy, it is not appropriate to apply a similar model of dysplasia to cells such as naevomelanocytes, because they are not naturally continuously proliferative[12]. Of course, the evolution of benign melanocytes into a melanoma does involve multiple stepwise mutations in an abnormal clone of cells, most commonly in normal skin and occasionally in a naevus[13]. What is incorrect is to assume that any morphologically identifiable type of naevus is proliferative and that the naevus goes through stepwise mutations from naevus to melanoma[13].

Langerhans cells

Langerhans cells are mobile cells located both in the epidermis (at all levels) and dermis. They are dendritic cells and have no desmosomes (in both respects similar to melanocytes) but are mesodermal, originating in bone marrow. They are best thought of as highly specialised macrophages.

Although Langerhans cells have a different derivation to melanocytes, they both commonly stain positive for S100 and therefore Langerhans cells can masquerade as melanocytes.

Langerhans cells ingest foreign antigens, process them into small peptide fragments, bind them with major histocompatibility complexes and present them to lymphocytes for activation of the immune system.

Sunlight reduces Langerhans cell numbers so this is a likely additional factor in skin tumour induction as well as that of sunlight causing mutations.

Merkel cells

Merkel cells are derived from the neural crest and are located in the basal layer of the epidermis. Located on the volar aspect of digits, in nail beds, genitalia and elsewhere on skin they act as transducers for fine touch.

The only nerve fibres that penetrate slightly into the epidermis are non-myelinated and they occur in proximity to Merkel cells.

2.3.2 Melanin production

The amino acid tyrosine is the precursor for the production of both eumelanin (the predominant melanin in skin phototypes 2–6) and pheomelanin (the predominant melanin in skin phototype 1) (see *Section 2.3.3* for more information on skin phototypes). Tyrosinase is the key enzyme in the melanin biosynthetic pathway and it catalyses the initial rate-limiting conversion of tyrosine to dihydroxyphenylalanine (DOPA). Once produced via tyrosinase activity, DOPA can spontaneously oxidise to form melanin.

Melanosomes are intracytoplasmic organelles within melanocytes that specialise in the synthesis and storage of melanin; they are the source of the vast majority of melanin in pigmented lesions (*Figure 2.8*). There is, however, another source of melanin and that is melanin which is formed by the oxidation of the organic (protein) substrate keratin. It is possible that this occurs by the same process whereby the exposed flesh of an apple darkens[14], explaining why keratin in seborrhoeic keratoses and congenital naevi, which is exposed, turns orange or brown, whereas keratin enclosed in the epidermis projects as white clods, dots or circles on dermatoscopy.

People with dark skin phototypes have more abundant and larger melanosomes which contain more melanin and which the melanocytes transfer to keratinocytes, via their more abundant dendrites. These larger melanosomes are individually dispersed whereas the smaller ones of fair-skinned phototypes are clustered in groups.

The melanin produced by a melanocyte at the basal layer of normal epidermis, after being concentrated in melanosomes, is transferred to approximately 60 neighbouring keratinocytes at all layers of the epidermis via extensions called dendrites; this association is referred to as the epidermal melanin unit (*Figure 2.8*). These melanosomes are positioned over the nuclei of the keratinocytes and as a result effectively protect the keratinocytes' genetic material from external radiation.

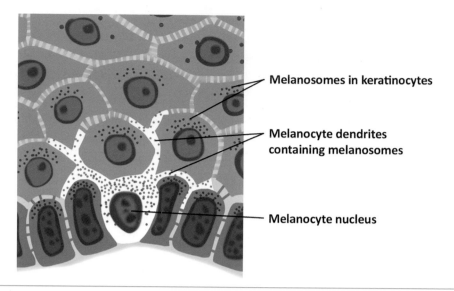

Melanosomes in keratinocytes

Melanocyte dendrites containing melanosomes

Melanocyte nucleus

Figure 2.8: *This schematic diagram of a portion of normal epidermis shows a melanocyte at the basal layer with dendrites weaving their way between keratinocytes and providing them with melanin-laden melanosomes.*

The majority of melanin in normal skin is located within the keratinocytes, mainly in the deeper part of the epidermis, having been transferred to them by melanocytes.

The melanocytes in naevi (naevomelanocytes) differ from the melanocytes distributed along the dermoepidermal junction.

- **Clark naevi** (so-called dysplastic naevi) comprise a limited proliferation of naevomelanocytes and may be junctional (flat macular) or compound (raised papular), having a dermal component limited to the superficial papillary dermis[9].

- **Congenital naevi**, defined as a histological subtype whether present at birth or not, are not neoplastic but rather are hamartomas, representing collections of melanocytes persisting following embryological migration. The presence of terminal hair in some congenital naevi is consistent with this hamartomatous origin. Congenital naevi differ from Clark naevi histologically, are raised (papular) and may have a dermal component which may extend into the reticular dermis[9].

- **Dermal naevi** (congenital type naevi confined to the dermis) are also composed of naevomelanocytes. Naevomelanocytes in the dermis are described as 'mature' which means that they have lost their melanin-producing capability, becoming small and compact.

- **Blue naevi** (also congenital-type naevi) are an exception to this and may continue to manufacture melanin in their dermally located naevomelanocytes.

While melanocytes are not naturally continuously proliferative, the melanocytes in naevi proliferate to form the naevus then stop proliferating. This is evidenced by the presence of mitotic figures and positive proliferation markers in naevi which are in a rapid growth phase, such as some Spitz naevi.

2.3.3 Skin phototypes

The Fitzpatrick phototyping scale was developed in 1975 by Thomas B. Fitzpatrick, a Harvard dermatologist, and is useful for stratifying the risk of certain disorders including sunburn and skin malignancy (*Table 2.2*)[15]. The differences between the different phenotypes relates to the quantity of melanin produced by melanocytes in the epidermis, as well as the type and quality of the melanin. The melanin in darker phenotypes is eumelanin, without a component of phaeomelanin, and it is contained in larger and more stable melanosomes. Fitzpatrick skin phototypes are referred to frequently in this book.

2.3.4 Melanocytic vs melanotic

A melanotic lesion is one which is pigmented by melanin (whether that lesion is melanocytic or not) (Figure 2.9A).

Table 2.2: *Fitzpatrick skin phototypes.*

Skin type	Skin colour	Reaction to sun exposure
I	Pale white	Always burns, never tans
II	White	Usually burns
III	Light brown	Burns mildly, tans relatively well
IV	Moderate brown	Rarely burns, tans well
V	Dark brown	Very rarely burns, tans easily
VI	Black	Least likely to burn, tans very easily

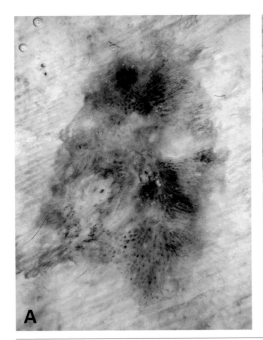 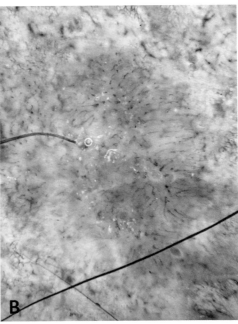

Figure 2.9: The pigmented (melanotic) lesion (A) is a squamous cell carcinoma in situ *which is not melanocytic. The non-pigmented (amelanotic) lesion (B) is an amelanotic melanoma and therefore it is melanocytic by definition.*

Table 2.3: *The definitions of melanotic and melanocytic.*

Melanotic: a lesion which is pigmented by melanin.
Melanocytic: a lesion which is comprised primarily of a proliferation of melanocytes.
'Melanotic' is about pigment and 'melanocytic' is about cells.

Lesions which contain melanin are melanotic (see *Table 2.3*) and they may be melanocytic or non-melanocytic (e.g. a solar lentigo is melanotic because it is pigmented with melanin, but it is not melanocytic because there is no proliferative increase in the number of melanocytes).

A melanocytic lesion *is one which is formed by a proliferation of melanocytes (whether it is pigmented or not)* (Figure 2.9B).

Lesions which contain a proliferation of melanocytes (melanocytic naevi and melanomas) are melanocytic but they are not necessarily melanotic (e.g. amelanotic melanomas are melanocytic but not melanotic).

2.3.5 Why does melanin appear as different colours at different depths in the skin?

Melanin is an efficient pigment and absorbs all light reaching it, so at the surface of the skin,

at the level of the stratum corneum, it effectively blocks the colour of haem from below, absorbs all light and appears black (*Figure 2.10A*). Melanin within the epidermis and at the dermoepidermal junction, still absorbs all light reaching it and blocks the colour of haem, but because some light is reflected from more superficial layers in the epidermis it appears near-black, which is brown (*Figure 2.10B*). Collagen fibrils scatter light as in a colloid solution, scattering short wavelength blue light more than long wavelength red light and, by the same process whereby the sky on earth appears blue due to scattering of light by atmospheric particles according to the Tyndall effect, melanin in the deep dermis appears blue (*Figure 2.10D*). In the superficial dermis the shift towards blue is reduced and melanin appears grey (*Figure 2.10C*).

This differential colour of melanin at various locations within the epidermis and dermis is extremely valuable because melanin, most commonly confined to the epidermis, can be carried to deeper levels by a limited number of

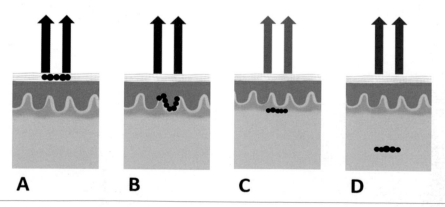

Figure 2.10: *Schematic illustration of dermatoscopic colours of melanin. (A) Melanin absorbs all incident light and it blocks the colour of haem so at the stratum corneum it appears black. (B) At the basal layer of the epidermis some light is reflected by the epidermal components superficial to it so melanin appears near-black, which is brown. (C) In the superficial dermis the Tyndall effect causes a shift towards blue, which is seen as grey. (D) In the deep dermis, with a major Tyndall effect, melanin appears blue.*

processes, including invasion of the dermis by pigment-laden malignant cells, which means that dermatoscopy can be used to recognise this behaviour of malignant tissue[16].

2.3.6 Epidermal appendages

Intradermal epidermal structures such as hair follicles and exocrine glands can be an important source of cells for re-epithelialisation following traumatic injury or surgical procedures such as cryotherapy or shave biopsy[8]. They can also be a source of tumour persistence after non-surgical treatment such as cryotherapy or topical therapy, or after superficial surgical treatment.

Both of these situations are particularly relevant on the face or scalp where these structures may lie in the subcutaneous fat beneath the dermis. A tumour can invade follicles and therefore be inadequately treated by non-surgical means or superficial excision, even on the non-hair-bearing scalp of male-pattern baldness (*Figure 2.11*).

Hair follicles

Hair follicles, being of both epidermal and dermal origin, are found over the entire surface of the body except the soles, palms, nail bed, nail matrix, glans penis, clitoris, labia minora, mucocutaneous junction, and portions of the fingers and toes.

Skin that does not contain hair follicles is known as *glabrous* ('shiny') skin. All other skin surfaces are *non-glabrous* (hair-bearing).

Sebaceous glands usually open into the hair follicle rather than directly onto the skin surface, and the entire complex is termed the pilosebaceous unit[17].

Figure 2.12 shows a pilosebaceous unit including the bulb (enlarged in *Figure 2.13*), suprabulbar portion, isthmus and infundibulum. A population of stem cells in the bulge, at the insertion of the erector pili muscle, may be a source of re-epithelialisation following injury[17].

Caucasian hair follicles are oriented obliquely to the skin surface, whereas the hair follicles of people with skin phototype 5

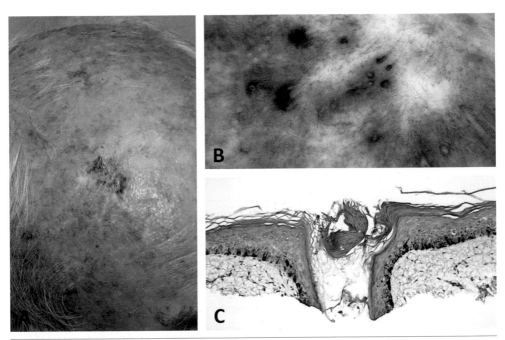

Figure 2.11: Dermatoscopy of the base of a shave biopsy of a pigmented skin lesion on bald scalp (B) reveals pigment lining follicular openings (pigmented circles). Histology (C) reveals that pigmented melanocytes are extending into these follicles (S100 melanocyte stain); melanoma in situ.

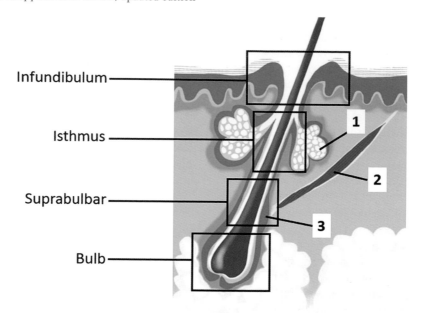

Infundibulum

Isthmus

Suprabulbar

Bulb

Figure 2.12: *Schematic diagram of a pilosebaceous unit showing the infundibulum, isthmus, suprabulbar portion and bulb. Also shown is a sebaceous gland (1), an erector pili muscle (2) and the stem cell bulge (3).*

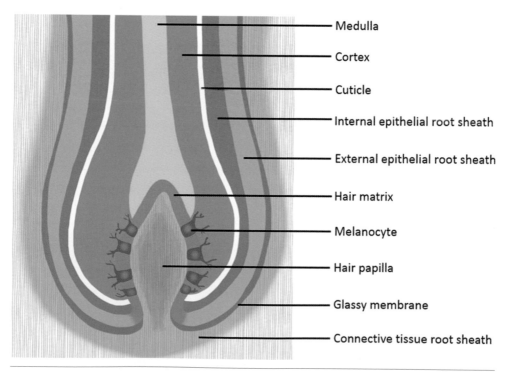

Medulla

Cortex

Cuticle

Internal epithelial root sheath

External epithelial root sheath

Hair matrix

Melanocyte

Hair papilla

Glassy membrane

Connective tissue root sheath

Figure 2.13: *Diagrammatic representation of the various layers of the hair follicle. The hair papilla is an extension of dermis being separated from the epidermal hair matrix, and from the melanocytes contained within it, by the basement membrane. The other layers are shown as labelled.*

and 6 are oriented almost parallel to the skin surface. Asian people have vertically oriented follicles that produce straight hairs[18]. These anatomic variations are an important consideration in avoiding alopecia when making incisions in the scalp.

The base of the hair follicle, or hair bulb, lies deep within the dermis and, on the face and scalp, may actually lie in the subcutaneous fat. This accounts for the remarkable ability of the face to re-epithelialise following even the deepest cutaneous wounds.

Exocrine glands

Sebaceous glands – present in all skin except palms, soles, nail bed and nail matrix, being very sparse on the dorsum of the feet. They are most concentrated on face, nose and scalp. Sebaceous glands produce and secrete sebum composed of complex oils including triglycerides and fatty acid breakdown products, wax esters, squalene, cholesterol esters and cholesterol (*Figure 2.14*). Sebaceous activity increases at puberty[17].

The function of sebum includes skin lubrication and waterproofing. A combination of sebum and sweat decreases pH of skin to 5.5 which is hostile to bacteria[1].

Sebaceous material is seen dermatoscopically as yellow or skin-coloured clods or structureless areas most commonly in sebaceous gland hyperplasia and also in sebaceous adenoma. Lipids are also commonly seen as yellow to skin coloured structureless areas in xanthomata and less commonly as yellow structureless areas in juvenile xanthogranuloma.

The lipid lipofuscin is seen in choroidal melanomas as an orange pigment and has been described as a dermatoscopic yellow structure in one non-choroidal cutaneous melanoma[19].

Eccrine (sweat) glands – located over the entire surface of the body except the vermillion border of the lips, the external ear canal, the nail beds, the labia minora, the glans penis and the inner aspect of the prepuce. They are most concentrated in the palms, soles and axillae.

Each gland consists of a coiled secretory intradermal portion that connects to the epidermis via a relatively straight distal duct (*Figure 2.14*)[17]. Eccrine glands produce sweat, which cools the body by evaporation and, in conjunction with dermatoglyphic ridges and furrows, increases grip strength on the palmar surface of the hands including fingers.

Dermatoscopically, eccrine openings are seen as white dots which facilitate the localisation of dermatoglyphic ridges on volar (palmar and plantar) skin onto which the eccrine ducts open[9]. This is of significance because a pattern of pigmented lines parallel on the ridges is a clue to melanoma[9].

Apocrine glands – are similar in structure, but not identical, to eccrine glands[17]. While eccrine glands open directly onto the skin, apocrine glands, like sebaceous glands, open into the hair follicle. They are found in the axillae, in the anogenital region and, as modified glands, in the external ear canal (ceruminous glands), the eyelid (Moll's glands), and the breast (mammary glands).

Apocrine glands are typically larger and more productive than eccrine glands. They are characterised by a simple cuboidal epithelium and widely dilated lumen that stores the secretory product (*Figure 2.14*). Apocrine secretions produce odour, and do not function prior to puberty. While eccrine glands secrete a clear, odourless fluid that serves to regulate body temperature, apocrine glands secrete a thick, milky sweat (secretion from apocrine glands contains protein, lipid, carbohydrate, ammonium and other organic compounds) that, once broken down by bacteria, is the main cause of body odour[17].

The mammary gland is considered to be a modified and highly specialised type of apocrine gland.

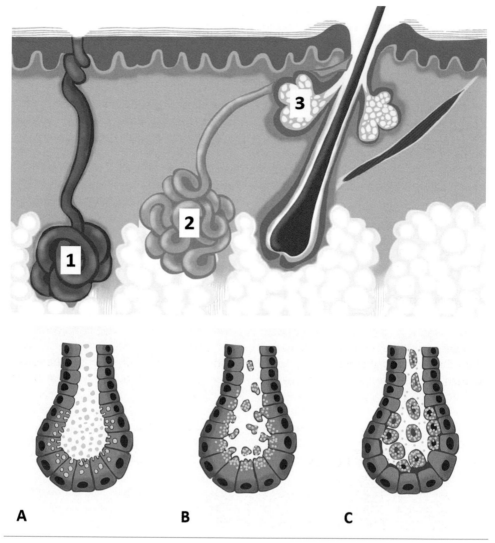

Figure 2.14: *(Upper image) Diagrammatic representation of skin demonstrating eccrine (1), apocrine (2) and sebaceous gland (3). (Lower image) Schematic diagram of exocrine glands of the skin. (A) Cuboidal cells lining eccrine glands secrete sweat into the lumen (merocrine secretion), this reaches the skin surface via the eccrine duct. (B) Apocrine glands secrete by pinching off vesicles which are secreted into hair follicles close to the skin surface where they mix with sebaceous secretions. (C) Holocrine glands (e.g. sebaceous glands) secrete by discharging the entire cytoplasm of their cuboidal cells into the lumen of the gland. Lower panel adapted from* Anatomy and Physiology Learning System *4e by E. Applegate, 2010, with permission from Elsevier.*

2.3.7 The basement membrane

The basement membrane which separates the epidermis from the dermis is an important structure both for the anatomy of normal skin and as a potential barrier for malignant cells between the epidermis and the dermis where their metastatic potential can be facilitated by blood and lymphatic vessels[20].

Basal cells of the stratum basale are connected to each other and to the layer of cells above them by desmosomes (see

Figure 2.4)[20]. Hemidesmosomes (collagen-containing structures) connect basal cells to the basement membrane[20].

2.3.8 The dermis

The functions of nutrition and excretion in the epidermis proceed by diffusion from the vascular layer of the dermis which primarily comprises collagen fibres formed by the predominant cell type, the fibroblast, all within a matrix of amorphous ground substance.

Fibroblasts – these produce and secrete procollagen and elastic fibres. Procollagen is converted into collagen that aggregates and becomes cross-linked.

Interwoven fibres of collagen – give tensile strength; collagen is approximately 75% of the dry weight of the dermis. Elastic fibres (comprising 3% of the dry weight of the dermis) return the dermis to the unstretched state[8]. Collagen, a structural protein, is composed of fibrils arranged into collagen fibres. The collagen fibres in the papillary dermis are finer than those in the reticular dermis, where they are arranged in coarse bundles in layers parallel to the surface (*Figure 2.15*).

Amorphous ground substance – mainly mucopolysaccharides (including hyaluronic acid) which bind water, allowing substances to move through the dermis. It acts as a lubricant between collagen and elastic fibres and provides bulk, enhancing the shock absorber function of dermis[8]. The deep margin of the dermis is highly irregular, bordering the subcutaneous layer.

Smooth muscle – present in arrector pili muscles and is vestigial in humans; originally it had the function of protection from cold by bringing the hair shaft into a vertical orientation.

Within the matrix of the dermis lie the adnexal structures of the skin including hair follicles,

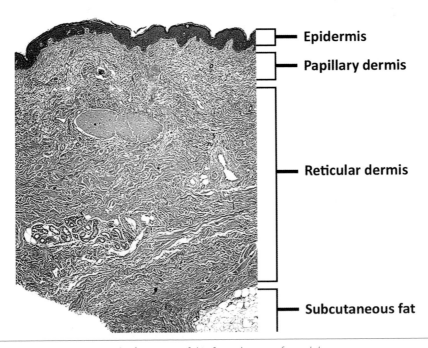

Figure 2.15: A photomicrograph of a section of skin from the arm of an adult.

Epidermis

Papillary dermis

Reticular dermis

Subcutaneous fat

eccrine, sebaceous and apocrine glands as well as blood and lymphatic vessels, nerves and organs of sensation.

Striated muscle – present in platysma and some facial expression muscles.

The dermis thickens from childhood until the fourth or fifth decade then thins in older age[20].

Lymphocytes – function in immunosurveillance and attack, and appear in higher numbers in pathological states including malignancy[17].

Mononuclear phagocytes – mobile cells functioning as scavengers that phagocytose and destroy bacteria and other debris. Melanophages contain scavenged melanin, and tattoo pigment is also scavenged and contained within these cells. When these cells phagocytose organic particles such as

bacteria they secrete cytokines that stimulate an immune response[17].

Mast cells – stimulated by antigens to release inflammatory mediators[17].

Polymorphs (polymorphonuclear leucocytes) – involved in the immune response, classically to bacterial infection.

Langerhans cells – mobile cells which are present in the dermis as well as at all layers of the epidermis[17].

2.3.9 Skin blood supply

A source vessel supplies a 3-dimensional vascular territory from bone to skin called an angiosome.

Cutaneous vessels originate from source vessels as perforating vessels which emerge from subcutaneous vessels in the deep fascia and travel towards the skin (*Figure 2.16*).

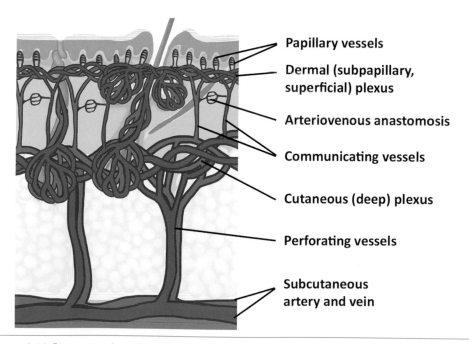

Papillary vessels

Dermal (subpapillary, superficial) plexus

Arteriovenous anastomosis

Communicating vessels

Cutaneous (deep) plexus

Perforating vessels

Subcutaneous artery and vein

Figure 2.16: Diagrammatic representation of blood vessels supplying the skin. Perforating vessels pass from source vessels in the muscle fascia to the cutaneous (deep) plexus which is connected by communicating vessels passing through the dermis to the (superficial) dermal plexus. Papillary vessels project vertically from the dermal plexus into each dermal papilla.

The cutaneous (deep) plexus and dermal plexuses are connected by communicating vessels oriented perpendicularly (*Figure 2:16*). The cutaneous plexus lies just above subcutaneous fat and supplies eccrine glands and hair papillae. The dermal plexus lies in between the papillary and reticular dermis and has arterioles going up into dermal papillae (*Figure 2.16*). Each such arteriole supplies an inverted cone of tissue with its base at the dermoepidermal junction[17].

2.3.10 Skin lymphatics

Skin lymphatics parallel the blood supply. Afferent lymphatics begin as blind-ended capillaries in the dermal papillae and pass to a superficial lymphatic plexus in the papillary dermis[17].

The two deeper horizontal dermal and subdermal plexuses parallel the corresponding vascular plexuses. Collecting lymphatics from the deeper plexus run with veins in the superficial fascia and course through filtering lymph nodes to join the venous circulation bilaterally near the junction of the subclavian vein and the internal jugular vein.

Lymphatic vessels are not expected to be visualised by dermatoscopy.

2.3.11 Skin innervation

Skin has an estimated 1 million nerve fibres concentrated most heavily on the face and extremities[1].

The cell bodies of sensory nerve cells lie in dorsal root ganglia.

Most free sensory nerves end in the dermis, but a few non-myelinated nerve endings penetrate the basal epidermis in proximity to Merkel cells which function as sensors of light touch, pressure and position (*Figure 2.17*).

All other nerve endings, nerve end-organs and receptors lie in the dermis or subcutaneous tissue.
- Free nerve endings in the dermis detect stimuli of pain, temperature and crude touch.
- Ruffini corpuscles detect skin stretch and heat.

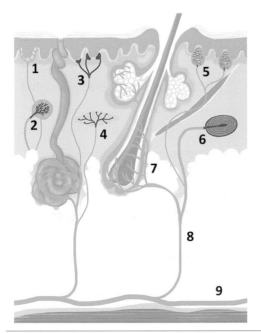

1 - Free nerve endings
  (pain, temperature, crude touch)

2 - Krause end-bulbs (cold)

3 - Merkel disks
  (light touch, pressure, position)

4 - Ruffini corpuscles
  (skin stretch, heat)

5 - Meissner's corpuscles
  (light touch, vibration)

6 - Pacinian corpuscles
  (deep touch, vibration)

7 - Hair root plexus

8 - Sensory nerve

9 - Cutaneous nerve

Figure 2.17: Diagrammatic representation of the nerve supply of the skin.

- Krause bulbs detect cold.
- Pacinian corpuscles detect deep touch and vibration.
- Meissner corpuscles detect light touch and vibration.

Autonomic nerves supply blood vessels, eccrine glands and arrector pili muscles[17].

Nerves and associated receptors are not expected to be visualised by dermatoscopy.

2.3.12 Anatomy of volar skin

Volar skin has a unique microanatomy related to the high concentration of eccrine ducts organised on dermatoglyphic parallel ridges with intervening furrows (*Figures 2.18* and *2.19*). This arguably increases traction when the skin is made wet by sweat production. The author's (CR) hypothesis for the dense concentration of eccrine glands on palmar/plantar surfaces is as a reservoir for re-epithelialisation following damage on these injury-prone and highly survival-critical surfaces. The evolutionary alternatives of hair folli-

cles (as on the face) or sebaceous glands (as on the nose) would not work well on volar surfaces.

2.3.13 Anatomy of the nail apparatus

The digital nails are derived from the stratum corneum of the germinal nail matrical epidermis. The nail apparatus includes both the dermis and epidermis of the nail matrix as well as the nail plate and nail bed.

An understanding of the anatomy of the nail apparatus is essential for the correct assessment of nail apparatus neoplasia (*Figures 2.20* and *2.21*). While virtually any skin tumour (BCC and adnexal tumours very rarely) can arise in the nail apparatus, melanoma almost invariably arises from the germinal nail matrix or from the adjacent skin of the digit, rather than from the nail bed[9].

The histological features of nail matrix and nail bed tissue are similar to those of other skin surfaces with the exception that there are no adnexal structures, and less subcutaneous

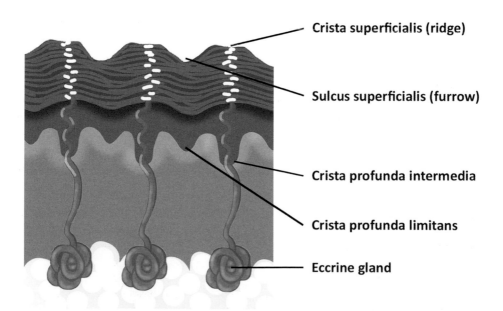

Figure 2.18: *Diagrammatic representation of volar skin in cross-section: dermatoglyphic ridges overlie the crista profunda intermedia which are rete ridges through which eccrine ducts traverse. Rete ridges, devoid of eccrine ducts, underlie the dermatoglyphic furrows and are designated crista profunda limitans.*

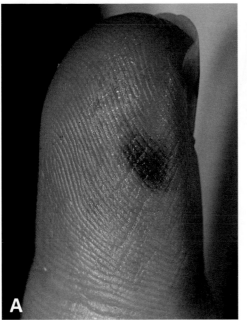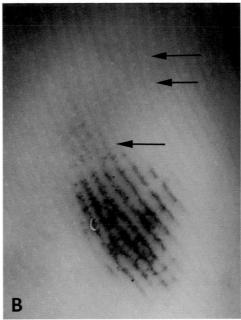

Figure 2.19: Clinical (A) and dermatoscopic (B) images of a volar naevus: fine brown parallel lines can be seen in the dermatoglyphic furrows, which overlie the crista profunda limitans, between the elevated ridges. Arrows point to the openings of eccrine ducts which are located in the centre of the dermatoglyphic ridges.

tissue. Another significant difference is that melanocytes may be difficult to recognise without special stains[21].

The germinative matrix extends distally to the level of the lunula but apart from that extension it is covered by the proximal nail fold. The stratum corneum of the nail matrix gives rise to, and is therefore continuous with, the overlying nail plate.

2.3.14 Anatomy of the eye in relation to melanocytic neoplasia

Although the eye is not part of the skin, it is a potential site for primary melanoma to develop and therefore an understanding of its microanatomy is relevant to clinicians who diagnose and manage skin malignancies.

A cross-section of the eye is illustrated in *Figure 2.22*. Melanocytes migrate to the eye during embryogenesis from the neural crest and are located in the uveal tract. *In vitro* studies have shown that they retain their

ability to make melanin throughout life. A separate population of retinal pigmented epithelial (RPE) cells is derived directly from the optic neuroepithelium. The majority of RPE cells do not play any significant role in active pigment production in the adult[22]. Uveal tract melanoma and conjunctival melanomas are the two types of melanoma that occur in the eye. Melanoma does not arise from RPE cells, which are not melanocytes.

The retina is composed of two layers: the (anterior) neural retina (abutting the cavity of the eye/vitreous humor) containing photoreceptor cells (rods and cones) and the (posterior) retinal pigment epithelium which separates the retina from the choroid (vascular) layer.

Unlike the skin, the retinal *epithelium*, although comprising pigment-producing retinal epithelial cells, does not contain melanocytes, which are all confined to the *vascular layer* (uveal tract).

The majority of cases of uveal tract

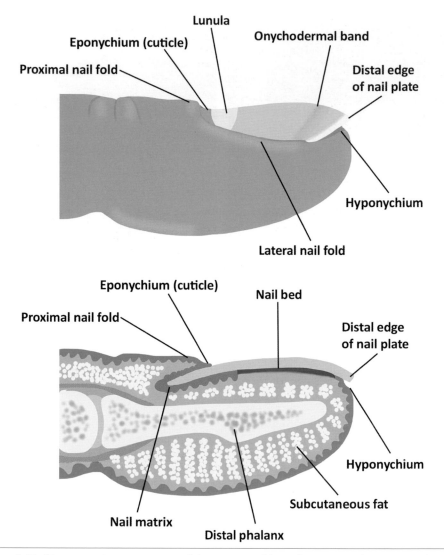

Figure 2.20: Diagrammatic representation of the anatomy of the nail apparatus: clinical (upper diagram) and cross-sectional (lower diagram).

melanoma (over 90%) involve the choroid. Approximately 7% involve the ciliary body and 3% involve the iris[23].

Conjunctival pigmentation can be a risk factor for melanoma. Primary acquired melanosis (PAM), without atypia or with mild atypia, shows 0% progression to melanoma, whereas PAM with severe atypia shows progression to melanoma in 13%. The greater the extent of PAM in 'clock-hours' is, the greater the risk is of transformation to melanoma[24].

Radiation which reaches the uvea in adults is all in the visible spectrum, with UV light being obstructed by the cornea, lens and retinal pigmented epithelium. Because of this, UV radiation exposure of the choroid in adulthood is not a risk factor for melanoma. In spite of this, for reasons which are not clear, individuals with light skin phototypes are at an increased risk for choroidal melanoma; the white:black incidence ratio of uveal melanoma being 18:1[25–28].

Other studies have shown that light

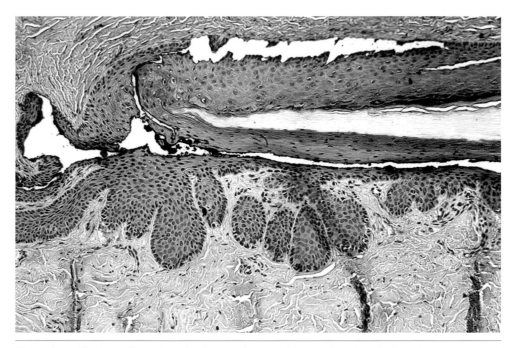

Figure 2.21: *Histology of a section of nail matrix showing the normal epidermal–dermal appearance with rete ridges. Note that the epidermis of the nail matrix wraps around the proximal extremity of the nail plate, being inverted above it. It is only the germinative matrix beneath the nail plate from which melanoma is expected to arise.*

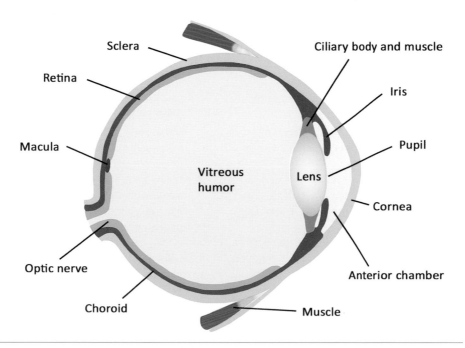

Figure 2.22: *Diagrammatic cross-section of the eye: the uveal tract comprises the iris, ciliary body and choroid and is the vascular, pigmented middle layer of the three concentric layers that make up the eye.*

coloured (blue, hazel) irises are associated with a higher risk of uveal melanoma[29].

Paradoxically, it has been reported that solar radiation causes a decrease in the incidence of uveal melanoma[28]. This is consistent with the reported effect of UV radiation on the occurrence of some other malignant tumours that are not exposed to sunlight, e.g. non-Hodgkin's lymphoma, and prostate, breast, colon and ovarian cancers. It is speculated that this may be due to a protective effect of increased vitamin D production[30].

References

1. Paul SP. *Skin: A Biography*, 2015. Fourth Estate.
2. Medzhitov R and Janeway CA, Jr. Decoding the patterns of self and nonself by the innate immune system. *Science*, 2002;296:298.
3. Silver DL and Pavan WJ. The origin and development of neural crest-derived melanocytes. In: *From Melanocytes to Melanoma*, Hearing VJ and Leong SPL (eds), 2006. Humana Press.
4. Adameyko I, Lallemend F, Aquino JB, *et al.* Schwann cell precursors from nerve innervation are a cellular origin of melanocytes in skin. *Cell*, 2009:139:366.
5. Nitzan E, Pfaltzgraff ER, Labosky PA, and Kalcheim C. Neural crest and Schwann cell progenitor-derived melanocytes are two spatially segregated populations similarly regulated by Foxd3. *PNAS*, 2013;110:12709.
6. Rigel S. *Cancer of the Skin, 2nd Edition*, 2011 (pp. 24 and 25). Elsevier.
7. Ackerman AB. *The Sun and the "Epidemic" of Melanoma: Myth on Myth*, 2nd Edition, 2008. Ardor Scribendi.
8. Robinson JK, Hanke CW, and Siegel DM. *Surgery of the Skin*, 3rd Edition, 2015. Elsevier Mosby.
9. Kittler H, Rosendahl C, Cameron A, and Tschandl P. *Dermatoscopy*, 2nd Edition, 2016. Facultas.
10. Halprin KM. Epidermal "turnover time" – a re-examination. *Br J Dermatol*, 1972;86:14.
11. Rosendahl C, Cameron A, Argenziano G, Zalaudek I, Tschandl P, and Kittler H. Dermoscopy of squamous cell carcinoma and keratoacanthoma. *Arch Dermatol*, 2012;148;1386.
12. Rosendahl CO, Grant-Kels JM, and Que SKT. Dysplastic nevus: fact and fiction. *J Am Acad Dermatol*, 2015;73:507.
13. Kittler H, and Tschandl P. Dysplastic nevus: why this term should be abandoned in dermatoscopy. *Dermatol Clin*, 2013;31:579.
14. Deutch CE. Browning in apples: Exploring the biochemical basis of an easily-observable phenotype. *Biochem Mol Biol Educ*, 2018;46:76.
15. Fitzpatrick TB. The validity and practicality of sun-reactive skin types I through VI. *Archives Dermatol*, 1988;124:869.
16. Rosendahl C, Cameron A, McColl I, and Wilkinson D. Dermatoscopy in routine practice – "Chaos and Clues." *Aust Fam Physician*, 2012;41:482.
17. Nouri K. *Skin Cancer*, 2008. McGraw-Hill Medical.
18. New Hair Institute Medical Group. Racial Variations [Internet; cited 4 Feb 2018]. Available from: https://newhair.com/fut/racial-variations/.
19. Jegou Penouil MH, Gourhant J-Y, Segretin C, Weedon D, and Rosendahl C. Non-choroidal yellow melanoma showing positive staining with Sudan Black consistent with the presence of lipofuscin: a case report. *Dermatol Pract Concept*, 2014;4:9.
20. Hunter J, *et al.* Function and structure of skin. In: *Clinical Dermatology*, 3rd Edition, Hearing R, *et al.* (eds), 2002. Blackwell Science.
21. Weedon D, Van Deurse M, and Rosendahl C. "Occult" melanocytes in nail matrix melanoma. *Am J Dermatopathol*, 2012;34:855.
22. Smith–Thomas L, Richardson P, Thody AJ, *et al.* Human ocular melanocytes and retinal pigment epithelial cells differ in their melanogenic properties *in vivo* and *in vitro*. *Curr Eye Res*, 1996;15:1079.
23. Australian Cancer Network Melanoma Guidelines Revision Working Party. *Clinical*

Practice Guidelines for the Management of Melanoma in Australia and New Zealand. Ocular and Periocular Melanoma: Supplementary Document, 2008. New Zealand Guidelines Group.

24. Shields JA, Shields CL, Mashayekhi A, *et al.* Primary acquired melanosis of the conjunctiva: risks for progression to melanoma in 311 eyes. The 2006 Lorenz E. Zimmerman lecture. *Ophthalmology*, 2008;115:511.

25. Hu, DN, Yu PG, McCormick SA, Schneider S, and Finger PT. Population-based incidence of uveal melanoma in various races and ethnic groups. *Am J Ophthalmol*, 2005;140:612.

26. Holly EA, Aston DA, Char DH, Kristiansen JJ, and Ahn DK. Uveal melanoma in relation to ultraviolet light exposure and host factors. *Cancer Res*, 1990;50:5773.

27. Pane AR, and Hirst LW. Ultraviolet light exposure as a risk factor for ocular melanoma in Queensland, Australia. *Ophthalmic Epidemiol*, 2000;7:159.

28. Weis E, Shah CP, Lajous M, Shields JA, and Shields CL. The association between host susceptibility factors and uveal melanoma: a meta-analysis. *Arch Ophthalmol*, 2006;124:54.

29. Vajdic CM, Kricker A, Giblin M, *et al.* Eye color and cutaneous nevi predict risk of ocular melanoma in Australia. *Int J Cancer*, 2001;92:906.

30. Yu GP, Hu DN, and McCormick SA. Latitude and incidence of ocular melanoma. *Photochem Photobiol*, 2006;82:1621.

CHAPTER 3

Dermatopathology for dermatoscopists

The dermatoscope is a low powered microscope which permits visualisation of the epidermis and dermis in the horizontal plane compared to the view in the vertical plane provided by a conventional microscope using vertically sectioned specimens. It is therefore not surprising that there are histological features which correlate with what is seen through the dermatoscope and an understanding of this correlation is critical both to the dermatoscopist and the dermatopathologist.

The dermatopathologist can only report based on the pathology slides presented by laboratory technicians; with standard processing, as little as 2% of the whole specimen is assessed[1]. As a result, structures seen by the dermatoscopist are not always displayed to the dermatopathologist, a situation which may result in an incorrect dermatopathological diagnosis being rendered.

It is a responsibility of the dermatoscopist to convey relevant information to the dermatopathologist, documented in writing and, ideally, by providing clinical and dermatoscopic images. This enables the pathologist to know what to search for and provides the opportunity of requesting additional material ('levels') from the technician if the expected features are not discovered. The dermatoscopist also has the opportunity to communicate directly with the dermatopathologist if the report does not correlate with the dermatoscopic findings, causing the rendered diagnosis to be in doubt. The corollary is that it is also an advantage if the dermatopathologist has an in-depth knowledge of dermatoscopy as it correlates with histology.

This chapter will provide an account of the fundamentals of dermatopathology including:
- specimen processing
- the histology of normal skin
- dermatopathological terminology
- basic dermatopathology of melanoma, BCC, benign keratinocytic lesions and SCC, along with important dermatoscopic–histological correlations.

 ## 3.1 From the scalpel to the microscope

The processing of an excised specimen to produce microscope slides suitable for diagnostic assessment by a dermatopathologist is both elaborate and critical. Not only is correct processing important for an accurate outcome, but so is expert examination and interpretation of the findings.

An example of typical specimen processing workflow is presented here.

3.1.1 Specimen processing workflow

1. **Integrity of specimen identification.**
   Specimen mix-up can occur anywhere

in the chain of specimen handling, starting with the operating room, and steps are necessary to avert that eventuality[2]. Protocols should be set in place; one example is for the clinician to be confronted with the specimen label at the time of placing the specimen in the formalin container, in response to which he or she vocalises the name and body site written on that label for verification by both the patient and surgical support staff.

2. **Transport to the laboratory.** Following the procedure, the specimen jar is placed into a plastic bag along with the pathology request form, and a courier, employed by the pathology provider, picks this up along with any other pathology specimens. The courier ideally also checks that the specimen container is labelled with patient and body site details and that there is actually a specimen in the container. They then sign for the specimen in a book filled out in advance by practice staff. This effectively ensures

a chain of possession which has now passed to the pathology provider.

3. **Specimen transferred to the laboratory.** The courier delivers the specimens to the laboratory where the specimen containers are checked again for contents, labelling and correctly matching paperwork.

4. **Measuring, cutting up (specimen grossing) and inking.** A labelled plastic cassette is prepared for each specimen. The specimen is now ready to be removed from the formalin and this is done on a cutting-up table on which the respective labelled plastic cassette has been placed ready to receive the cut-up tissue (*Figure 3.1*). It is important that no material remains on this surface from previous specimens.

The specimen, having been removed from the formalin, is measured, as is any visible lesion, and the dimensions are recorded. The location of any orientating suture or other marker is also noted and recorded. The specimen then has ink

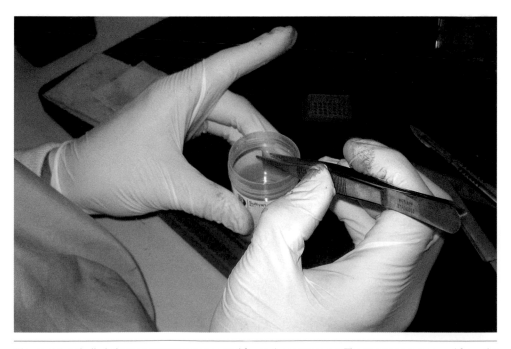

Figure 3.1: *Labelled plastic cassettes are prepared for each specimen jar. The specimen is removed from the jar on a bench on which sits its unique plastic cassette.*

applied to the lateral and deep margins to indicate the original surgical margins prior to cutting up at the laboratory. If the specimen has been orientated, different coloured ink is applied to identify the orientation, because any marking suture used by the clinician will be removed before the specimen is further processed and any other marking method may be altered during processing.

The specimen is now ready to be cut up. One processing technique is called 'bread-loafing' due to the way the specimen is cut into slices like a loaf of bread. Typically, an elliptical specimen will be cut transversely in this fashion every 3mm producing tissue samples approximately 3mm thick (*Figure 3.2*).

5. **Impregnation with paraffin wax in solution.** The 3mm thick tissue samples are then placed in the labelled plastic cassette and covered with a spring-loaded stainless steel or plastic lid in preparation for the next step in processing which involves immersing

the cassettes in a series of solvents to remove water and lipids and to replace them with paraffin wax.

6. **Embedding of tissue and formation of a solid paraffin block.** Portions of tissue are placed together in a stainless steel mould and liquid paraffin is poured over them. This container is placed on a refrigerated cold plate which causes the paraffin to solidify (*Figure 3.3*). It is critical that each tissue sample is correctly orientated in the solidifying paraffin so that the face of the specimen to be sectioned, which is at the base of the stainless steel mould, will be presented correctly to the microtome blade. While the paraffin is solidifying, the original labelled plastic cassette is pressed onto it and this, along with the attached paraffin block, is lifted free of the stainless steel mould.

7. **Shaving the tissue block.** The cassette is clamped into a vice and a microtome is moved up and down over the face of the paraffin block, shaving off thin layers of paraffin wax with embedded tissue

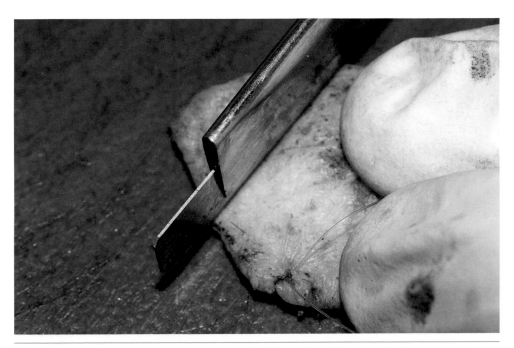

Figure 3.2: *The specimen is cut up (at 3mm intervals if elliptical) and the 3mm thick tissue specimens are placed in the labelled plastic cassette.*

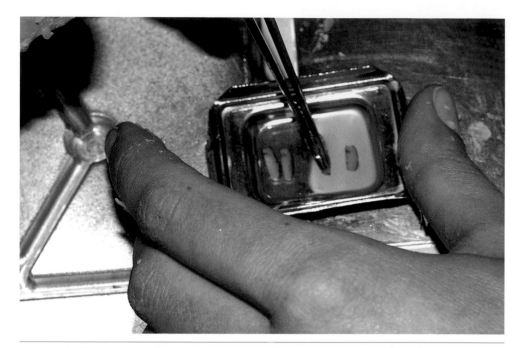

Figure 3.3: *After processing, to replace tissue-water with wax, the specimens are placed in a stainless steel mould and liquid paraffin wax is added. As this wax solidifies, the position of each of the tissue pieces is adjusted so that the face of the lesion to be presented to the microtome for sectioning, being at the base of the mould, will be orientated appropriately.*

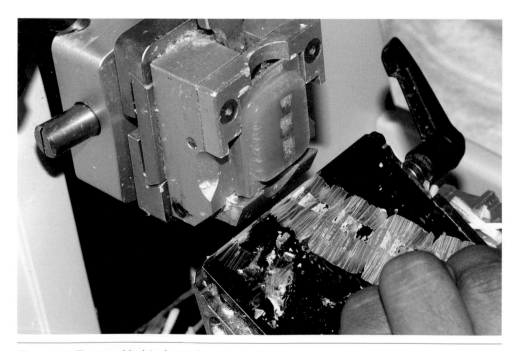

Figure 3.4: *The tissue block is clamped in a vice and a microtome moves up and down shaving very thin ribbons of wax with embedded tissue.*

3–6μm thick (*Figure 3.4*). A micron (μm) is one millionth of a meter (one thousandth of a millimetre) – for perspective, the diameter of a red blood cell is around 7μm.

8. **Transfer of tissue to the microscope slide.** The shaved 'ribbons' of tissue-embedded paraffin wax are floated in a water bath. To avoid a risk of specimen mix-up it is essential that no ribbons from any previously processed specimen remain in the water bath. A microscope slide, complete with patient and specimen identification details, is slipped under a selected ribbon of tissue-embedded wax and the extremely thin and fragile ribbon is deftly scooped onto the slide.

9. **Staining the specimen.** Stains are used in dermatopathology to enhance structural detail in the histology specimen. Unstained slides can be examined, but differentiation of cellular structures can be difficult to appreciate (*Figure 3.5*). Various stains are employed for

different purposes and some of these are described below.

Haematoxylin and eosin (H&E) stain. Hematoxylin is a natural product used as a dye in laboratories throughout the world to stain nuclei in microscope slide preparations. This chemical compound is extracted from the logwood tree, *Haematoxylum campechianum*, discovered by Spanish explorers in the Yucatan in 1502. A vigorous trade soon developed after this discovery, related to growing the logwood tree and preparing hematoxylin for use in dyeing fabrics in Europe. It was amateur microscopists who first used hematoxylin to stain cellular components[3].

Eosin, a synthetic derivative of coal tar, is used as a counterstain to haematoxylin. Tissue stained with haematoxylin and eosin shows pink–orange cytoplasmic staining and either blue or purple staining of nuclei. Eosin also stains red blood cells intensely red.

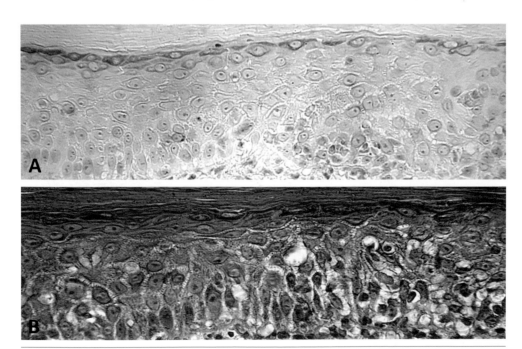

Figure 3.5: A photomicrograph of unstained tissue (A) presents a challenge in the differentiation of structures which is facilitated by staining with haematoxylin and eosin (B).

Melanin stains. Melanin appears brown on H&E staining, but if only a small amount is present it may not be clearly evident. Masson Fontana (stains melanin black) and Schmorl's stain (stains melanin blue–green) are just two stains that can be used to demonstrate the presence of melanin more clearly (*Figure 3.6*). These stains do not distinguish melanin within melanocytes from melanin within keratinocytes.

Melanocyte stains. There are varieties of immunoperoxidase stains that selectively stain melanocytes whether melanin is present or not; these can be useful when distinction from keratinocytes is difficult (*Figures 3.7* and *3.8*). These stains include SOX10 (a nuclear specific stain) as well as S100 which also stains the dendritic Langerhans cells. Because these mobile cells can be present at all layers of the epidermis as well as in the dermis, they can easily be confused with melanocytes. This is not a problem with

a significant proliferation of melanocytes because Langerhans cells are not expected to form aggregates.

One stain which is employed to detect whether or not melanocytes have retained the ability to produce melanin is HMB45. This stains premelanosomes regardless of whether melanin is being produced and so can detect whether melanocytes in the dermis have matured as expected in naevi and lost their melanin-producing capability. Naevi generally exhibit an HMB45 gradient with staining fading out at deeper levels, whereas melanomas may not have this gradient[4].

Proliferation stains. Stains for proliferation such as MIB-1 and Ki67 are useful for revealing tumour proliferative activity and, in some situations, they may do this with even more sensitivity than is provided by assessment of mitotic figures. If a melanocytic lesion has cells in the dermis with positive

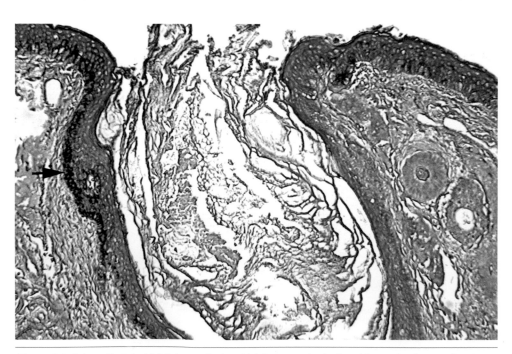

Figure 3.6: Schmorl's stain highlights melanin which is present in the basal layer of cells extending into a follicle (arrow) in this photomicrograph of an in situ melanoma on the nose.

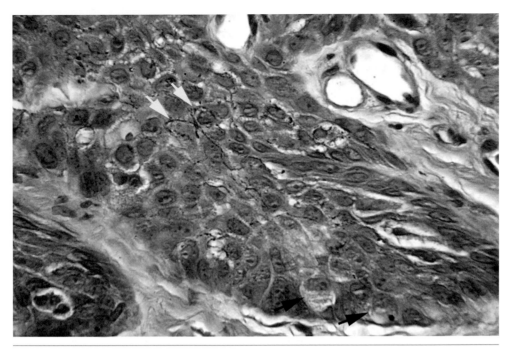

Figure 3.7: *Some heavily pigmented dendrites (yellow arrows) can be seen in this photomicrograph of a nail matrix biopsy stained with H&E, but melanocytes are not easily distinguished from other cells. Two melanocytes, identified by their abundant pale cytoplasm, are indicated (black arrows).*

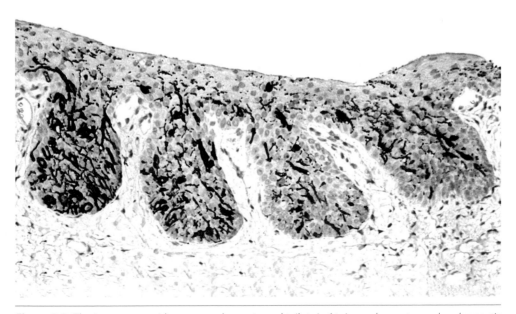

Figure 3.8: *The immunoperoxidase pan melanocyte cocktail stain (stains melanocytes and melanocytic dendrites red) reveals the full extent of the melanocytic proliferation in this photomicrograph of the lesion shown in* Figure 3.7; *nail matrix melanoma.*

staining for a proliferation marker this provides evidence against the diagnosis of naevus as opposed to melanoma[4]. An exception is Spitz naevus which can show active proliferation[5]. The other proliferating cell type which may stain positive and cause confusion is the lymphocyte.

Other stains. Other commonly used stains include stains for keratinocytes (Cytokeratin – CK stains), for Merkel cell carcinoma, for vascular tumours and for fungal hyphae (PAS stains).

10. **Attaching the cover slip.** After the process of staining is completed a cover slip is attached to the microscope slide with adhesive to provide a flat optical surface.
11. **Slide checking and collation.** Finally the slides are inspected visually in conjunction with the wax blocks to ensure the integrity of the slide labelling process and that all of the tissue is present on the stained slide. All of the slides for an individual case are collated with the request form and the macroscopic description and delivered to the dermatopathologist.

3.2 The histology of normal skin

The structure of normal skin, including its histology, was described in *Chapter 2* and the reader should be familiar with the contents of *Section 2.3* before proceeding, but here is a brief summary.

The skin is composed of two layers: the outermost epidermis and the dermis, beneath which lies the subcutis (*Figure 3.9*). The epidermis consists of approximately 7 rows of living cells covered by a layer of keratin-

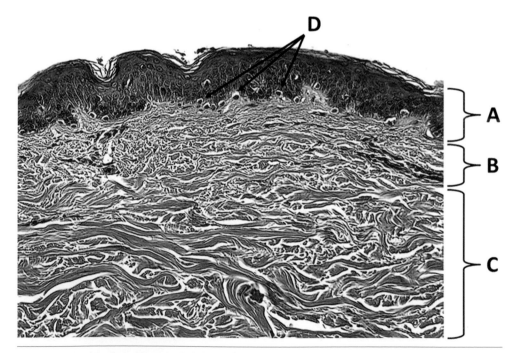

Figure 3.9: In this photomicrograph (H&E) of normal skin on the shoulder, the epidermis is displayed as a deeply stained cellular layer (A) below which is seen the more lightly stained papillary dermis (B) overlying the coarse horizontally oriented collagen fibres of the reticular dermis (C). Melanocytes are seen as cells with dark nuclei and a distinct pale cytoplasm (D), interspersed along the basal layer of keratinocytes (arrows).

rich non-viable cells, the stratum corneum. Although largely located within the dermis, the adnexal structures are epidermal.

- **The main cell type of the epidermis is the keratinocyte** – these cells arise at the basal layer as basal cells, maturing into squamous cells as they are displaced upwards by the formation of new basal cells.
- **Melanocytes** – distributed among basal cells at the basal layer of the epidermis in a ratio of 1:10 -30 depending of the degree of sun exposure of the skin[6].
- **Other cells found in the epidermis** include Langerhans cells and Merkel cells.
- **The epidermis has no blood or lymphatic vessels** – it relies for nutrition on

diffusion from the blood vessels in the dermis from which it is separated by the basement membrane, a structure not normally visible with H&E staining[7] but highlighted by some stains including the PAS stain.

- **The dermal vascular plexus** – runs horizontally between the papillary and reticular dermis and sends vessels vertically into the dermal papillae which lie between the epidermal rete ridges.
- **The dermis is composed mainly of the structural protein collagen** – this, as well as elastin, is produced by fibroblasts, within a matrix of amorphous ground substance comprising polysaccharide–protein complexes called proteoglycans[8].

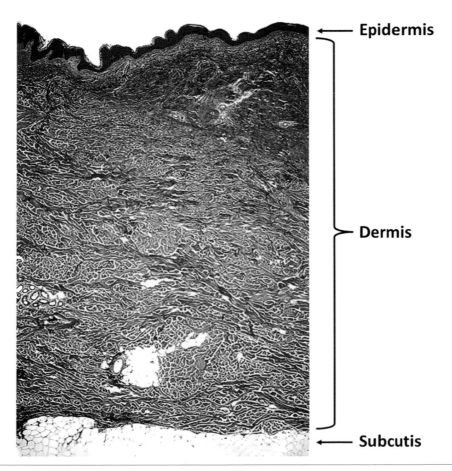

Figure 3.10: *The main feature of skin on the back is the thickness of the dermis which can be several millimetres. In this photomicrograph (H&E) the dermis is more than 20 times the thickness of the epidermis.*

The collagen of the deep reticular dermis is structurally coarser and it is this property, and the horizontal versus vertical orientation of the fibres, which distinguishes the reticular dermis from the more superficial papillary dermis.

- **The dermis contains the vessels and nerves that supply the skin, as well as adnexal structures** – these include hair follicles and eccrine, sebaceous and apocrine glands. Apart from fibroblasts and the cells of vessels, nerve structures and adnexae, the cell types commonly found in the dermis include histiocytes (macrophages/melanophages) and lymphocytes.

- **The subcutis is composed mainly of fat** – this can be the location of vessels and nerves as well as the deeper portions of terminal hair follicles.

The skin at all locations has the same basic structure of epidermis and dermis overlying the subcutis but there are site-specific variations which have functional implications. Histological images of skin at various body sites, all stained with H&E, are displayed (*Figures 3.10–15*).

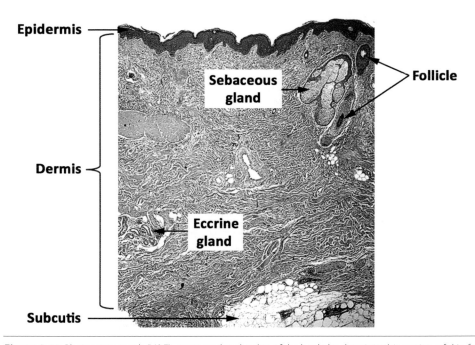

Figure 3.11: *Photomicrograph (H&E): compared to the skin of the back the dermis in this section of skin from the arm is only about 10 times as thick as the epidermis. Portions of a hair follicle and two other adnexal structures are annotated.*

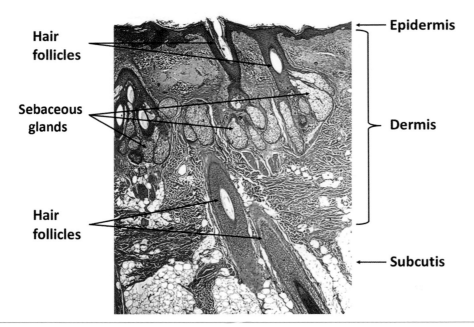

Hair follicles

Sebaceous glands

Hair follicles

Epidermis

Dermis

Subcutis

Figure 3.12: *Photomicrograph (H&E): a distinguishing feature of the skin on the scalp is that terminal hair follicles plunge deeply, penetrating the subcutaneous fat. This has significance with respect to treatment of malignancies at this location. Because of the increased presence of terminal hair, sebaceous glands are more abundant.*

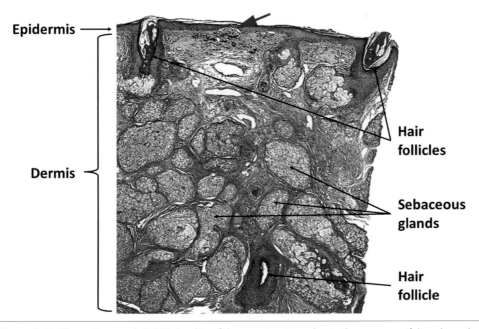

Epidermis

Dermis

Hair follicles

Sebaceous glands

Hair follicle

Figure 3.13: *Photomicrograph (H&E): the skin of the nose is unique due to the presence of densely packed sebaceous glands without associated terminal hairs. These glands provide sebum but are also rich sources of epidermal cells for re-epithelialisation following injury. There is a small melanoma* in situ *in the central epidermis of this punch biopsy specimen (blue arrow).*

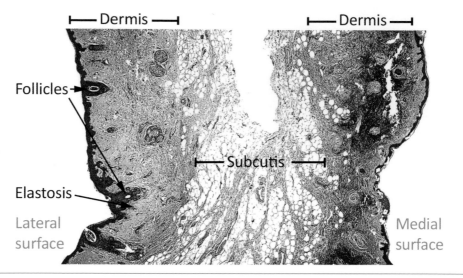

Figure 3.14: *Photomicrograph (H&E): histology of a section of skin through the full thickness of the ear lobe shows the differences between the lateral and medial surfaces with the subcutis shared between both.*

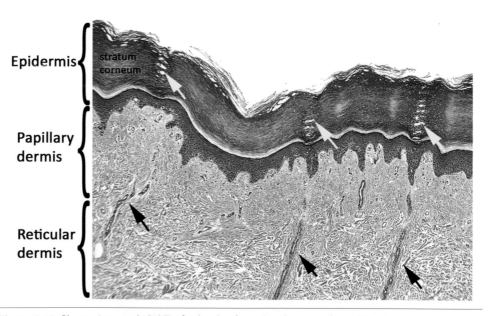

Figure 3.15: *Photomicrograph (H&E) of volar skin from the plantar surface of the foot demonstrates the thick stratum corneum which in this case is more than three times as thick as the remainder of the epidermis. The coarse collagen bundles in the reticular dermis are easily distinguishable beneath the fine fibrils of the papillary dermis and several eccrine ducts are seen traversing the dermis (black arrows), epidermis (where the duct is known as the acrosyringium) and stratum corneum (yellow arrows).*

3.3 Terminology used in dermatopathology

In this section some commonly used terms will be defined and illustrated in alphabetical order.

Acantholysis: a process characterised by loss of cell-to-cell adhesion which can occur in:

- inflammatory conditions such as the bullous diseases where it results in blister formation
- certain neoplasms, such as acantholytic actinic keratosis, which may resemble BCC and acantholytic SCC (*Figure 3.16*) where it probably results from abnormal desmosome function in tumour cells.

When the acantholysis is such that clefts appear superior to the basement membrane, this is designated **suprabasal cleft formation**, a feature seen in some actinic keratoses (*Figure 3.17*).

Acanthosis: refers to the process of thickening of the stratum spinosum of the epidermis. The prefix *'acanth-'* is applied to a number of different epidermal structures and entities. For example, an acanthoma is a neoplasm of keratinocytes and includes seborrhoeic keratosis (*Figure 3.18*), clear cell acanthoma, large cell acanthoma, melanoacanthoma and keratoacanthoma. All acanthomas are benign neoplasms with the exception of keratoacanthoma, which is probably a benign-behaving variant of SCC[9].

Clefting: when clear spaces are seen at the edges of aggregates of tumour cells this processing artefact is known as cleft formation or *'clefting'* and it is a feature seen in BCC, Spitz naevi and melanoma (*Figures 3.19–21*). Clefting may be noted at scanning magnification (low power) and, when this is seen in a melanocytic lesion which does

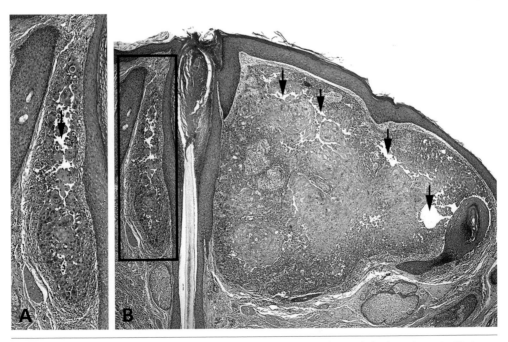

Figure 3.16: *Photomicrograph (H&E) of an acantholytic pigmented SCC, with the boxed area in (B) shown enlarged in (A). The acantholysis is seen as white fissuring between aggregates of tumour cells (arrows).*

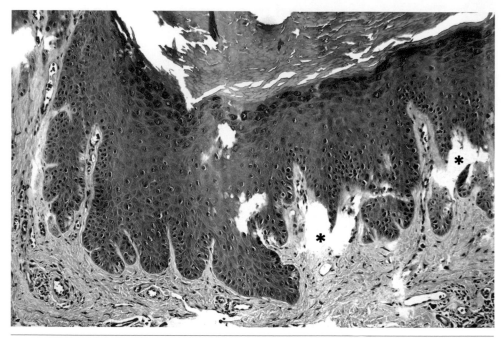

Figure 3.17: *Photomicrograph (H&E) of an actinic keratosis displaying suprabasal cleft formation (asterisks).*

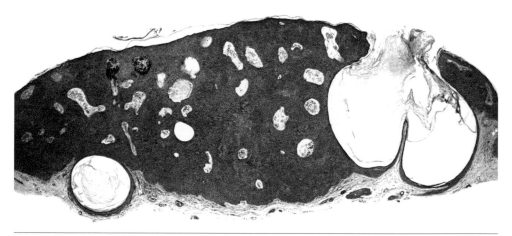

Figure 3.18: *Photomicrograph (H&E) showing acanthosis in a seborrhoeic keratosis with marked thickening of the epidermis.*

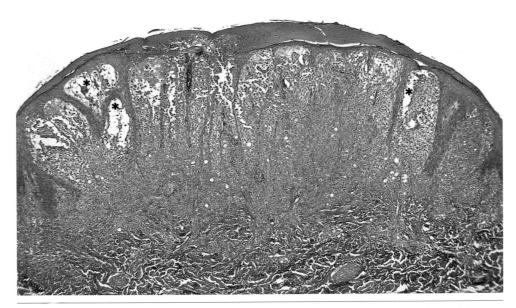

Figure 3.19: *Photomicrograph (H&E) showing prominent clefting in a nodular melanoma (asterisks).*

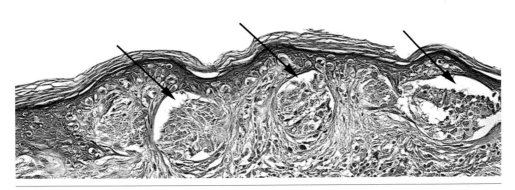

Figure 3.20: *Photomicrograph (H&E) showing clefts at the periphery of nests of melanocytes (arrows); melanoma.*

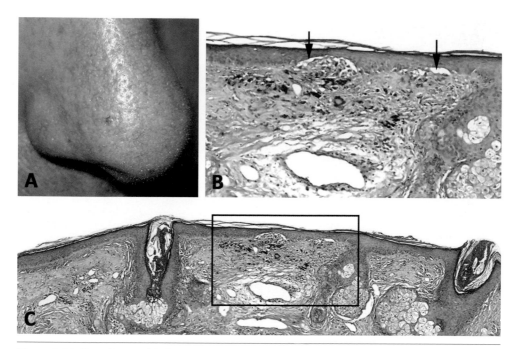

Figure 3.21: Clinical image (A) of a 1.5mm lesion on the nose. Photomicrographs (H&E) with clefting (boxed area (C) and indicated by arrows in a higher power view of the boxed area (B)), which attracted attention to the abnormal melanocytic proliferation; melanoma in situ[10].

not have the morphology of a Spitz naevus, it warrants a careful search for evidence of melanoma.

Desmosomes: the intercellular projections that connect keratinocytes (*Figure 3.22*), the loss of which may be responsible for acantholysis.

Elastosis: caused by a breakdown of elastic tissue in the dermis due to damage by solar radiation resulting in an increase in elastotic tissue (*Figure 3.23*).

Epidermal consumption: is atrophy of the epidermis overlying a melanocytic lesion and it may be seen in *in situ* or invasive melanomas in which the proliferation of the malignancy has displaced and/or degraded the overlying epidermis, causing it to become thin (*Figure 3.24*). Ultimately this can lead to ulceration.

Follicular extension: refers to the presence of lesional cells in infundibular structures including hair follicles (*Figure 3.25*).

Grenz zone: a zone of uninvolved dermis separating a lesion from the epidermis (*Figure 3.26*).

Kamino bodies: consist of pink basement membrane material within the epidermis, typically seen in a Spitz naevus (*Figure 3.27*).

Lentiginous proliferation: with regard to melanocytes, this is a proliferation of predominantly single melanocytes at the dermoepidermal junction (*Figure 3.28*). When they are lined up 'shoulder to shoulder' in contact with each other that is termed 'confluent'. The word lentiginous is derived from the word lentil, a metaphor for the clinical appearance of the pigmented macule lentigo. Lentiginous refers to the histological appearance of malignant melanocytes in

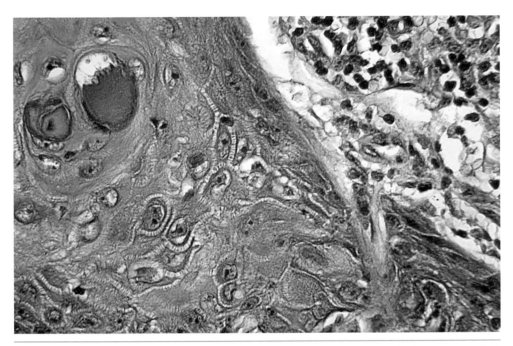

Figure 3.22: *Photomicrograph (H&E) of a squamous cell carcinoma clearly showing the desmosomes which connect adjacent keratinocytes. In this image adjacent desmosomes in linear array resemble the structure of segmented worms.*

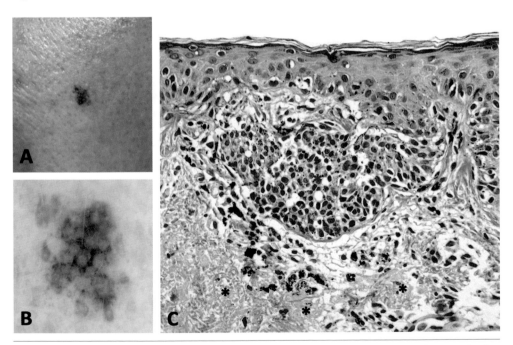

Figure 3.23: *In the photomicrograph (H&E) shown in (C) black asterisks mark areas of elastosis. The fact that this is present beneath a pigmented melanocytic proliferation (red asterisk) supported the 50-year-old patient's assertion that this lesion on her cheek (A) was new. Images courtesy Drs Agata Bulinska and Leonard Gross.*

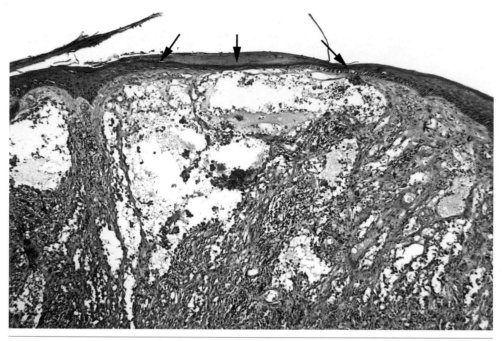

Figure 3.24: *Photomicrograph (H&E) of a portion of a nodular melanoma showing epidermal consumption (arrows) with incipient ulceration.*

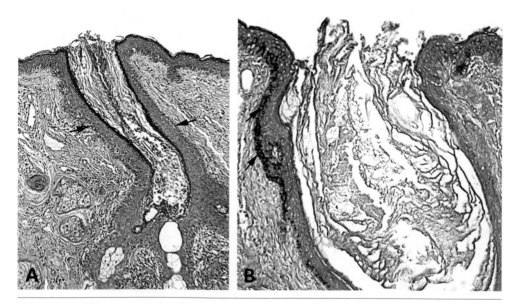

Figure 3.25: *Photomicrographs showing extension of pigmented malignant melanocytes down hair follicles (arrows) in a lentigo maligna on the nose. In this case while the melanocytes contain melanin, this is not evident with H&E staining (A) but is clearly seen with Schmorl's stain (B).*

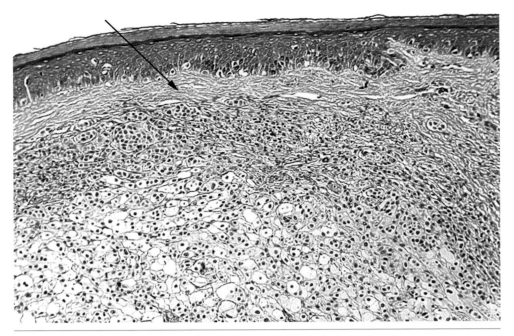

Figure 3.26: A grenz zone (arrow) in a photomicrograph (H&E) of a balloon cell melanoma.

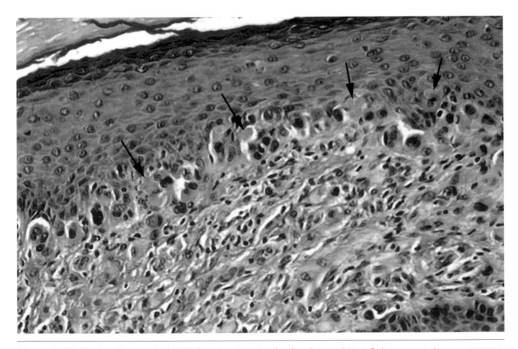

Figure 3.27: Photomicrograph (H&E) showing Kamino bodies (arrows) in a Spitz naevus. Image courtesy Dr Leonard Gross.

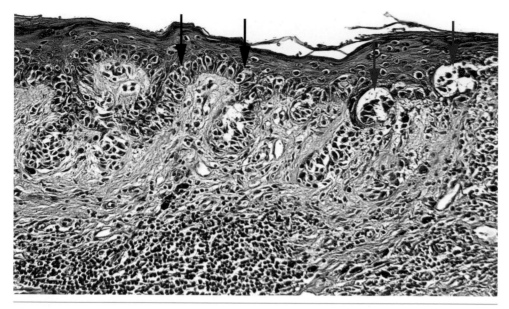

Figure 3.28: Photomicrograph (H&E) of a melanoma showing nesting (red arrows), as well as a confluent lentiginous proliferation of malignant melanocytes (black arrows). The aggregated small cells at the central lower part of the lesion represent an infiltrate of lymphocytes.

the variant of melanoma *in situ* called lentigo maligna. The origin of the word is related to the appearance of pigmented keratinocytes and/or pigmented melanocytes lined up along the basal layer of a lentigo.

Lymphocytic infiltrate: refers to a collection of lymphocytes within a lesion (*Figure 3.29*) and it is part of the host's response to abnormal cells. The immune attack may be on a benign lesion (e.g. LPLK) but it is also frequently a marker for a malignant lesion.

Lymphovascular and vascular invasion: characterised by the presence of tumour cells in blood or lymphatic vessels (*Figure 3.30*).

Maturation: in compound and dermal naevi the dermal melanocytes usually lose their melanin-producing capability and become small and compact (*Figure 3.31* black box). One speculative explanation is that melanin in the dermis performs no biological function and biological entities tend to avoid expending unnecessary energy. As well as being small,

these melanocytes, because of the maturation process, actually have a high nuclear–cytoplasmic ratio but their benign nature is evident due to their small size and uniformity. No melanin pigment can be seen. This process as it relates to melanocytes is termed '*maturation*'. In invasive melanoma, melanocytes typically do not 'mature' as they descend into the dermis which means that they remain large and retain their melanin-producing capability, whether or not they actually produce melanin (*Figure 3.32*).

Melanin incontinence: refers to the presence of melanin in the dermis where it appears to be extracellular but has actually been taken up by histiocytes (macrophages) known as melanophages (*Figure 3.33*). This heterotopic melanin results from an immune attack on a pigmented lesion which may in fact be confined to the epidermis and it is the explanation for the common presence of dermatoscopic grey colour in both benign (e.g. LPLK) and malignant (e.g. melanoma *in situ*, pigmented BCC and pigmented SCC *in situ*) lesions.

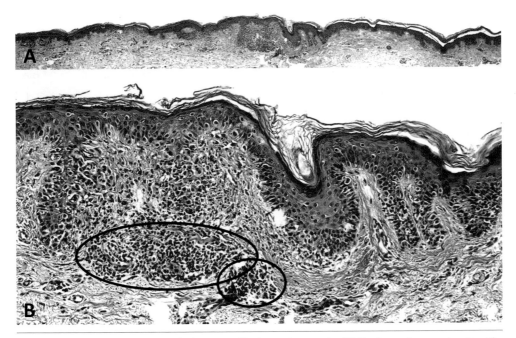

Figure 3.29: *Low power (A) and high power (B) photomicrographs (H&E) of a melanoma in situ. The dense proliferation of uniformly small, hyperchromatic (dark-staining) lymphocytes (encircled) led to closer inspection, revealing the presence of a proliferation of melanocytes in the adjacent epidermis (cells with abundant clear cytoplasm); melanoma in situ.*

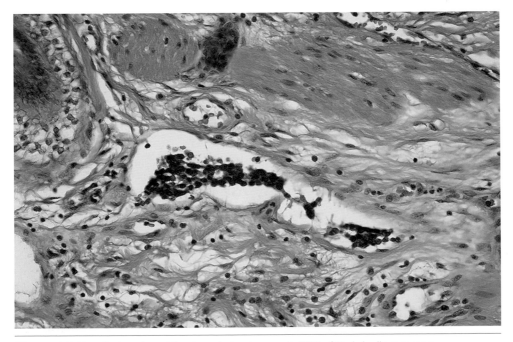

Figure 3.30: *Vascular invasion evident in a photomicrograph (H&E) of Merkel cell carcinoma.*

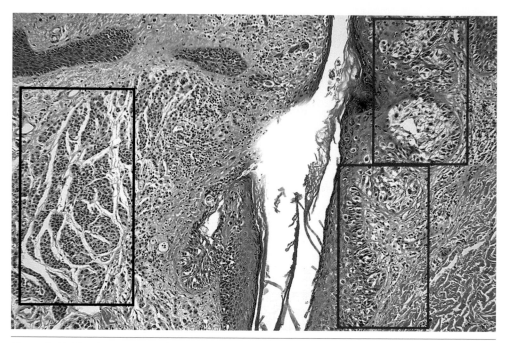

Figure 3.31: *This photomicrograph (H&E) shows a melanoma (red boxes) arising in association with a dermal naevus (black box). The melanocytes in the naevus are mature: uniformly compact and monomorphic. The malignant melanocytes are larger (compared to both the benign melanocytes and the adjacent keratinocytes) and pleomorphic.*

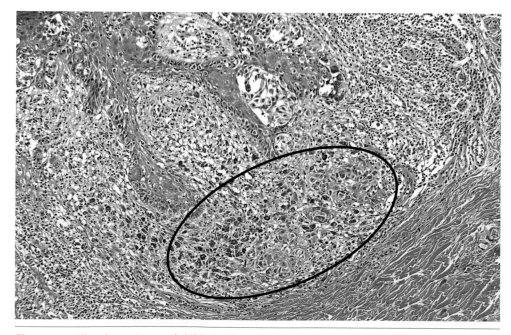

Figure 3.32: *This photomicrograph (H&E) shows a different section from the same melanoma displayed in* Figure 3.31. *The deep dermal malignant melanocytes (circle) have not matured. They are large, pleomorphic and heavily pigmented.*

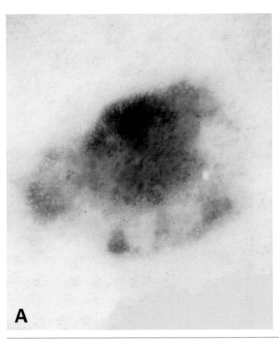
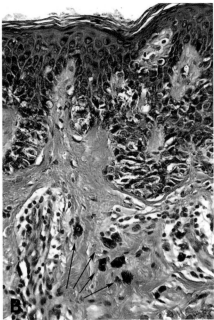

Figure 3.33: Dermatoscopic (A) and histological (B) (H&E) images of a melanoma in situ. The melanin in the dermis (arrows) is not within melanocytes but it is within macrophages (the macrophages are not visible with H&E staining). This accounts for the presence of melanin in the papillary dermis, which correlates with dermatoscopic grey dots (A).

Mitotic figures and apoptosis: mitotic figures represent cells in the stage of mitosis and are a marker of cellular proliferation in cutaneous malignancies (*Figures 3.34–37*). Apoptosis, representing programmed cell death, also reflects increased cell turnover and therefore proliferation (*Figure 3.36*).

Nesting: an architectural feature in which proliferating cells are aggregated together as 'nests' (*Figure 3.38*). With respect to melanocytic lesions, uniform nesting is a feature of naevi while single cell proliferation is a feature of melanoma. Nests in melanomas tend to be irregular in size, shape, cellularity and distribution, with confluence and bridging (*Figure 3.38*).

Pagetoid spread: refers to the presence of cells with abundant cytoplasm surrounding the nucleus, located in the epidermis above the level of the dermoepidermal junction (*Figures 3.39–41*). It is named after this feature which can be seen in the distribution of malignant cells in Paget's disease of the nipple but is most frequently used to describe the appearance of malignant melanocytes at all layers of the epidermis as an early feature in many melanomas.

Papillomatosis: characterised by hypertrophy of dermal papillae resulting in a verrucous (wart-like) contour as seen in some seborrhoeic keratoses and dermal naevi, as well as in warts (*Figure 3.42*).

Psoriasiform hyperplasia: like acanthosis, also involves thickening of the epidermis but preferentially involving the rete ridges (*Figure 3.43*).

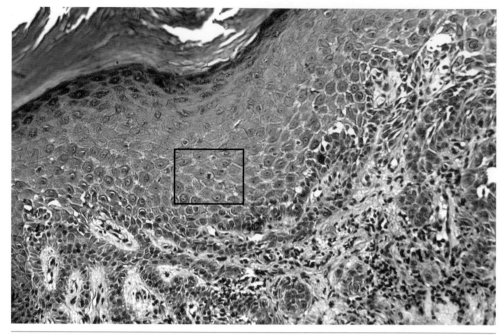

Figure 3.34: A mitotic figure in a photomicrograph (H&E) of an SCC seen at scanning power (centre of boxed area).

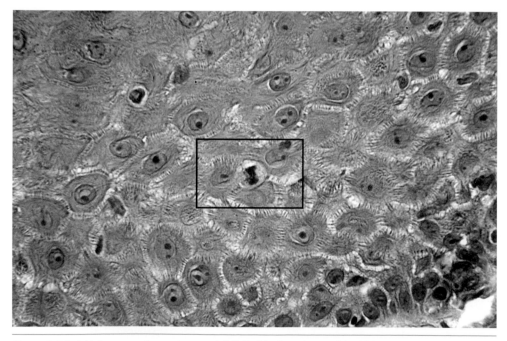

Figure 3.35: A high-power photomicrograph (H&E) of the boxed area of the SCC in Figure 3.34 confirms the low-power impression of a mitotic figure.

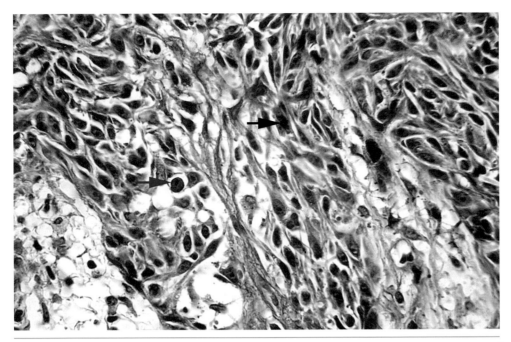

Figure 3.36: *A mitotic figure (black arrow) and apoptotic figure (red arrow) in a photomicrograph (H&E) of an invasive melanoma. Apoptosis (programmed cell death) is a marker for high cell turnover just as mitotic figures are (H&E).*

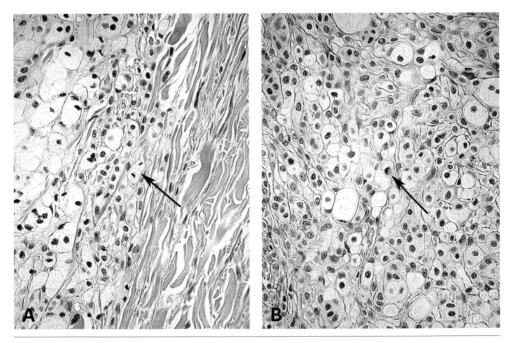

Figure 3.37: *Mitotic figures in two photomicrographs (H&E) of a balloon cell melanoma[11].*

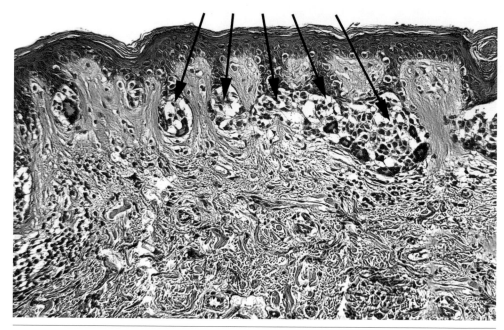

Figure 3.38: Photomicrograph (H&E) of a melanoma with nests (arrows) showing variability of size and distribution with some confluence (bridging).

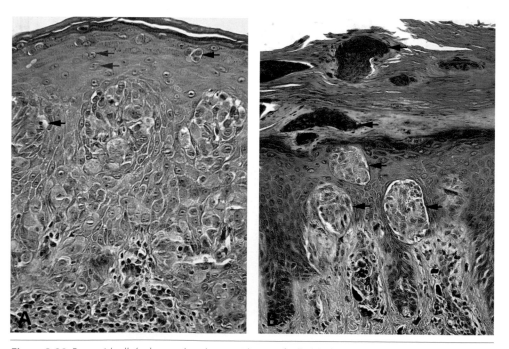

Figure 3.39: Pagetoid cells (red arrows) and pagetoid nests of cells (black arrows) in photomicrographs (H&E) of extra-mammary Paget's disease of the labia minora (A) and a Reed naevus (B).

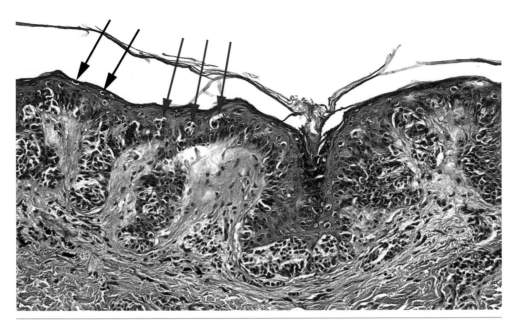

Figure 3.40: *Pagetoid spread of cells (black arrows) and small nests (red arrows) in a photomicrograph (H&E) of a melanoma.*

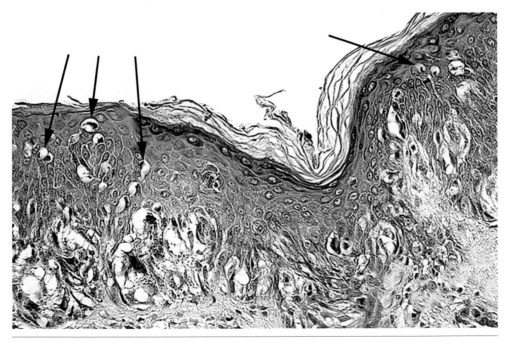

Figure 3.41: *Pagetoid spread of melanocytes (arrows) in a photomicrograph (H&E) of a melanoma.*

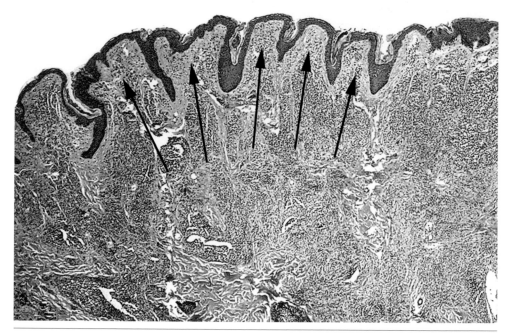

Figure 3.42: *Photomicrograph (H&E) of a dermal naevus exhibiting papillomatosis with the hypertrophic dermal papillae indicated by arrows.*

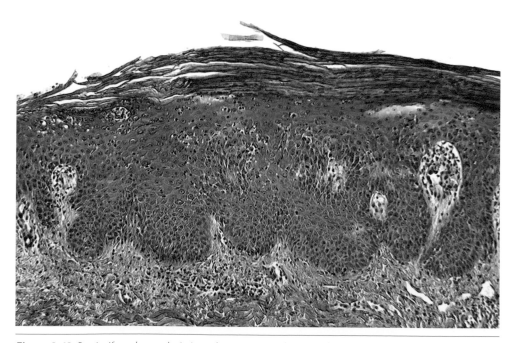

Figure 3.43: *Psoriasiform hyperplasia in a photomicrograph (H&E) of psoriasis.*

3.4 Dermatoscopic histological correlation of neoplastic lesions

This section will first outline the principles by which neoplastic skin lesions are assessed dermatopathologically. It will then describe and illustrate the significant histological features and dermatoscopic correlations of the three major skin malignancies: melanoma, BCC and SCC, as well as the histological features of the major benign keratinocytic lesions.

3.4.1 The assessment of lesions

A lesion is a discrete entity recognisable as distinct from normal skin and it may be submitted, in part or whole, for dermato-pathological examination for the purpose of diagnosis. Although such diagnosis might be made by histological pattern recognition, there are features which must be present for a specific diagnosis to be made, and it is these features and their correlation with dermato-scopic features that will be considered in this section.

With dermatoscopy the assessment of a lesion involves a stepwise assessment of patterns, colours and finally clues (see *Chapter 8*). With dermatopathology the first assessment is that of architecture followed by cytology.

In a systematic dermatopathological examination the initial assessment is performed at low power, in some cases by holding the microscope slide up to a light, and it is an assessment of the architecture, including the organisation, symmetry, circum-scription and contour of the lesion.

Architecture

This refers to the arrangement of the cells and structures on the histology slide and relates to the degree of internal orderliness of the lesion. *Figure 3.44* is a low power view of three skin specimens from one mature Australian patient, all excised on the same day. *Figure 3.44A* shows histology of 'normal'

sun-damaged skin from beside a melanoma on the arm. At the surface the layered stratum corneum can be seen displaying a basket-weave pattern. The rest of the epidermis is seen as a similarly purple layer of cells in an orderly arrangement with each other. On the far right there is some brown pigment in the cells of the basal layer consistent with an ephilis (freckle). Beneath the cells of the basal layer of the epidermis is the papillary dermis, composed mainly of collagen, in which vessels can be seen. The dermis is essentially normal apart from some evidence of elastosis (seen as a pale mauve or grey colour) and ectasia of vessels due to sun damage. The general orderliness of the various structures is consistent with 'normal' architecture.

Parts (B) and (C) in *Figure 3.44* are photo-micrographs of a melanoma *in situ* and an invasive melanoma, respectively, and the increasing disorder of the cellular and pigment arrangement compared to the upper image, is evident. To assess the other aspects of architecture: symmetry, circum-scription and contour, it is ideal to view the lesion in its entirety (see *Section 3.4.2* and *Figure 3.46*).

Cytology

While architecture refers to the arrangement of the cells and other structures, cytology refers to the features of the individual cells. *Figure 3.45* shows a higher power view of a portion of *Figure 3.44A*. The individual cells are uniformly similar in size with no significant variation in their nuclei with respect to size or colour. The cytology is normal.

3.4.2 Histology of melanoma

Clinically and dermatoscopically melanoma can be in the differential diagnosis of benign melanocytic lesions (naevi) as well as benign and malignant non-melanocytic lesions (e.g. LPLK, BCC and pSCC *in situ*). Histologically, once

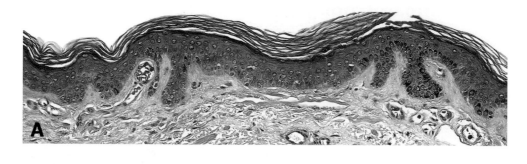

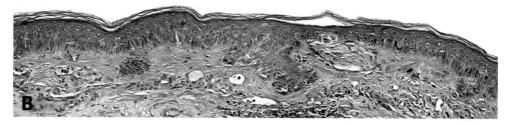

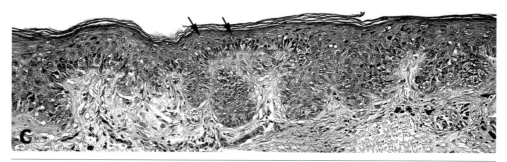

Figure 3.44: Photomicrographs (H&E): sections of skin from the same patient on the same day demonstrating the increasing architectural disarray moving from normal perilesional skin (A), to melanoma in situ (B) and invasive melanoma (C). The evident atypia includes pagetoid melanocytes (arrows), as well as disordered keratinocytes and melanin distribution.

the melanocytic nature of a lesion is identified the decision comes down to distinguishing a melanoma from a naevus. While there is no single criterion that reliably distinguishes a melanoma from a naevus, the distinction is not difficult in the majority of cases if the following accepted diagnostic criteria for a diagnosis of melanoma are applied[12].

Diagnostic criteria for the diagnosis of melanoma

Architecture:

- Asymmetry with poor circumscription, epidermal consumption, clefting.

- Confluent junctional proliferation of melanocytes or full-thickness pagetoid spread. Single cells exceed nests in some high-power fields.
- Nests varying in size, shape and interval with confluence and bridging.
- Nests remain pigmented at the base and fail to disperse.

Cytology (in some melanomas cytology may be normal):

- Cytological atypia (melanocyte nuclei larger, with prominent nucleoli, abnormal chromatin distribution and varying morphology).

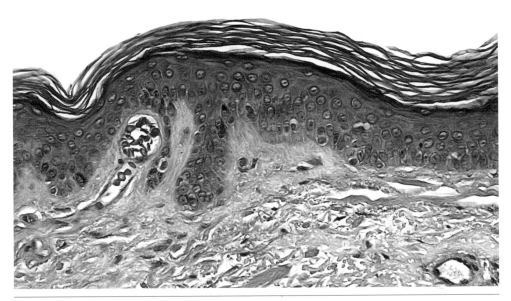

Figure 3.45: *A higher power view of part of the slide displayed in* Figure 3.44A. *Examination of the features of the individual cells shows no significant deviation from normal, consistent with normal cytology.*

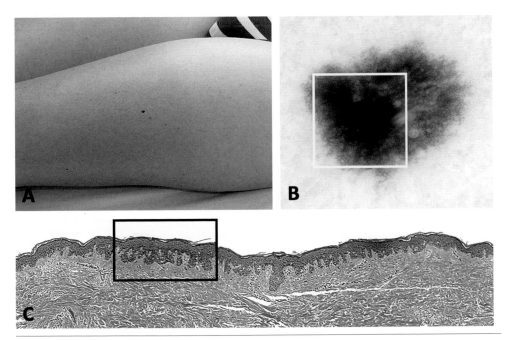

Figure 3.46: *Clinical (A), dermatoscopic (B) and histological (H&E) (C) views of a pigmented skin lesion on the thigh. Apparent dermatoscopic chaos and thick reticular lines (yellow box) lead to excision biopsy to exclude melanoma. Histologically (C) the lesion is sharply circumscribed and symmetrical except for slightly broader rete ridges on one side (black box) correlating with the dermatoscopically thickened lines; Clark (acquired) naevus. In retrospect the dermatoscopy is reasonably biologically symmetrical, the peripheral brown completely surrounding the darker centre and with no chaos of border abruptness.*

- Mitoses and apoptosis.
- Melanocytes fail to mature as they descend into the dermis.

The histological features which identify a melanoma have dermatoscopic correlates and communication of these to the dermatopathologist will ensure that the relevant expected features are identified or excluded.

Architecture

Once a melanocytic proliferation has been identified, the first assessment is of architecture. Just as clinically and dermatoscopically a naevus is expected to be non-chaotic with a uniform gradual border over the entire periphery, histologically it should be symmetrical and well circumscribed (*Figure 3.46*). The presence of histological asymmetry and of poor and/or variable circumscription can raise suspicion for melanoma, just as dermatoscopic chaos of pattern, colour or border abruptness can (*Figure 3.47*). It should be noted that while dermatoscopic symmetry is assessed on pattern, colour and border-abruptness, histological symmetry is defined geometrically.

The organisation of melanocytes in naevi: expected to be in nests, cords, fascicles or strands. The nests may be at the tips of rete ridges and/or spread along the dermoepidermal junction. They are expected to be distributed symmetrically, correlating with either a brown non-chaotic reticular pattern or a brown symmetrical clod pattern respectively[13]. Melanocytes in both naevi (compound, dermal or blue) and invasive melanomas can also be found in the dermis. In a compound naevus or dermal naevus they are expected to be arranged symmetrically, with the nests tending to disperse to single cells at the base of the lesion.

The organisation of melanocytes in melanomas: tends to be arranged in a chaotic manner with significant single cell proliferation at the dermoepidermal junction; in places confluent and with the nesting that

does occur, varying in size, shape and interval often with confluence and bridging. To the extent that the melanocytes are pigmented, this correlates with chaos of both structure and colour.

Areas that are lightly pigmented or non-pigmented often have enhanced pink or red colour due to the hyperaemia of tumour tissue with its enhanced metabolic demand. When an immune attack by lymphocytes has resulted in regression and subsequent fibrosis, the collagen may correlate with dermatoscopic white structureless areas.

Pagetoid spread: another architectural feature of melanoma is the spread of single malignant melanocytes and nests of melanocytes away from the dermoepidermal junction to higher layers of the epidermis in the phenomenon designated as pagetoid spread. While this can occur to a limited extent centrally in an irritated naevus, more extensively following UV irradiation and commonly in Spitz naevi, it can be a notable feature in melanomas and, when combined with asymmetry and poor circumscription, it favours the diagnosis of melanoma rather than naevus. When the pagetoid small clusters of melanocytes and of nests are pigmented they will appear dermatoscopically as dark brown or black dots or clods (the human eye cannot discriminate single cells dermatoscopically, the limit of dermatoscopic resolution being approximately 0.05mm – the diameter of about 5 melanocytes). When black dots or clods are peripherally located that fulfills one of the nine clues to melanoma in the 'Chaos and Clues' algorithm (see *Chapter 6*) (*Figure 3.48*)[14].

Lymphocytic infiltrate: the features seen through a dermatoscope and microscope not only reflect the behaviour of malignant tissue but also the body's response to that tissue. A lymphocytic infiltrate is frequently seen adjacent to, or even within, a melanoma and while this can also be a feature of benign lesions including a naevus (e.g. halo naevus), the infiltrate is expected to be asymmetrical

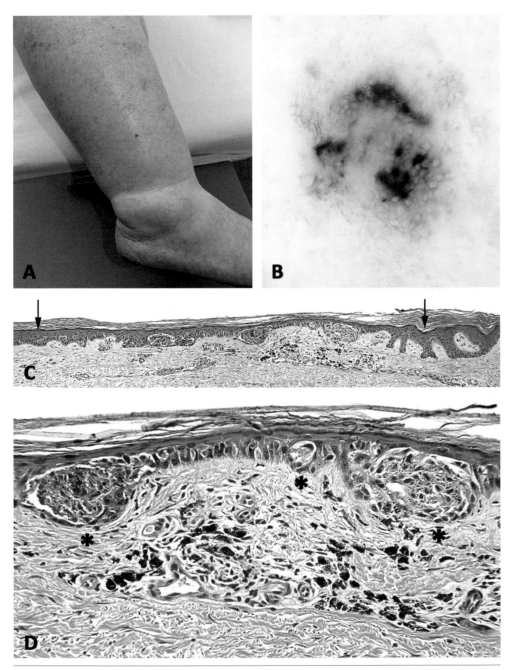

Figure 3.47: *Clinical (A), dermatoscopic (B) and histological (H&E) (C, D) images of a pigmented skin lesion on the leg. The lesion is poorly circumscribed and asymmetrical both dermatoscopically and histologically (approximate borders marked with arrows (C)). Nests vary in size and interval (asterisks) and numbers of single cells, which are confluent (between nests) exceed the number of nests (D). The epidermis is too atrophic to make room for any pagetoid spread; melanoma in situ.*

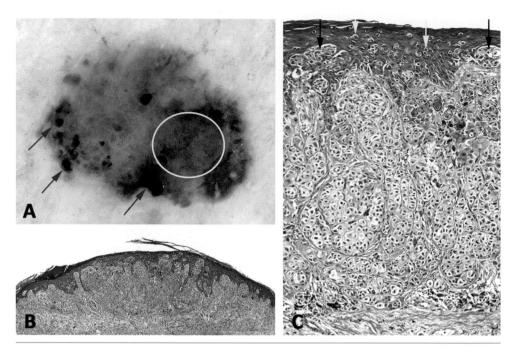

Figure 3.48: *Dermatoscopic (A) and histological images (H&E) (B, C) of a pigmented skin lesion in the popliteal fossa. Dermatoscopic black clods (red arrows) correlate with pagetoid pigmented melanocyte nests (black arrows). Black dots (yellow circle) correlate with pagetoid pigmented small clusters of melanocytes. Single pagetoid melanocytes (yellow arrows) would not be visible dermatoscopically. Dermatoscopic structureless blue correlates with abundant pigment in deep dermal nested melanocytes (C).*

in relation to a melanoma (*Figure 3.49*)[15]. The asymmetrical lymphocytic proliferation may be noticed by the dermatopathologist and draw attention to a subtle melanoma, there being an aphorism among pathologists that 'lymphocytes are better than pathologists at recognising melanoma'.

Melanin incontinence: lymphocytes are colourless so a lymphocytic proliferation is not visible dermatoscopically. But, one of the common sequelae of an immune attack is melanin incontinence whereby melanin particles, remaining after cellular destruction in the immune attack, are taken up by macrophages (melanophages) and carried into the dermis where they produce the dermatoscopic feature of grey dots[10]. Fortunately for the dermatoscopist, this immune response produces the clue of grey dots for many pigmented malignancies, including most *in situ* melanomas.

Maturation of melanocytes: as mentioned above, dermal melanocytes in compound and dermal naevi are often arranged in symmetrical nests, dispersing to single cells at the base. These melanocytes change as they descend into the dermis. They no longer produce melanin, presumably because there is no function for melanin below the epidermis, and they lose their melanin-producing function, becoming smaller and more compact with a reduction in the amount of cytoplasm. The corollary of this process, known as 'maturation', is the fact that with the exception of the superficial dermal component of some congenital naevi, the dermal component of all other naevi, except blue and combined naevi, is non-pigmented.

In contrast to the melanocytes in compound and dermal naevi, the malignant melanocytes that invade the dermis in melanomas rarely undergo maturation, and as a result they tend to retain the same size and

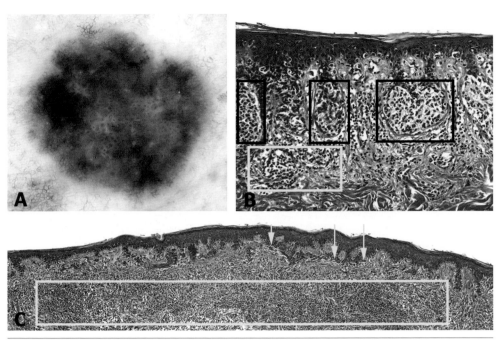

Figure 3.49: *Dermatoscopic (A) and histological images (H&E) (B, C) of a pigmented skin lesion on the chest. In (C) a dense lymphocytic infiltrate (yellow box) attracts attention and a melanocytic proliferation can just be seen above it at low power (yellow arrows). In the high power view (B) single melanocytes are seen throughout the epidermis and melanocyte nests are also confined to the dermoepidermal junction (black boxes). In high power view (B) a yellow box indicates the dermal infiltration of lymphocytes; melanoma in situ.*

pigment-producing activity as their epidermal counterparts (see *Figure 3.32*). Melanin in the dermis appears grey or blue dermatoscopically and, while symmetrical blue is expected in blue and combined naevi, the presence of asymmetrical blue colour due to melanin is a clue that melanin is located where it should not be, pointing to invasive neoplasia (*Figure 3.50*). If that neoplasia is melanocytic then invasive melanoma will be the expected cause.

Cytology

It is a fact that cytology can be normal in some melanomas and that is why it is essential that any biopsy, preferably an elliptical excision biopsy, is sufficient to demonstrate the architecture of the lesion.

Abnormal cytology can be expressed in several ways, some or all of which may be present in a melanoma.

- **The malignant melanocytes may be larger than normal** (*Figure 3.51*): but a more significant marker of cytological atypia is the presence of pleomorphic (variable size) hyperchromatic (dark-coloured) nuclei and prominent nucleoli (*Figure 3.52*).
- **Mitotic figures:** another significant marker of cytological atypia is the presence of mitotic figures (evidence of proliferation) as well as apoptotic figures (caused by programmed cell death), both being markers of high cell turnover. These are regarded as even more significant when present near the base of the lesion[12].
- **Lack of maturation of melanocytes as they descend into the dermis:** this is a cytological feature which may be associated with the presence of melanin deep in the dermis in nested melanocytes which can be present at the base of the lesion, failing

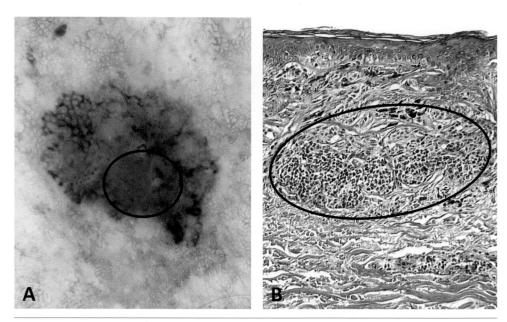

Figure 3.50: *Dermatoscopic (A) and histological (H&E) (B) images of a pigmented skin lesion. Dermatoscopic structureless blue (circle in A) correlates with heavily pigmented and nested melanocytes deep in the dermis (circle in B). A lentiginous proliferation of single melanocytes can be seen at the dermoepidermal junction and some pagetoid melanocytes are visible in the epidermis. Dermatoscopic structureless blue in a chaotic lesion is a clue to malignancy; melanoma invasive.*

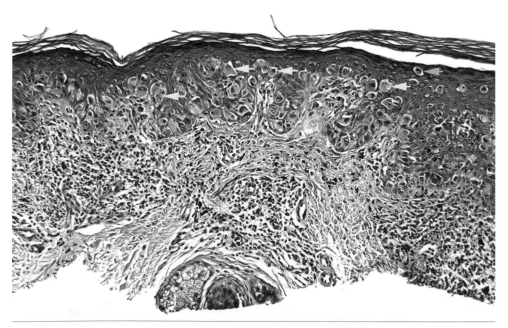

Figure 3.51: *Photomicrograph (H&E) showing a proliferation of epithelioid melanocytes (yellow arrows) at the dermoepidermal junction and at all layers of the epidermis, including one exhibiting almost full-thickness pagetoid spread (blue arrow); melanoma invasive.*

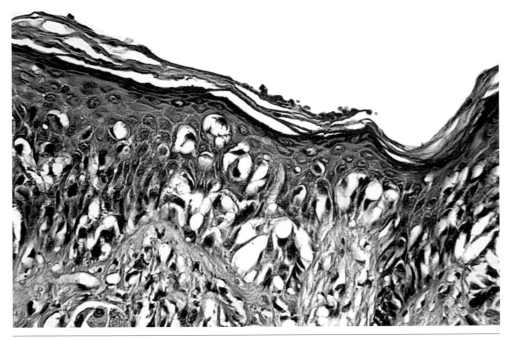

Figure 3.52: *Pleomorphic and hyperchromatic melanocyte nuclei are seen in this photomicrograph (H&E) of a melanoma.*

to disperse to single cells as expected in a naevus (*Figure 3.50*).

3.4.3 Histology of basal cell carcinoma

Basal cell carcinoma is a malignancy probably derived from cells in hair follicles rather than from basal cells[16]. Compelling indirect evidence for this comes from the fact that BCC almost exclusively occurs on non-glabrous (hair-bearing) skin. Notwithstanding this, BCC generally extends from the dermoepidermal junction into the dermis. There is no intraepidermal form of BCC, so it should be regarded as an invasive cutaneous malignancy.

Architecture

The architecture of BCC typically presents as an island or clusters of basaloid cells attached to the undersurface of the epidermis, projecting into the dermis. The clusters may exhibit palisading of nuclei at the periphery with haphazard cellular arrangement centrally (*Figure 3.53*). The clusters and

islands are surrounded by newly formed BCC-specific stroma which is different from that of the surrounding dermis. Clefting at the stromal tumour interface is common.

Cytology

Cytologically the lesional cells have hyperchromatic nuclei and scanty cytoplasm. Desmosomes are not present. Numerous mitotic figures are seen, sometimes atypical and there is a correspondingly high number of apoptotic tumour cells. This probably accounts for the generally slow growth rate of BCC even though there are many mitoses.

Starting from the basic criteria listed above, the histological features of BCC vary according to the subtype, as do the dermatoscopic features.

Superficial BCC: characterised by clusters of BCC cells hanging down from the dermoepidermal junction (*Figure 3.53*). If the lesion is not pigmented the dermatoscopic features of erythema and fine serpentine vessels relate to the associated increased vascularity, although

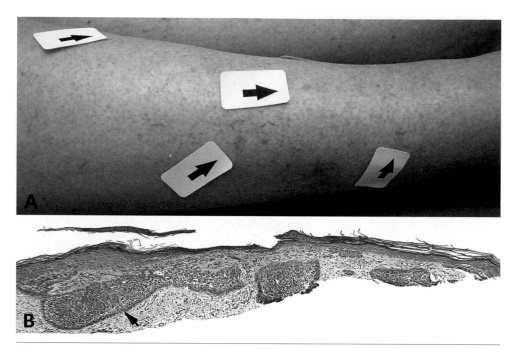

Figure 3.53: *Clinical image of multiple superficial BCCs (A) and a histological image (H&E) (B) of one of them. The proliferation of neoplastic cells hangs down from the undersurface of the epidermis. Palisading of the outer layer of cells is evident (arrow in image B).*

BCC stroma may also accentuate the clarity of the vessels. If the lesion is pigmented, this may present dermatoscopically as brown, grey or blue dots or clods, or as light brown structureless pigmentation. Characteristic structures such as radial converging lines and clods with a central dot can be present in all BCC subtypes, including superficial BCC.

Nodular or nodulocystic BCC: circumscribed nodular proliferations of 'solid' clusters of BCC cells, the individual clusters being separated by stroma (*Figure 3.54*). The solid tumour mass is supported by a vascular network, and large bore vessels set in translucent stroma can present dermatoscopically as sharply defined, thick, branched, serpentine vessels.

Micronodular BCC: characterised by smaller nodules and, if the lesion is circumscibed, this subtype can be managed in a similar manner to nodular BCC. But if it is poorly circumscribed and the micronodules extend into

surrounding tissue, this should be managed as an aggressive BCC and excision with appropriately wider margins should be considered. Designation as micronodular is histological, there being no clinical or dermatoscopic features which identify this subtype.

Aggressive subtypes include infiltrative and morphoeic BCC: the features of these are often combined, infiltrating BCC being characterised by strands of tumour tissue invading adjacent dermis and sometimes even fat, with the addition of bands of fibrosis in morphoeic (sclerosing) types (*Figure 3.55*). These aggressive subtypes have less BCC stroma and the associated vessels tend to be finer and this, as well as less likelihood of pigmentation, makes them less evident clinically so that they may be advanced when diagnosed. Their identification may rely on just a subtle clinical difference from surrounding skin to prompt careful dermatoscopic examination, with the discovery of white structureless scar-like tissue with fine vessels as the predominant clue.

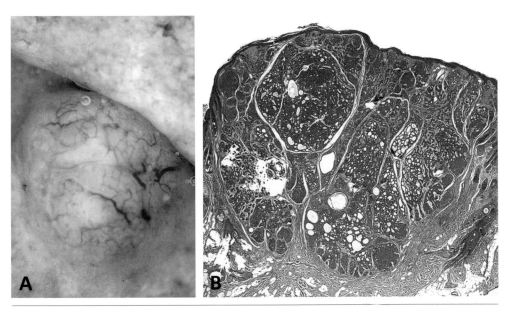

Figure 3.54: *Dermatoscopic (A) and histological (H&E) (B) images of a nodulocystic BCC on the nasolabial groove. The lesion is well circumscribed.*

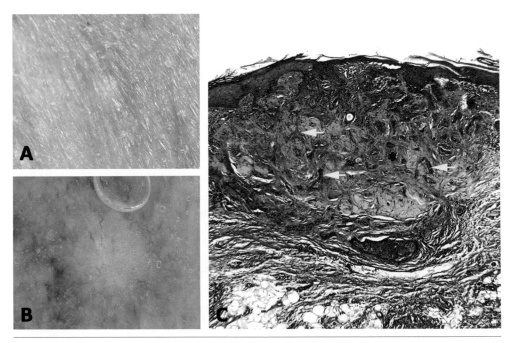

Figure 3.55: *Close up (A), dermatoscopic (B) and histological (H&E) (C) images of an infiltrating and sclerosing BCC on the cheek. Clinically and dermatoscopically the lesion is subtle but histologically it is infiltrating deeply (yellow arrows), the thin cords being separated by extensive collagenous fibrous tissue (asterisk).*

3.4.4 Histology of common benign keratinocytic lesions

The most relevant benign keratinocytic lesions in the differential diagnosis of skin malignancies are solar lentigo, seborrhoeic keratosis and LPLK.

Solar lentigo

Architecture: the architecture of solar lentigo is characterised by elongated rete ridges which may be joined by finger-like projections. Although there may be a slight increase in the density of melanocytes, this does not constitute melanocytic neoplasia. The characteristic and common reticular appearance of solar lentigines is due to pigment in keratinocytes in rete ridges (*Figure 3.56*). On the face, rete ridge hyperplasia may not be present and follicles may give a pattern of structureless pigmentation interrupted by follicular openings or occasionally there may be a pattern of brown circles.

Cytology: the cytology of the keratinocytes which make up solar lentigo is normal.

Seborrhoeic keratosis

Architecture: the architecture of seborrhoeic keratosis varies according to the subtype, but acanthosis is the most evident feature; the degree of acanthosis is variable. Collections of orthokeratotic keratin occur in horn cysts correlating with dermatoscopic white clods and dots. Where accumulations of this loose laminar keratin are exposed to the atmosphere in surface invaginations the normally white keratin becomes discoloured, correlating with dermatoscopic yellow, orange or brown clods (*Figure 3.57*). Nests of keratinocytes known as squamous eddies may also be seen. The keratin on the surface of seborrhoeic keratoses is typically in the form of loosely laminated orthokeratin and it is commonly thickened: hyperkeratosis (*Figure 3.58*).

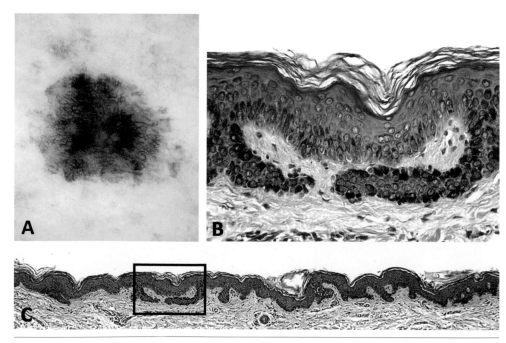

Figure 3.56: Dermatoscopic (A) and histological (H&E) (B, C) images of a solar lentigo. The boxed area in (C) is shown enlarged in (B). Rete ridges are predominantly bulb-like with heavy pigmentation of basal keratinocytes giving a prominent reticular pattern.

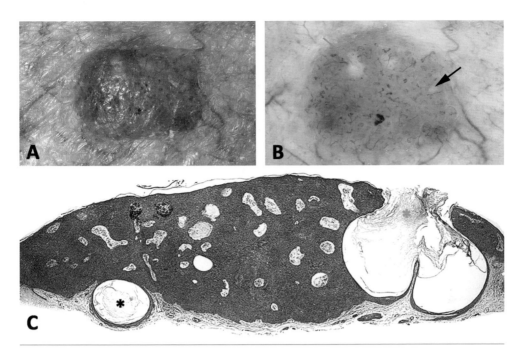

Figure 3.57: *Clinical (A), dermatoscopic (B) and histological (H&E) (C) images of a seborrhoeic keratosis. The epidermis is marked by acanthosis (purple-coloured cellular mass). An enclosed keratin cyst (black asterisk in C) correlates with a white clod (black arrow in B) and an open keratin crypt (blue asterisk in C) correlates with an orange clod (blue arrow in B).*

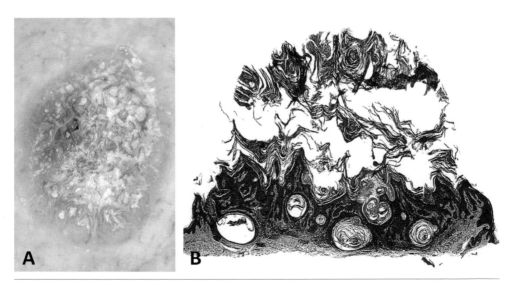

Figure 3.58: *Dermatoscopic (A) and histological (H&E) (B) images of a seborrhoeic keratosis. Extensive surface keratin is evident in both images and this obscures the keratin horn cysts seen histologically, from the dermatoscopic view.*

Cytology: the cytology of seborrhoeic keratoses is composed of basaloid cells with a varying mixture of squamoid cells, lacking atypical cytological features.

Lichen planus-like keratosis

Lichen planus-like keratosis (LPLK) is the term given for a benign keratinocytic lesion, typically a solar lentigo or seborrhoeic keratosis which is undergoing, or has undergone, immune regression. In the early stages the precursor lesion will be evident both dermatoscopically and histologically, with clinical and dermatoscopic erythema due to inflammation, correlating with a brisk lymphocytic proliferation histologically (*Figures 3.59* and *3.60*). A more mature LPLK may only present melanin incontinence, as evidence of a pigmented precursor lesion, correlating with dermatoscopic grey dots. If the precursor lesion was not pigmented

there may well be very little either dermatoscopically or histologically to reveal its nature, such non-pigmented LPLK commonly being mistaken dermatoscopically for BCC or thin amelanotic melanoma.

3.4.5 Histology of squamous cell carcinoma

Actinic keratosis

Actinic keratosis (AK) is regarded by some as the earliest form of SCC[17]. The fact that most AK do not progress to the point where the cells have gained 'immortality' would seem inconsistent with malignant status. However, to the extent that AK is at least a precursor to SCC, it is relevant to give an overview of its histological features.

Architecture and cytology: AK is characterised by epidermal dysplasia including

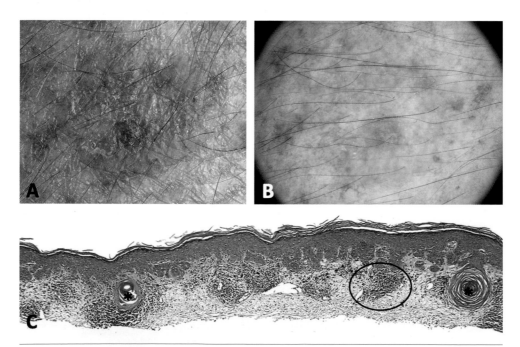

Figure 3.59: Clinical (A), dermatoscopic (B) and histological (H&E) (C) images of an LPLK on the forearm. Clinically there is a poorly defined pigmented lesion. Dermatoscopically there is extensive structureless erythema with a central remnant of seborrhoeic keratosis and peripheral remnants of solar lentigo. Histologically there is some acanthosis with prominent non-pigmented rete ridges correlating with the structureless dermatoscopic pattern. Two keratin cysts (asterisks) are further evidence of the seborrhoeic keratosis precursor. There is a heavy infiltration of lymphocytes in the dermis (one example circled).

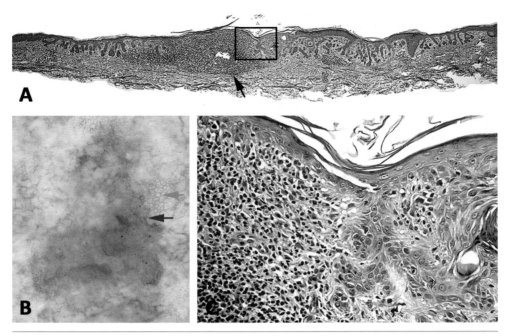

Figure 3.60: *Dermatoscopic (B) and histological images (H&E) (A, C) of an LPLK. A remnant sharp scalloped border (red arrow in B) and an area of reticular pattern (blue arrow in B) are evidence of a precursor solar lentigo, the fine reticular lines correlating with accentuated fine pigmented rete ridges (blue circle in A). There is a marked lymphocytic infiltrate (black arrow in A) over which the epidermal rete ridges are attenuated, correlating with a dermatoscopic structureless area. The boxed area in (A) is shown at high power in (C).*

architectural disorder with sparing of just a few layers of cells beneath the stratum granulosum (*Figures 3.61* and *3.62*). There is also cytological atypia of these dysplastic cells. Associated features include discontinuous disruption of the stratum granulosum as well as parakeratosis due to retention of nuclei by rapidly proliferating squamous cells as they pass into the stratum corneum (*Figure 3.61*). This same rapid proliferation can cause an accumulation of cells in the stratum corneum appearing as surface keratin scale. The dense parakeratotic scale overlying AK is more compact than the loose laminar keratin produced by seborrhoeic keratosis, which may be the reason that it remains white compared to exposed keratin on seborrhoeic keratoses.

Dermatoscopic histological correlation: dermatoscopy is designed to render the normal stratum corneum invisible, but the presence of significant surface scale can challenge this so all that may be seen dermatoscopically is structureless white. Subcorneal epidermis and dermis which is visible may be pink due to increased blood flow in the dermis resulting from the increased metabolic demand of neoplastic tissue. Fine serpentine or coiled blood vessels may be seen, characteristically lacking the clarifying effect of BCC-type stroma. In facial skin, involvement of hair follicle epidermis by highly keratinised keratinocytes can lead to the dermatoscopic feature of white circles[18]. This combined with background erythema has led to an appearance described in metaphorical terminology as a 'strawberry pattern'[19].

Pigmented actinic keratosis
Actinic keratoses may be pigmented in which case the pigment, seen histologically in keratinocytes, or as melanin incontinence following immune attack, can correlate dermatoscopically

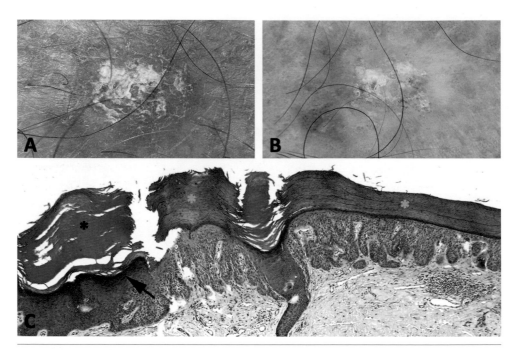

Figure 3.61: Clinical (A), dermatoscopic (B) and histological images (H&E) (C) of a solar keratosis on the dorsal hand. Dysplasia of the epidermis spares a few layers of cells just beneath the stratum corneum. Hyperkeratotic parakeratosis (blue asterisks) and focal disruption of the stratum granulosum is prominent above abnormal epithelium, while hyperkeratotic orthokeratosis (black asterisk) and an intact stratum granulosum (arrow) overlies relatively normal epithelium.

with brown or grey dots respectively; more rarely with angulated lines (polygons)[20]. Pigmented grey dots may be randomly distributed or on the face they may be orientated around white circles correlating with melanin incontinence from neoplastic follicular epithelium.

Four-dot clods: the dermatoscopic feature of polarising specific 4-dot clods resolves to follicular structures with non-polarised dermatoscopy (*Figure 3.62*). Their morphology may be due to an interaction between polarised light and its selective reflection from laminated keratin surrounding follicles.

Squamous cell carcinoma *in situ*

Architecture and cytology: SCC *in situ* differs histologically from AK with dysplasia involving the full thickness of the epidermis (*Figure 3.63*), in contrast to AK in which

several layers of cells beneath the stratum granulosum are spared. Apart from that, the dermatopathology is similar even though SCC *in situ*, Bowenoid-type, presents typically as a broad plaque with sharply defined borders.

Dermatoscopic histological correlation: dermatoscopically there are significant differences from AK, with a characteristic monomorphous pattern of coiled vessels typically in a clustered or linear arrangement.

Pigmented variants of SCC *in situ*

Pigmented variants make up 3–5% of SCC *in situ* and the pigment may be present in the epidermis as basal hyperpigmentation of keratinocytes, scattered in keratinocytes at all levels of the epidermis, or as melanin incontinence in the dermis, correlating dermatoscopically with structureless brown, brown dots and grey dots, respectively (*Figure 3.64*)[21].

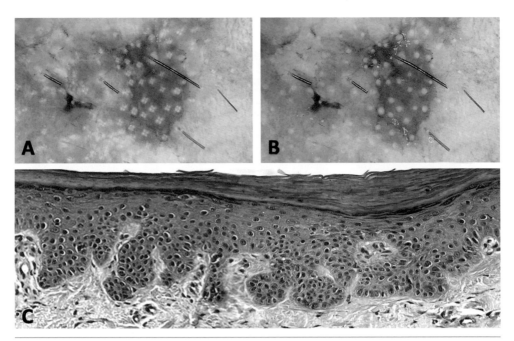

Figure 3.62: *Polarised (A) and non-polarised (B) dermatoscopic and histological (H&E) (C) images of a pigmented solar keratosis on the dorsal hand. Four-dot clods (A) correlate with white clods (B) seen in non-polarised dermatoscopy. Histologically the dysplasia spares about 3 layers of cells below an intact stratum granulosum. Limited parakeratosis is evident in the stratum corneum. Heavy basal hyperpigmentation of keratinocytes correlates with dermatoscopic structureless brown.*

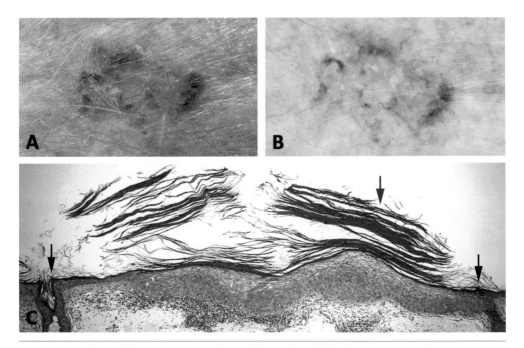

Figure 3.63: *Clinical (A), dermatoscopic (B) and histological (H&E) (C) images of a lightly pigmented squamous cell carcinoma in situ. There is very evident full-thickness dysplasia of the epidermis with overlying parakeratosis (red arrow). Basket-weave orthokeratin overlies normal epidermis on each side (black arrows).*

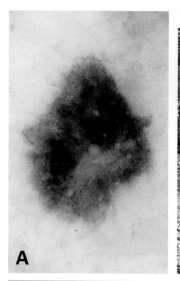
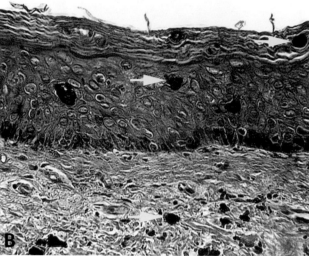

Figure 3.64: *Dermatoscopic (A) and histological (H&E) (B) images of a pigmented squamous cell carcinoma in situ on the arm. A heavily pigmented flat basal layer correlates with dermatoscopic brown structureless pigment and melanin particles (yellow arrows) at all layers of the epidermis, as well as in the dermis, correlate with dermatoscopic brown, black and grey dots.*

Dermatoscopic histological correlation: the coiled vessels of SCC *in situ* correlate with dilated and tortuous dermal papillary vessels in linear arrangement. Angiocentric melanin can result in red dots correlating with these vessels blending into pigmented dots in linear array, a very specific dermatoscopic clue to pSCC *in situ* (see *Figure 4.38*)[21].

Squamous cell carcinoma

Squamous cell carcinoma is an invasive malignancy which extends from the epidermis through the basement membrane into the dermis. Unlike BCC, SCC may metastasise while relatively small, albeit rarely. Although metastasis is more likely with poorly differentiated or large lesions, any SCC greater than 2mm thick has this potential[22] and therefore the histological measurement of Breslow thickness of SCC has prognostic significance.

Architecture: the architecture of SCC is characterised by tumour nests which arise

from the epidermis and extend into the dermis. One corollary of this is that any SCC without an epidermal component must be considered as a potential manifestation of metastatic disease.

SCCs display variable central keratinisation and horn pearl formation depending on the degree of differentiation. The degree of differentiation in the tumour nests is used to grade SCCs into well, moderately or poorly differentiated.

SCC occasionally infiltrates along nerve sheaths, the adventitia of blood vessels, lymphatics, fascial planes, and embryological fusion planes. Symptomatic perineural infiltration is an adverse prognostic indicator[23]. Perineural lymphocytes are an important clue to the likely presence of perineural invasion.

Cytology: the cytology of SCC varies according to the degree of differentiation. With well differentiated forms, individual cells have abundant eosinophilic cytoplasm and a large, often vesicular, nucleus. Cell keratinisation is often present. SCCs have keratin of a higher molecular weight than BCCs and stains can be used to differentiate if necessary.

Dermatoscopic histological correlations:

- Surface keratin can accumulate on the surface of an SCC for the same reason as it does on an AK but, due to the volume of the underlying mass of malignant keratinocytes, the amount of surface keratin can be much greater (*Figure 3.65*). Like the keratin over an AK, the keratin over an SCC is usually parakeratotic and dense and therefore not liable to exposure-related discoloration, retaining its

white colour[24]. Surface keratin on a raised non-pigmented lesion is one of the three major clinical/dermatoscopic clues to SCC and KA, the other two being white structureless areas and white circles (*Figures 3.65* and *3.66*)[18].

- White structureless areas correlate with the histological feature of massed highly keratinised malignant keratinocytes beneath the epidermis.
- White circles, as with AK, correlate with highly keratinised keratinocytes in the epithelium of infundibula. In a raised lesion, raised other than due to surface keratin, this is a clue to invasive SCC or KA[18].

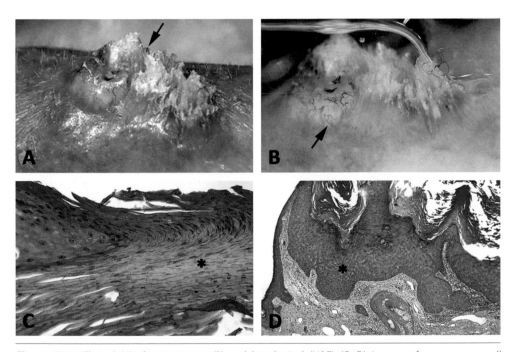

Figure 3.65: *Clinical (A), dermatoscopic (B) and histological (H&E) (C, D) images of a squamous cell carcinoma on the superior rim of the ear. White surface keratin (arrow in A) correlates with compact parakeratosis (asterisk in C) overlying malignant keratinocytes, and dermatoscopic structureless white (arrow in B) correlates with a mass of keratinised malignant keratinocytes (asterisk in D).*

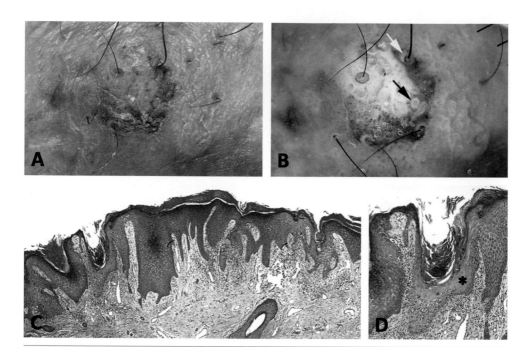

Figure 3.66: *Clinical (A), dermatoscopic (B) and histological images (H&E) (C, D) of a squamous cell carcinoma on the dorsal hand. White circles (arrows in B) correlate with keratinised malignant keratinocytes in follicles (asterisk in D). Oblique orientation of a follicle (yellow arrow in B) displays an emerging hair shaft surrounded by a white cylinder, correlating with invasion of the infundibulum by malignant keratinocytes.*

References

1. Jackson JE, Kelly B, Petitt M, Uchida T, and Wagner RF. Predictive value of margins in diagnostic biopsies of nonmelanoma skin cancers. *J Am Acad Dermatol*, 2012;67:122.

2. Weyers W. Confusion—specimen mix-up in dermatopathology and measures to prevent and detect it. *Dermatol Pract Concept*, 2014;4:27.

3. Titford M. The long history of hematoxylin. *Biotech Histochem*, 2005;80:73.

4. Ivan D, and Prieto VG. Use of immunohistochemistry in the diagnosis of melanocytic lesions: applications and pitfalls. *Future Oncol*, 2010;6:1163.

5. Penneys N, Seigfried E, Nahass G, and Vogler C. Expression of proliferating cell nuclear antigen in Spitz nevus. *J Am Acad Dermatol*, 1995;32:964.

6. Hendi A, Brodland DG, and Zitelli JA. Melanocytes in long-standing sun-exposed skin: quantitative analysis using the MART-1 immunostain. *Archives Dermatol*, 2006;142:871.

7. Henrikson RC, and Mazurkiewicz JE. *Histology*, 1997. Lippincott Williams & Wilkins.

8. Robinson JK, Hanke CW, Sengelmann RD, and Siegel DM. *Surgery of the Skin*, 2005. Mosby.

9. Mandrell JC, and Santa Cruz D. Keratoacanthoma: hyperplasia, benign neoplasm, or a type of squamous cell carcinoma? *Semin Diagn Pathol*, 2009;26:150.

10. Rosendahl C, Cameron A, Bulinska A, Williamson R, and Kittler H. Dermatoscopy of a minute melanoma. *Aust J Dermatol*, 2011;52:76.

11. Maher J, Cameron A, Wallace S, Acosta-Rojas R, Weedon D, and Rosendahl C. Balloon cell melanoma: a case report with polarized and non-polarized dermatoscopy and dermatopathology. *Dermatol Pract Concept*, 2014;4:11.

12. Weedon D. *Weedon's Skin Pathology*, 3rd Edition, 2002. Churchill Livingstone.

13. Kittler H, Rosendahl C, Cameron A, and Tschandl P. *Dermatoscopy*, 2nd Edition, 2016. Facultas.

14. Rosendahl C, Cameron A, McColl I, and Wilkinson D. Dermatoscopy in routine practice – "Chaos and Clues". *Aust Fam Physician*, 2012;41:482.

15. Mihm MC, and Mulé JJ. Reflections on the histopathology of tumor-infiltrating lymphocytes in melanoma and the host immune response. *Cancer Immunol Res,* 2015;3:827.

16. Peterson SC, Eberl M, Vagnozzi AN, *et al*. Basal cell carcinoma preferentially arises from stem cells within hair follicle and mechanosensory niches. *Cell Stem Cell,* 2015;16:400.

17. Lober A, and Lober W. Actinic keratosis is squamous cell carcinoma. *Southern Med J,* 2000;93:650.

18. Rosendahl C, Cameron A, Argenziano G, Zalaudek I, Tschandl P, and Kittler H. Dermoscopy of squamous cell carcinoma and keratoacanthoma. *Arch Dermatol*, 2012;148:1386.

19. Peris K, Micantonio T, Piccolo D, and Concetta M. Dermoscopic features of actinic keratosis. *J Deutsch Dermatol Gesellsch, *2007;5:970.

20. Tschandl P, Rosendahl C, and Kittler H. Dermatoscopy of flat pigmented facial lesions. *J Eur Acad Dermatol Venereol*, 2015;29:120.

21. Cameron A, Rosendahl C, Tschandl P, Riedl E, and Kittler H. Dermatoscopy of pigmented Bowen's disease. *J Am Acad Dermatol*, 2010;62:597.

22. Breuninger H, Schaumburg-Lever G, Holzschuh J, and Horny HP. Desmoplastic squamous cell carcinoma of skin and vermilion surface. A highly malignant subtype of skin cancer. *Cancer,* 1997;79:915.

23. Jennings L, and Schmults CD. Management of high-risk cutaneous squamous cell carcinoma. *J Clin Aesthet Dermatol*, 2010;3:39.

24. Rizk M, Alian M, Tschandl P, *et al*. A prospective diagnostic study on povidone-iodine retention in lesions suspected to be squamous cell carcinoma or keratoacanthoma. *Aust J Dermatol*, 2019; in press (https://doi.org/10.1111/ajd.12897).

CHAPTER 4

The language of dermatoscopy: naming and defining structures and patterns

4.1 The evolution of metaphoric terminology for dermatoscopic structures and patterns

The advent of dermatoscopy created the need for a vocabulary and not surprisingly this evolved and flourished rapidly, parallel to the publication of research into this novel science. Dermatoscopy is a colourful and totally visual science and the proliferation of graphic metaphorical terms to describe structures created a blend of science and art which, although appealing to many, was problematic at the same time. The vocabulary became large which was a problem for students in itself, but more concerning was the manner by which metaphoric terms appeared and came into use, each carrying inbuilt preconceived diagnostic implications. For example, if segmental radial lines were seen in a lesion believed to be a melanoma they would be labelled 'radial streaming', but if the lesion was believed to be a BCC they would be called 'leaf-like' or even 'maple leaf-like' structures. In no other field of medicine does diagnosis precede description, but that is what happened with the evolution of metaphoric terminology in dermatoscopy.

In 2007 Kittler introduced revised pattern analysis (RPA) and with it, geometric descriptive terminology[1]. Then in 2008 Kittler *et al.* introduced a classification of vessel morphology also based on pattern analysis[2]. A consensus meeting in Vienna in 2015 found that the descriptive geometric terminology was preferred over metaphorical terminology by a margin, although the majority stated that they used both languages[3].

4.1.1 Structures in revised pattern analysis

Revised pattern analysis can be applied to all skin lesions and involves an analysis of pigmented structures as well as white, skin-coloured and vessel structures[4]. Structureless areas have the same significance as patterns formed by structures.

Pigmented structures can be pigmented by melanin (black, brown, grey or blue) or by other pigments which can mimic melanin, including keratin exposed to the atmosphere (yellow, orange, brown) and blood or its breakdown products (red, purple and black). As a general rule if blue, purple or black are seen in association with any brown colour they should be interpreted as colours of melanin rather than of blood[5].

White structures are defined as being *whiter than perilesional skin* and include lines (polarising-specific and non-polarising-specific), circles, clods (including dots) and structureless (including surface keratin/scale)[5].

 ## 4.2 Revised pattern analysis of lesions pigmented by melanin

4.2.1 Basic structures

In the language of RPA, there are only three basic pigmented structures: lines (including pseudopods), circles and clods (including dots) (*Figures 4.1* and *4.2*). Because lines are a very specific structure they are further subdivided into six different types: reticular, branched, angulated, parallel, radial and curved (*Figure 4.3*). A pattern is an area made up of multiple repetitions of a basic structure. Lines (reticular and branched), circles, and clods can be white as well as pigmented. Any area large enough to form a pattern, with no basic structure predominating, is termed structureless. A structureless area, just like a structure, can have any colour.

The terms used for structures are clearly defined[4] and are described in the sections which follow.

4.2.2 Lines

A **line** is a structure with length usually greatly exceeding width.

Reticular lines: a group of straight lines which intersect sensibly at right angles to form a net-like pattern (*Figure 4.4*). With respect to pigmented reticular lines, they are the surface projection of a pattern produced by pigmented rete ridges and non-pigmented dermal papillae (*Figure 4.5*). The pigment on the rete ridges may be in keratinocytes or melanocytes.

Reticular lines can be found in naevi,

melanomas, solar lentigo, seborrhoeic keratosis and dermatofibroma. Significantly they effectively rule out a diagnosis of BCC or SCC.

Branched lines: a group of straight lines similar to reticular lines, intersecting but not as regular and not always at right angles (*Figure 4.6*). Their significance generally coincides with that of reticular lines.

Angulated lines: straight pigmented lines, not reticulated or branched, meeting at angles of 90° or more, but not crossing (*Figure 4.7*). These lines may join to form complete or incomplete polygons[6].

Parallel lines: straight pigmented lines arranged in a parallel pattern, found on volar skin and nails (*Figure 4.8*). On volar skin they may be arranged on ridges, in furrows, or crossing the ridges and furrows.

Radial lines: a group of pigmented lines which converge at a central point or would do so if extended (for example, at a point at the centre of a lesion) (*Figure 4.9*). Radial lines may radiate from a location within a lesion or from the perimeter of a lesion at which location they can either be circumferential or segmental. A pseudopod is one type of radial line which is defined as a radial line with a terminal clod (*Figure 4.10*).

Curved lines: pigmented lines which are not straight, have few intersections and may be parallel or distributed randomly (*Figure 4.11*). Parallel curved lines usually occur in pairs.

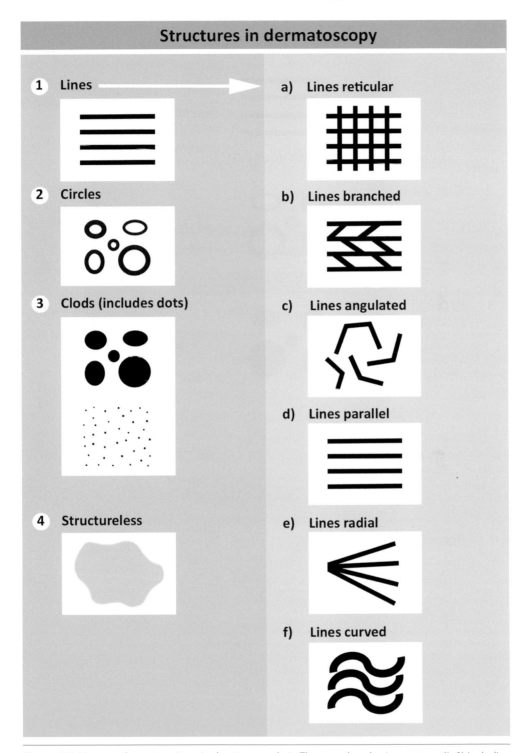

Figure 4.1: *Non-vessel structures in revised pattern analysis. There are three basic structures (1–3) including six types of lines (a–f). An area with no basic structure predominating is termed structureless.*

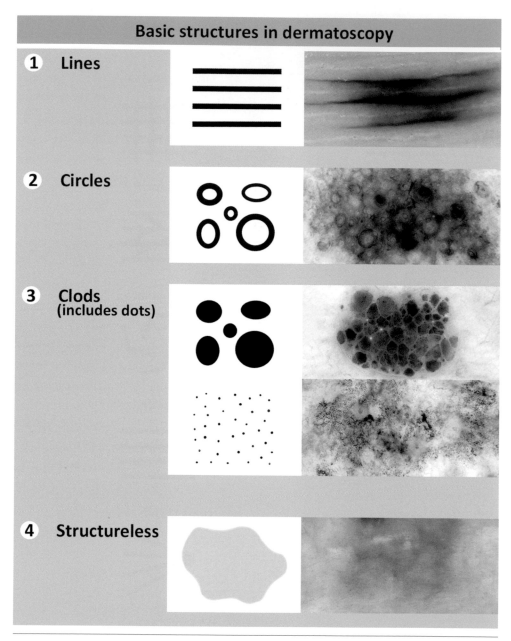

Figure 4.2: *Diagrammatic representations (left column) and representative images (right column) of the various dermatoscopic basic structures as defined in revised pattern analysis.*

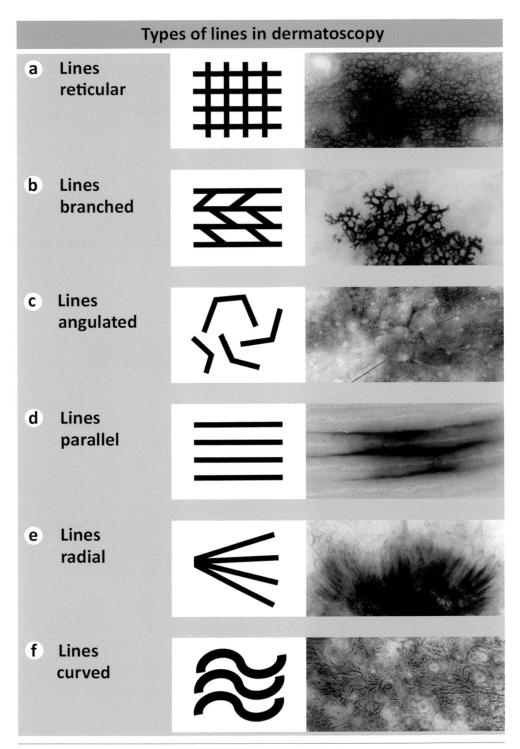

Figure 4.3: *Diagrammatic representations (left column) and representative images (right column) of the various dermatoscopic lines as defined in revised pattern analysis.*

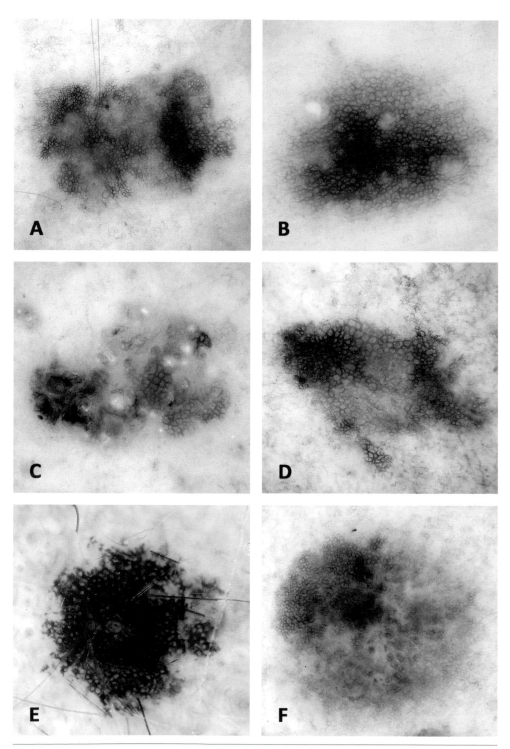

Figure 4.4: *Six lesions each exhibiting a pattern of reticular lines: (A) melanoma* in situ; *(B) naevus; (C) seborrhoeic keratosis; (D) solar lentigo; (E) ink spot lentigo; (F) dermatofibroma.*

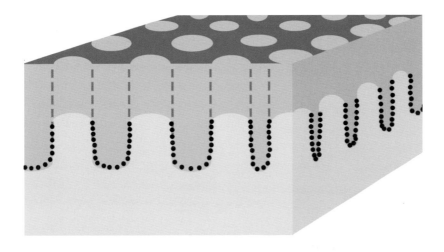

Figure 4.5: *Diagrammatic representation of a pattern of reticular lines formed by pigmented rete ridges alternating with dermal papillae.*

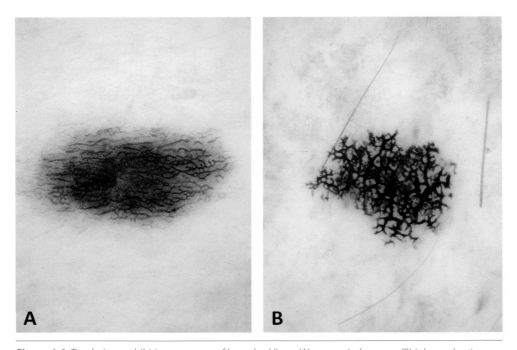

Figure 4.6: *Two lesions exhibiting a pattern of branched lines: (A) congenital naevus; (B) ink spot lentigo.*

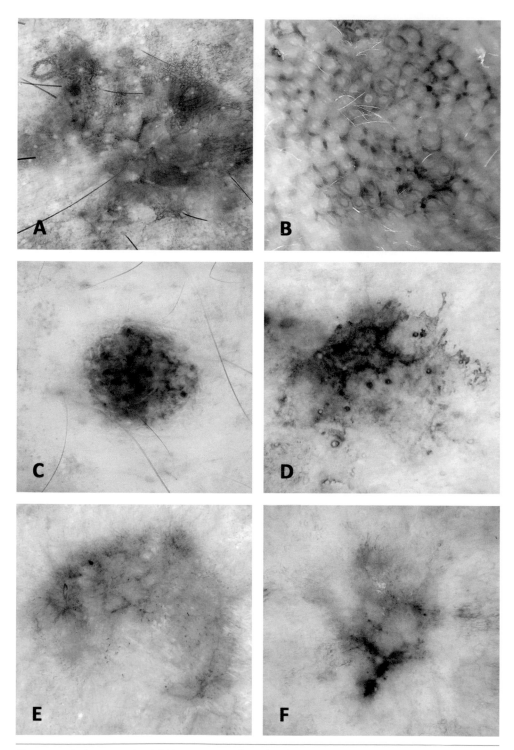

Figure 4.7: *Six lesions each exhibiting a pattern of angulated lines: (A and B) melanoma; (C) naevus; (D) solar lentigo; (E) basal cell carcinoma; (F) squamous cell carcinoma in situ.*

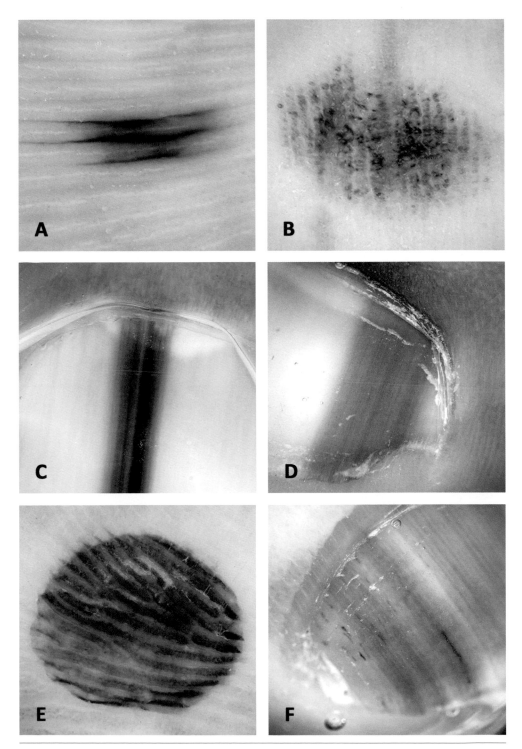

Figure 4.8: *Six lesions exhibiting a pattern of parallel lines: (A) volar naevus; (B) volar melanoma; (C) nail matrix melanoma; (D) nail matrix naevus; (E) volar corneal haemorrhage; (F) nail matrix melanotic macule.*

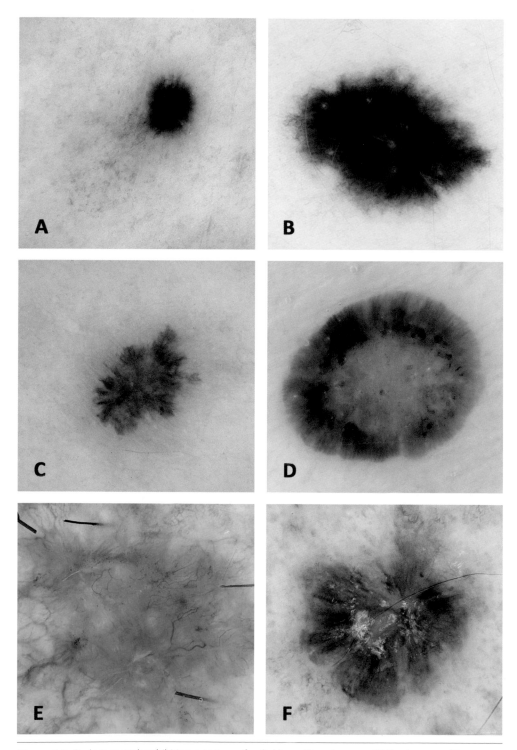

Figure 4.9: *Six lesions each exhibiting a pattern of radial lines: (A) melanoma; (B) Reed naevus; (C) recurrent naevus; (D) seborrhoeic keratosis; (E) basal cell carcinoma; (F) squamous cell carcinoma in situ.*

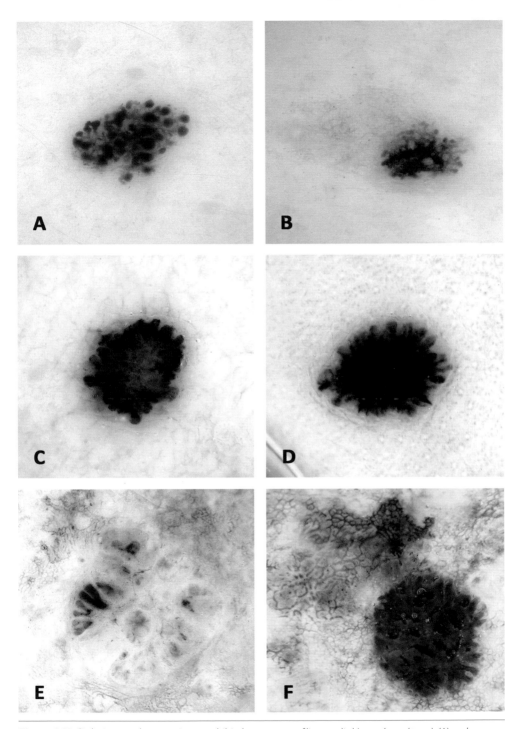

Figure 4.10: *Six lesions each appearing to exhibit the presence of lines radial (pseudopod type): (A) melanoma; (B) naevus; (C) spitzoid melanoma; (D) Reed naevus; (E) basal cell carcinoma; (F) seborrhoeic keratosis. Note that the radial lines in (E) radiate from a hypopigmented area as is specific for basal cell carcinoma.*

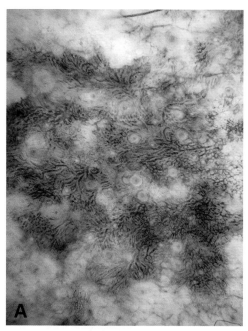
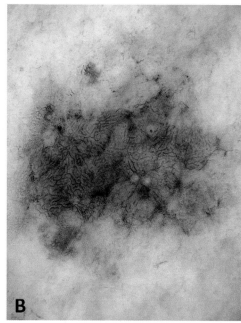

Figure 4.11: Two lesions each exhibiting a pattern of curved lines: (A) solar lentigo; (B) melanoma – note that angulated lines are also evident.

4.2.3 Circles

A circle is a curved line sensibly equidistant from a central point (this includes ellipses). It may be the colour of melanin or white. Skin-coloured circles have no diagnostic significance and neither do follicular openings in a pigmented background, unless there is a defined circular line, defined by pigment or white.

If the centre of the structure is paler than the periphery and the periphery is characterised by a circular line, then the structure is correctly described as a circle rather than a clod, a clod being defined as a solid object (*Figure 4.12*).

Pigmented circles defining an adnexal structure

When melanin is present in cells lining adnexal structures, dermatoscopic pigmented circles can be seen. While brown circles might be expected, the oblique orientation of follicles can carry the melanin pigment below dermis, even when the pigmented cells are confined to follicular epidermis, causing dermatoscopic grey circles to be seen (*Figure 4.13*)[7]. This is an explanation for dermatoscopic grey circles in *in situ* melanomas on the face. Brown and grey circles defining follicles can also be seen in benign conditions such as solar lentigo and seborrhoeic keratosis, and even on normal skin with phototypes 5 and 6. But in lighter skin phototypes, when the compelling morphology of such a benign lesion is not present, pigmented circles on the head or neck, related to follicular openings, are a clue to melanoma[8]. Pigmented circles, not relating to adnexal structures, represent a pattern of reticular lines modified by acanthosis and are a clue to seborrhoeic keratosis.

4.2.4 Clods

A clod is a well-defined, solid object and it can be of any colour and shape (*Figures 4.14–4.16*).

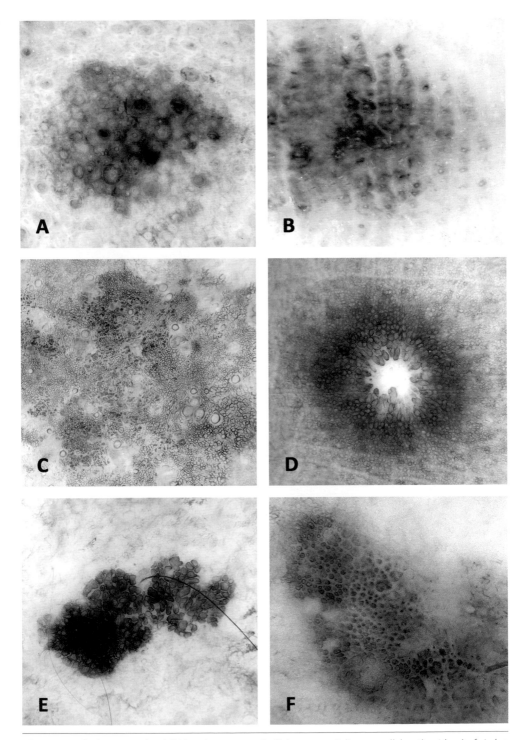

Figure 4.12: *Six lesions each exhibiting the structure (in B the pattern is lines parallel on the ridges) of circles: (A) melanoma; (B) melanoma (volar); (C) solar lentigo; (D) dermatofibroma; (E) seborrhoeic keratosis; (F) squamous cell carcinoma in situ. Note that a discrete structure with the centre lighter in colour than the periphery fulfils the definition of a circle rather than a clod.*

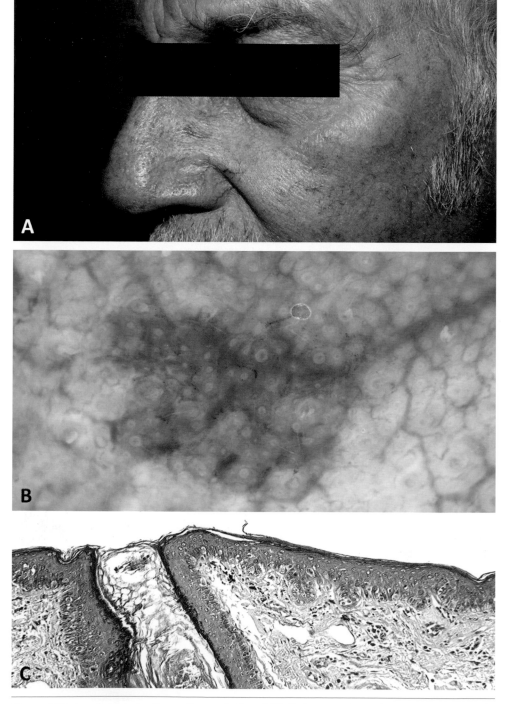

Figure 4.13: *A melanoma in situ on the nasal sidewall (A) displays prominent dermatoscopic grey circles (B). Although the melanoma is confined to the epidermis, pigmented melanocytes lining the follicle are seen through dermal collagen because the follicle is oblique (C). Due to the scattering of light by dermal collagen (Tyndall effect) this melanin is seen as grey[7].*

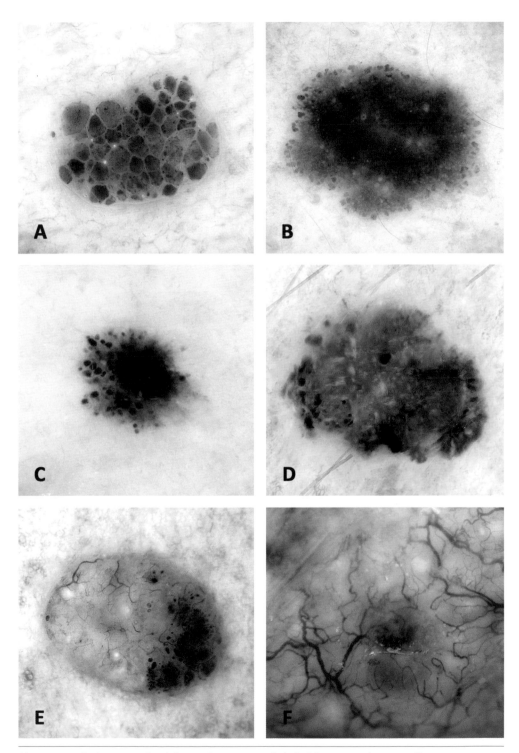

Figure 4.14: *Six lesions each exhibiting the presence of clods: (A) congenital naevus; (B) growing naevus; (C, D) melanoma; (E, F) basal cell carcinoma.*

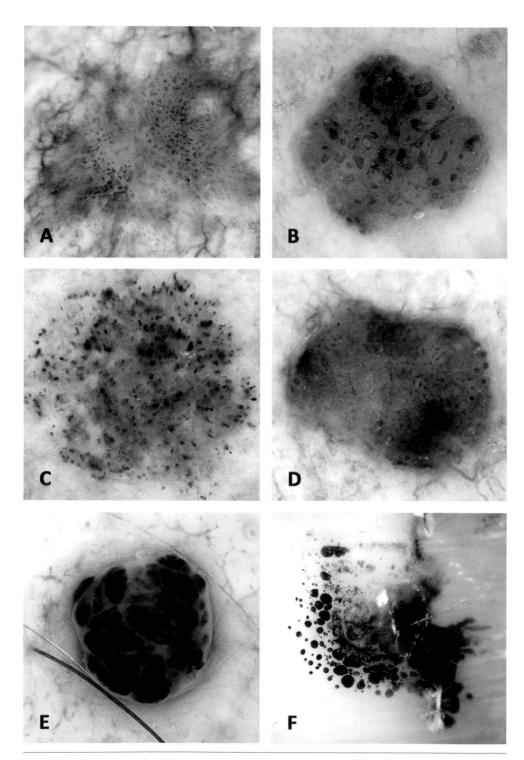

Figure 4.15: *Six lesions each exhibiting a pattern of clods: (A) squamous cell carcinoma* in situ; *(B) seborrhoeic keratosis; (C) lichen planus-like keratosis; (D) clonal seborrhoeic keratosis; (E) haemangioma; (F) subungual haemorrhage.*

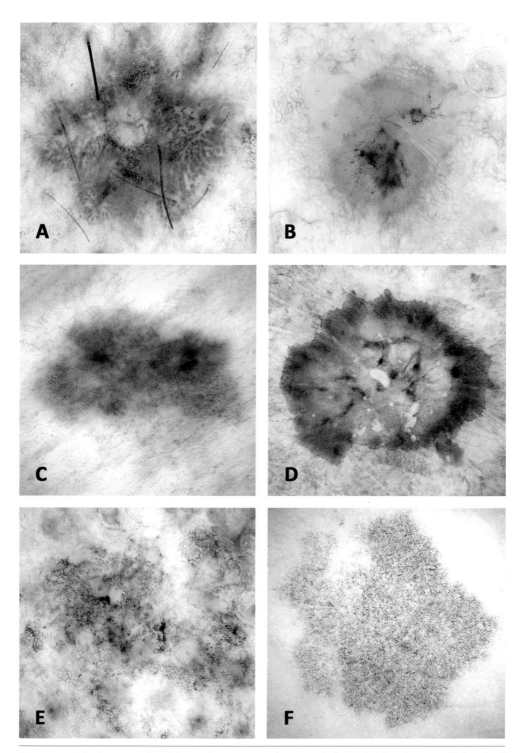

Figure 4.16: *Six lesions each exhibiting the structure of minute clods (dots): (A) melanoma; (B) basal cell carcinoma; (C) squamous cell carcinoma in situ; (D) seborrhoeic keratosis; (E) lichen planus-like keratosis; (F) tinea nigra.*

A dot is a minute clod too small to have a discernible shape (at 10 times magnification) (*Figure 4.16*). A dot is a structure as small as or smaller than the diameter of a hair shaft (1/20mm – the limit of resolution of the human eye)[4].

4.2.5 Structureless

A structureless area is an area covering a significant portion of a lesion with no basic structure predominating (*Figure 4.17*). Note that structureless does not necessarily equate to featureless.

 ## Patterns in revised pattern analysis

A pattern is formed by multiple repetitions of a basic structure and it must cover a significant portion of a lesion to be regarded as a pattern[4]. For example, a few lines covering 5–10% of a lesion with an otherwise structureless pattern would constitute a clue (see *Section 4.4*) rather than a pattern. If, however, reticular lines covered 30% of an otherwise structureless lesion then the lesion would be regarded as having two patterns (*Figure 4.18*). So, while arbitrary rules of degree are best avoided, for the purpose of consistency it is reasonable to define the minimum area of a pattern as 20% of the surface area of a lesion[9]. However, the dermatoscopist is not a robot and the exercise of discretion in the allocation of a pattern is acceptable. Revised pattern analysis allows for variations of perception and such variations are not regarded as right or wrong. Two dermatoscopists whose descriptions vary in detail should arrive at the same conclusion if patterns, colours and clues are evaluated sequentially and objectively, although the pathways to those conclusions may vary[4].

Patterns should be assessed as such and a few structures out of synchrony do not destroy a pattern. For example, looking at the right side of *Figure 4.18* you may recognise a few circles, but that does not interfere with the description of a pattern of reticular lines. It must be remembered that we are describing biological material rather than an architect's design and it is appropriate to tolerate reasonable variation.

4.3.1 Why the 2-step method of dermatoscopy is not used in revised pattern analysis

The 2-step method of dermatoscopy requires that melanocytic status be determined by dermatoscopy as a first step before the lesion is assessed for clues to melanoma as a second step[10,11]. The so-called *melanocytic* criteria (network, pseudonetwork, aggregated brown globules, radial streaming, pseudopods, homogenous blue pigmentation and parallel lines on volar skin) are not melanocytic criteria at all. They are just *melanotic* criteria and can occur in any *pigmented* lesion whether it has a proliferation of melanocytes or not. The lesion in *Figure 4.18* has a definite pigment network but it is a solar lentigo in collision with a pSCC *in situ*, neither of which are melanocytic. So-called pseudonetwork is commonly seen in solar lentigo and pAK, and they also are not melanocytic. Lines radial segmental are seen in pSCC *in situ* (*Figure 4.19A*) and in pBCC (*Figure 4.19B*), both of which are not melanocytic. The sensitivity and specificity of the first step of the 2-step process were evaluated in a study on consecutive lesions in a practice in Europe, compared to a practice in Australia[12]. The specificity was found to be 67.9% in Europe and 33.6% in Australia, due to the relatively high prevalence in Australia of lesions on sun-damaged skin including solar lentigo, lichen planus-like keratosis (LPLK) and pSCC *in situ*.

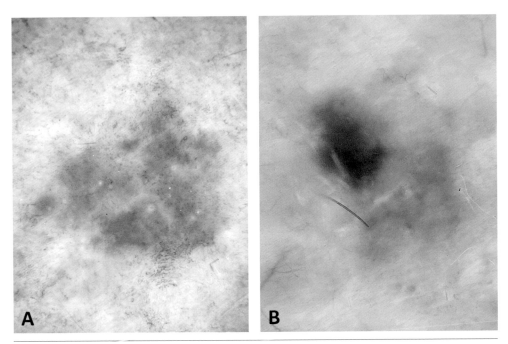

Figure 4.17: *Two lesions each exhibiting a structureless pattern: (A) lichen planus-like keratosis; (B) melanoma (invasive). Note that even if you wanted to describe the large pigmented structure in the melanoma (B) as a clod, you can't have a pattern of a single clod.*

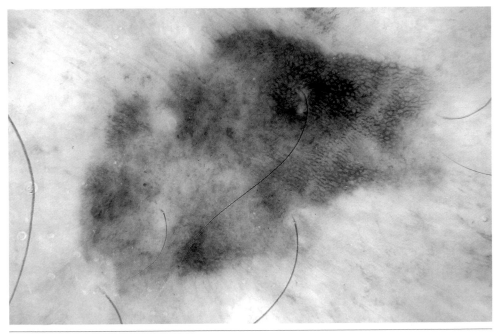

Figure 4.18: *A lesion with a pattern of lines reticular on the right and an area on the left which has many structures but with no single structure predominating. Although this area is not featureless it is regarded as a structureless area, i.e. an area with a structureless pattern.*

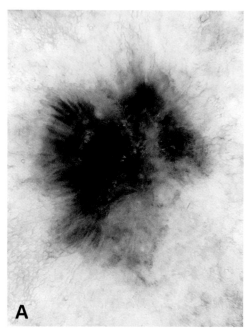
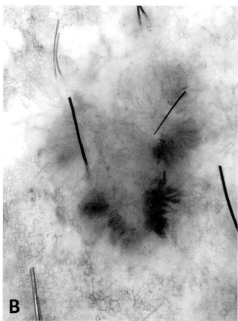

Figure 4.19: *Dermatoscopy of a squamous cell carcinoma in situ (A) and a basal cell carcinoma (B) shows that both lesions have lines radial segmental. Assessed by the 2-step process these lesions would incorrectly be regarded as melanocytic.*

4.4 The process of revised pattern analysis

Pigmented structures (and white structures, whiter than perilesional skin) are far more specific as diagnostic clues than non-pigmented structures such as blood vessels and should always be given priority when present[1]. RPA involves a stepwise assessment of pattern, colours and finally clues to determine a specific provisional diagnosis or a limited differential diagnosis (*Figure 4.20*).

Step 1
The first step in RPA is to assess the pattern(s) and colour(s) with a decision made as to whether there **is one pattern or more than one pattern** and in the case of a single pattern whether there is **one colour or more than one colour** (*Figure 4.20*). Defining a

precise number of patterns and colours does not additionally assist the diagnostic process and so the simple decision on whether there is one pattern and colour or more than one is adequate[4].

The colours seen in dermatoscopy include the:
• colours of melanin – black, brown, grey and blue
• colours of keratin – yellow, orange and white
• colour of collagen – also white
• colours of blood – red, blue, purple and black.

Shades of brown (dark brown and light brown) are only recognised if there is an abrupt transition with a high degree of variation[4].

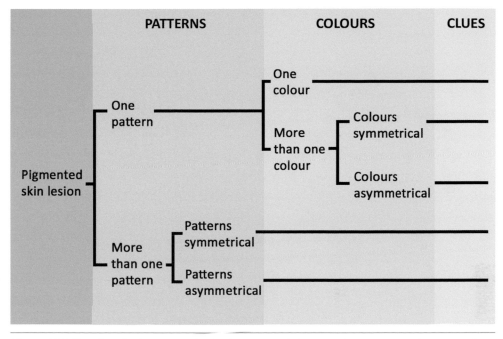

Figure 4.20: *Flowchart for the process of revised pattern analysis: a stepwise assessment of patterns colours and clues.*

Step 2

The second step in RPA involves an assessment of symmetry which is decided on the basis of pattern and colour, regardless of shape.

- If there is one pattern and one colour then by definition the lesion is symmetrical.
- If there is more than one pattern then symmetry is determined by whether the patterns are combined symmetrically, regardless of colour. If there is only one pattern, symmetry is decided on the basis of colour[4].

The lesion shown in *Figure 4.21A* has two patterns: a central structureless pattern and peripheral clods combined symmetrically in a concentric arrangement. It does not matter that there are a few clods missing at the top.

Such variation is acceptable in biological tissue. Another way of understanding this is to realise that such a degree of variation is not consistent with the disorganised behaviour of malignant tissue.

The lesion shown in *Figure 4.21B* has a pattern of clods. There is one pattern and two colours (yellow and white, combined symmetrically). The background does not constitute a structureless pattern because it is overlaid by the pattern of clods which takes priority.

Step 3

Having assessed the patterns and symmetry of a skin lesion, RPA then proceeds in a stepwise fashion according to **clues**.

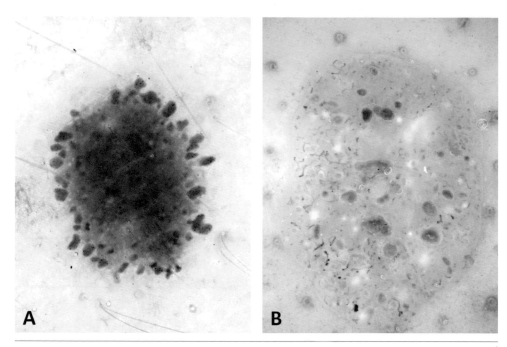

Figure 4.21: Dermatoscopic images of two pigmented lesions. Lesion (A) has two patterns, central structureless and peripheral clods, combined in a symmetrical concentric pattern (growing naevus). Lesion (B) has one pattern, clods, and two colours, yellow and white, symmetrically combined (seborrhoeic keratosis).

Revised pattern analysis applied to lesions with white structures

A general principle of RPA is that pigment defines structure. White structures, in which white colour is *whiter than surrounding perilesional skin*, are an exception to this rule and such white structures have the same significance as pigmented structures. If white structures are located on a structureless pigmented background they actually have priority over that pigmented background, just as pigmented structures would, and they define the pattern.

4.5.1 White lines

White lines are of two different types:
- Polarising-specific: only seen with polarising mode; shiny, whiter than surrounding skin, orientated at right angles to each other but not crossing.
- Non-polarising-specific: seen with both polarising and non-polarising modes; whiter than surrounding skin, linear morphology including linear straight, linear serpentine and reticular.

Polarising-specific white lines are only seen with dermatoscopes in polarising mode and are orientated perpendicularly to each other but do not cross (*Figure 4.22*)[9]. When the dermatoscope is rotated they may shift in orientation. When the dermatoscope is switched between polarised and non-polarised mode they will appear and disappear, respectively. Any lines which have these polarising-specific features, even if of another

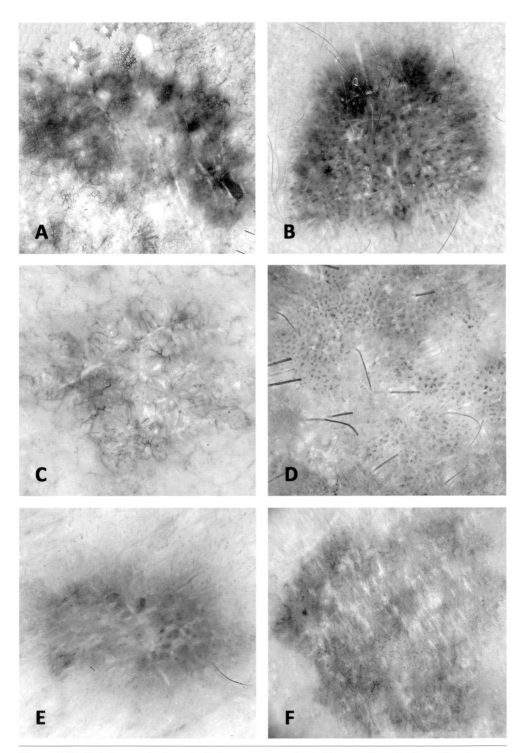

Figure 4.22: *Six lesions each of which displays a pattern of polarising-specific white lines: (A) melanoma; (B) Spitz naevus; (C) basal cell carcinoma; (D) squamous cell carcinoma in situ; (E) dermatofibroma; (F) lichen planus-like keratosis.*

colour such as blue, have the same significance as polarising-specific white lines[9].

Polarising-specific white lines are seen in the two malignancies of melanoma and BCC as well as the two benign (symmetrical) lesions of dermatofibroma (DF) and Spitz naevus[13]. They are also seen in some SCC *in situ*, LPLK and scar tissue and their interpretation depends on the context. For example, a lesion with the morphology of a naevus, seborrhoeic keratosis or haemangioma should be considered for biopsy if this feature is seen. With respect to BCC it is a supporting feature and may draw attention to a non-pigmented lesion leading to a careful search for other vascular and stromal clues.

Polarising-specific white structureless areas, often seen over BCC and sometimes over melanoma[13] have a similar significance as polarising-specific white lines, but they are not expected over Spitz naevus or DF.

Polarising-specific structures, including polarising-specific white lines, may alter with rotation of the dermatoscope and because of this they are always rated as a clue and not as a pattern.

White lines seen with non-polarised (as well as polarised) dermatoscopy are a compelling clue to malignancy, in particular melanoma (*Figure 4.23*). These white lines may or may not be in a reticular pattern. A reticular pattern of white lines generally excludes BCC[4] and SCC.

4.5.2 White clods (including white dots)

These structures, correlating with keratin aggregations within the epidermis, are commonly seen in seborrhoeic keratoses, congenital naevi, SCC and BCC (*Figure 4.24*). They may also be seen in a melanoma. The diagnostic interpretation depends on the context and as an isolated clue they have a low specificity.

4.5.3 White structureless areas in flat lesions

White structureless areas in flat lesions correlate either with keratin or collagen (*Figure 4.25*).

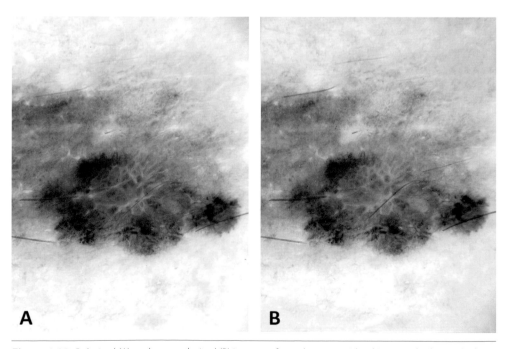

Figure 4.23: *Polarised (A) and non-polarised (B) images of a melanoma with white reticular lines which are not polarising-specific.*

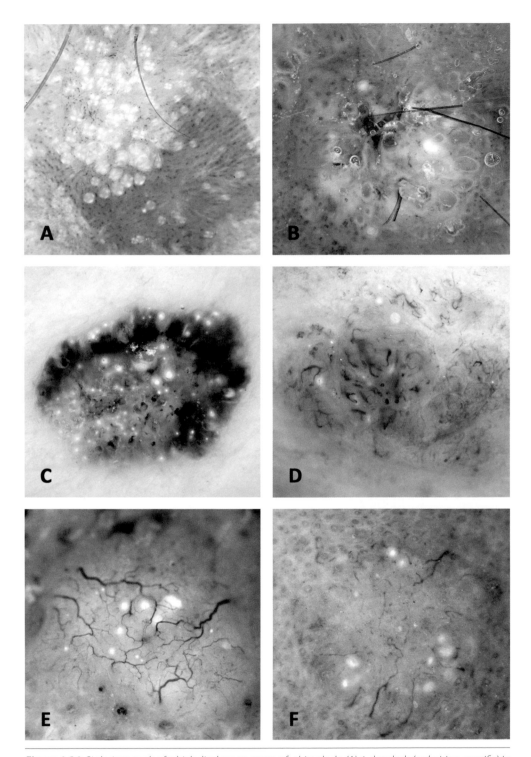

Figure 4.24: *Six lesions each of which displays a pattern of white clods. (A) 4-dot clods (polarising-specific) in a squamous cell carcinoma in situ. White clods in (B) squamous cell carcinoma; (C) seborrhoeic keratosis; (D) dermal naevus; (E) basal cell carcinoma; (F) desmoplastic trichoepithelioma.*

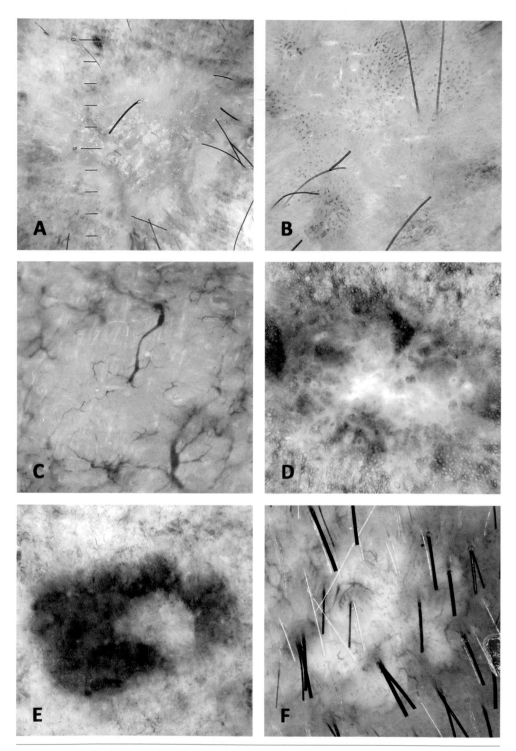

Figure 4.25: *Six flat lesions each of which displays a white structureless area: (A) keratin scale over an actinic keratosis; (B) squamous cell carcinoma* in situ; *(C) basal cell carcinoma; (D) dermatofibroma; (E) melanoma; (F) amelanotic blue naevus.*

If due to keratin they will be evident as surface scale, best appreciated clinically by visual inspection and palpation. Orthokeratotic keratin scale is generally yellow rather than white, so structureless white scale is more likely to be compact parakeratotic keratin as seen over an AK. Erythema of the underlying dermis supports this diagnosis[4].

A white structureless area in a flat lesion without evident surface scale is likely to correlate with collagen. A lesion with one pattern structureless, one colour white, can be seen with lichen sclerosus et atrophicus, morphea (localised scleroderma), morphoeic BCC, amelanotic blue naevus, or a scar.

A white structureless area in a flat pigmented or pink lesion, without keratin scale is likely to correlate with an area of collagen deposition which may follow traumatic scarring or immune regression and this can happen in benign or malignant lesions. Such an area may be seen symmetrically surrounding a pigmented skin lesion in the case of halo naevus or centrally in a DF. When present asymmetrically, other than due to (including therapeutic) scarring, malignancy should be suspected[9].

4.5.4 White circles in flat lesions

White circles correlate with highly keratinised epithelium surrounding adnexal openings and in a flat lesion on the face are a clue to AK (*Figure 4.26*). Background erythema due to the increased metabolic demand of neoplastic tissue often accentuates the white circles

and this has led to the metaphor 'strawberry pattern'[14]. This metaphoric term can only be applied selectively to non-pigmented AKs on the face. The geometric descriptor of 'white circles' applies equally to pigmented and non-pigmented facial AKs[4].

4.5.5 White keratin clues in raised lesions

White clues due to keratin (white circles, white structureless areas and surface keratin) have a special significance when a lesion is visibly or palpably raised[15] or where there is the dermatoscopic clue to a raised lesion of looped vessels[9]. This is because white clues due to keratin are a clue to squamous neoplasia and, if the lesion is raised (other than due to keratin scale), invasive malignancy must be suspected, making ablative therapy (e.g. cryotherapy) without biopsy inappropriate.

The correlation of white circles is as for flat lesions: the presence of highly keratinised neoplastic squamous cells in the adnexal lining epithelium, but in a raised lesion this is a clue to SCC and KA[15].

The correlation of a white structureless area in a raised lesion is usually an aggregated mass of highly keratinised neoplastic squamous cells, with exceptions including collagen as in a DF and cyst contents (*Figure 4.27*).

The correlation of white surface keratin is compact parakeratotic keratin overlying neoplastic epithelium.

4.6 Revised pattern analysis applied to lesions with orange, yellow and skin-coloured structures

There are some structures seen in dermatoscopy which do not fall into the category of pigmented by melanin (not brown, black, grey or blue), are not vascular (red, blue, purple, black) and are not white. These include orange,

yellow and skin-coloured structures (*Figure 4.28*). It should be realised that the differentiation between orange and yellow may not be clear-cut and the attributions to each colour below are to a large extent interchangeable.

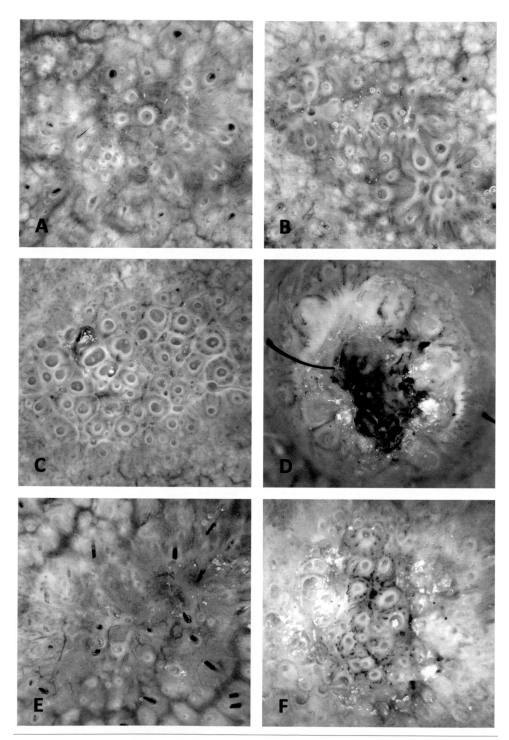

Figure 4.26: *Six lesions, some flat and some raised, each of which displays a pattern of white circles: (A) actinic keratosis; (B) squamous cell carcinoma in situ; (C) squamous cell carcinoma; (D) keratoacanthoma; (E) basal cell carcinoma; (F) lichen simplex chronicus. If a lesion with dermatoscopic white circles is raised invasive malignancy should be suspected.*

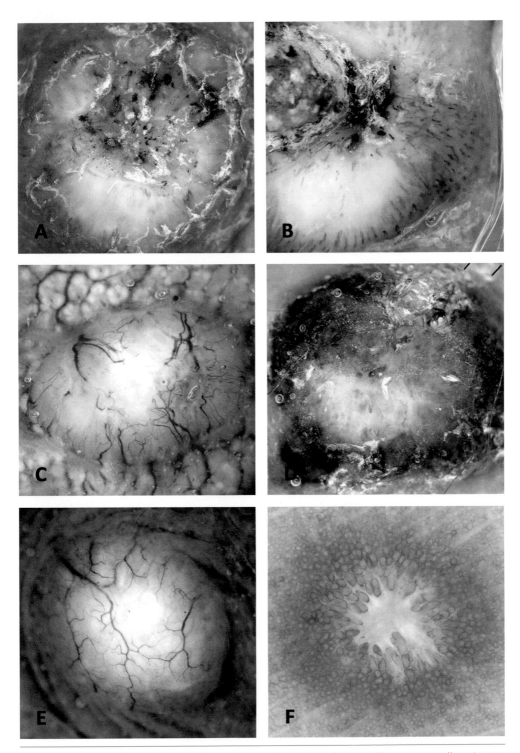

Figure 4.27: *Six raised lesions each of which displays a white structureless area: (A) squamous cell carcinoma; (B) keratoacanthoma; (C) basal cell carcinoma; (D) melanoma; (E) benign epidermal cyst; (F) dermatofibroma.*

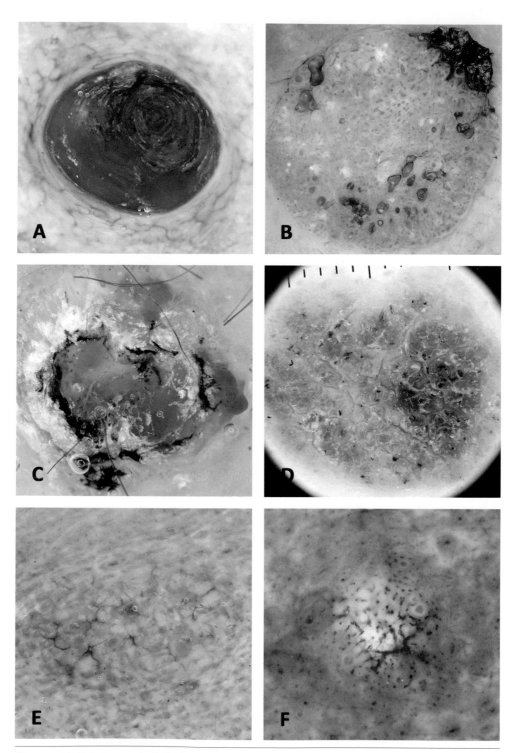

Figure 4.28: *Six lesions each of which displays orange or yellow structures: (A) keratin in a comedo; (B) keratin crypts in a seborrhoeic keratosis; (C) serous exudate from ulceration of a basal cell carcinoma; (D) keratin on a seborrhoeic keratosis; (E) sebaceous gland hyperplasia; (F) pus in a follicular infundibulum (folliculitis).*

Yellow structures

Correlates of dermatoscopic yellow structures include:

- **Keratin:** e.g. yellow clods in a seborrhoeic keratosis[16] and in some BCCs[17]
- **Ulceration:** surface serum exudate from ulceration (e.g. BCC)[4]
- **Lipids:** e.g. skin-coloured to yellow clods in sebaceous gland hyperplasia[18], naevus sebaceous[19], xanthogranuloma, sebaceous adenoma and lipofuscin in choroidal and non-choroidal melanoma[20]
- **Hemosiderin:** e.g. lichen aureus
- **Balloon cells:** e.g. balloon cell naevus and balloon cell melanoma[21]
- **Pus**[4] **and granulomas.**

Orange structures

Dermatoscopic orange clods are seen in seborrhoeic keratoses and congenital naevi where keratin aggregations are exposed. The fact that enclosed keratin collections in the same lesions are white suggests that either environmental contaminants or oxidation results in the orange colour. We speculate that oxidation of exposed keratin leads to conversion of organic DOPA (see *Section 2.3.2*) to melanin in the same way that oxidation causes the brown discoloration on the exposed portion of a partly eaten apple[22].

Skin-coloured structures

Skin-coloured clods are a structure frequently seen in dermal naevi in which they correlate with nests of non-pigmented melanocytes in hypertrophic dermal papillae (*Figure 4.29*).

Skin-coloured reticular lines are often termed negative or inverse network, although these terms are not included in the geometric terminology of RPA. This pattern may catch the eye and as such is a valuable clue, but the correct interpretation is that it represents a pattern of pigmented clods, correlating with pigmented dermal papillae, separated by non-pigmented epidermal rete ridges (*Figure 4.30*).

Such skin-coloured lines may be seen in congenital naevi, but in a chaotic lesion with more than one pattern other clues to melanoma should be sought.

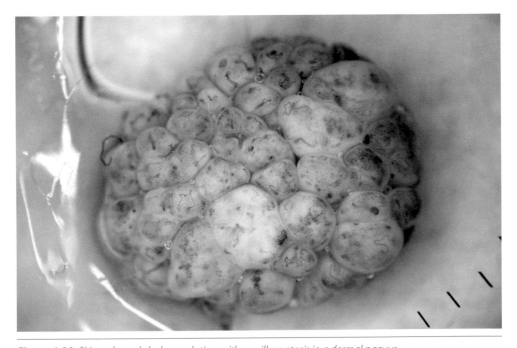

Figure 4.29: Skin-coloured clods correlating with papillomatosis in a dermal naevus.

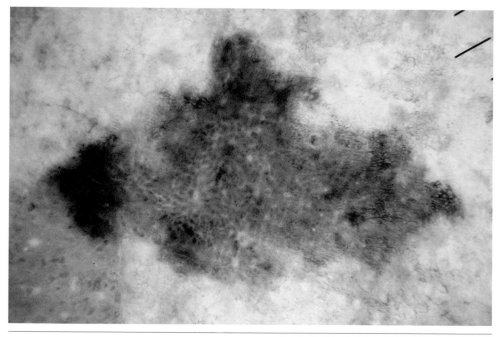

Figure 4.30: *Pigmented clods in a melanoma separated by skin-coloured lines creating a pattern referred to by some as a so-called 'negative' or 'inverse' network.*

4.7 Revised pattern analysis applied to vessel structures and patterns

4.7.1 Vessel structures

Revised pattern analysis precisely defines eight types of vessel structures and eight vessel arrangements[4].

Vessel structures occur as dots, clods (clods and dots are regarded as separate structures in the case of vessels) and lines of which there are six types: straight, looped, curved, serpentine, helical and coiled (*Figures 4.31* and *4.32*). Vessel types are defined as follows[4]:

- **Dot:** a vessel structure (red) too small to have a discernible shape (at 10× magnification).
- **Clod:** a well circumscribed solid vessel structure (red or purple) larger than a dot, any shape.
- **Linear:** a vessel structure with length greatly exceeding width.

Linear vessels may be:
- **Linear straight:** linear vessels without a bend.
- **Linear looped:** linear vessels with one sharp bend resulting in a reversal of direction (U-turn).
- **Linear curved:** linear vessels with one gentle bend.
- **Linear serpentine:** linear vessels with more than one bend and shaped in a snake-like fashion.
- **Linear helical:** linear vessels with multiple bends twisted along a central axis.
- **Linear coiled:** linear vessels with multiple bends and convoluted compactly.

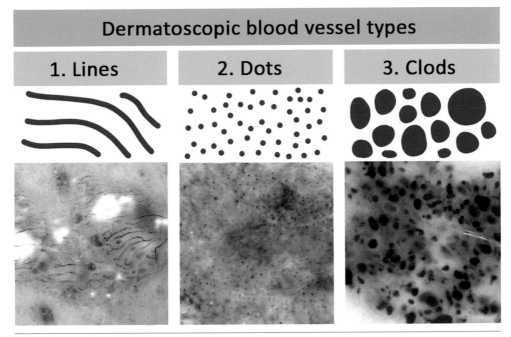

Figure 4.31: *Diagrammatic representation (upper) and dermatoscopic images (lower) of vessel types: 1. linear (example seborrhoeic keratosis); 2. dots (example Clark naevus); 3. clods (example haemangioma).*

4.7.2 Vessel patterns

Multiple vessels of one type may form a pattern and that pattern may be monomorphous (if one vessel type predominates), or polymorphous (if either *more than one vessel type is present in significant numbers within a pattern* or alternatively if there are *separate patterns of more than one vessel type*) (*Figure 4.33*). If there is, for example, a pattern of linear serpentine vessels with a couple of dot vessels, that is not a polymorphous pattern. There would need to be enough dot vessels either to clearly interfere with the pattern of serpentine vessels or as a separate cluster making a pattern of their own.

The eight types of vessel arrangement are: random, clustered, serpiginous, linear, centred, radial, reticular and branched (*Figure 4.34*) and the vessel *arrangements* which form patterns are defined as follows[4]:

- **Random:** vessels not arranged in any of the following seven specific ways below.
- **Clustered:** vessels which are concentrated in certain areas of a lesion.
- **Serpiginous:** dot or coiled vessels arranged in a linear snake-like pattern (this is different to the linear serpentine vessel *type*).
- **Linear:** dot or coiled vessels arranged in straight lines.
- **Centred:** vessels centred in *skin-coloured* clods.
- **Radial:** linear vessels in a group orientated from the periphery towards the centre of a lesion but not crossing it.
- **Reticular:** linear vessels crossing at right angles to form a net-like pattern.
- **Branched:** linear serpentine vessels which divide into consecutively thinner serpentine vessels from a central main stem.

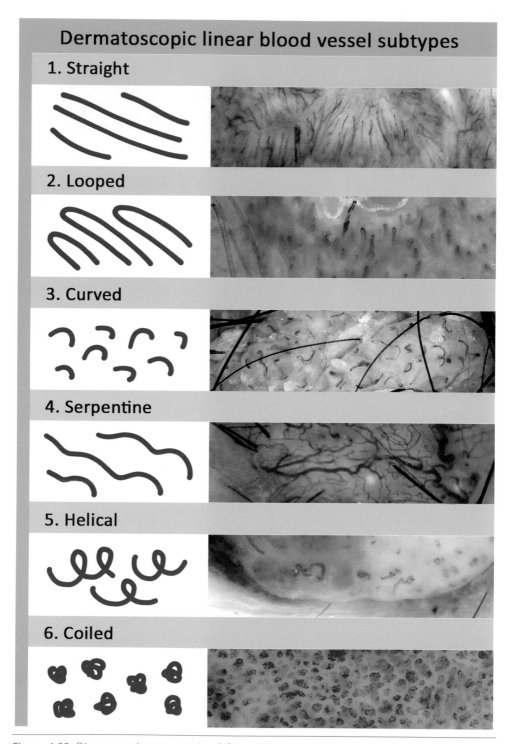

Figure 4.32: *Diagrammatic representation (left) and dermatoscopic images (right) of linear vessel types: 1. straight (example basal cell carcinoma); 2. looped (example squamous cell carcinoma); 3. curved (example dermal naevus); 4. serpentine (example basal cell carcinoma); 5. helical (example melanoma); 6. coiled (example squamous cell carcinoma in situ).*

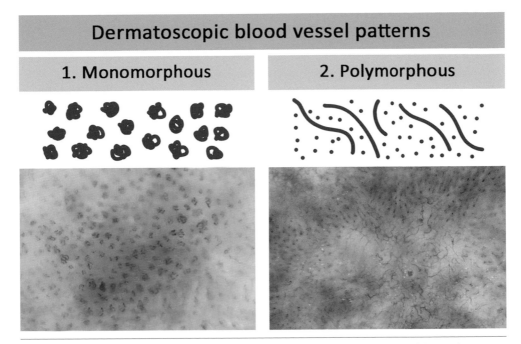

Figure 4.33: *Diagrammatic representation (upper) and dermatoscopic images (lower) of the two basic types of vessel pattern: 1. monomorphous (example monomorphous coiled vessels in a squamous cell carcinoma in situ) and 2. polymorphous (example a pattern of linear vessels and dot vessels forming a polymorphous pattern in an amelanotic melanoma).*

4.7.3 The anatomical correlation of vessel structures and patterns

Vessels seen on dermatoscopy include vessels of the horizontally orientated dermal plexus, seen as serpentine branched (*Figure 4.35*) or reticular vessels, as well as vessels extending vertically from the dermal plexus up into the dermal papillae, seen as dot or coiled vessels, unless a lesion becomes raised in which case they are seen as curved or looped vessels (*Figures 4.36* and *4.37*). The significance of this is that the presence of looped vessels is a dermatoscopic clue to a 'raised' lesion. In the context of malignancy, looped vessels suggest invasive status (*Figure 4.37*)[9].

Although vessels are not expected to be seen dermatoscopically on normal skin, they can become visible in situations of increased blood flow (e.g. inflammation or infection), atrophy of the epidermis (e.g. chronic solar atrophy) and increased metabolic demand

(e.g. neoplasia). Angioneogenesis, also associated with malignancy, typically results in polymorphous vessels. Because dot vessels depend on an intact dermal papillae architecture they are not expected in any raised portion of a melanoma, although they are frequently seen in hypopigmented macular portions.

The branched serpentine pattern of vessels associated with BCC is seen more clearly and more sharply focused in BCC because these vessels are set in a jelly-like translucent stroma (*Figure 4.35*). Similar vessels can be seen over any raised lesion, benign or malignant, solid or cystic, which displaces the horizontal dermal plexus towards an attenuated epidermis[4].

Dermatoscopic patterns formed by angiocentric melanin

It is known that dots, both pigmented and red, in linear arrangement are a dermatoscopic clue to pigmented Bowen's disease (pSCC *in*

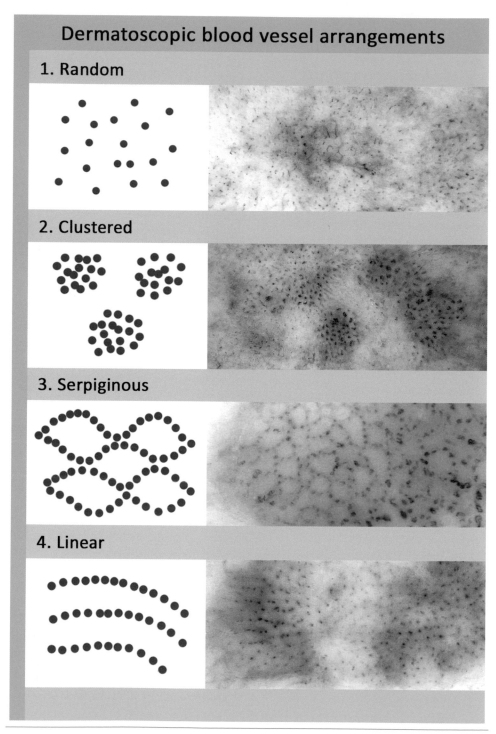

Figure 4.34: *Diagrammatic representation (left) and dermatoscopic images (right) of dermatoscopic blood vessel arrangements: 1. random (example squamous cell carcinoma in situ); 2. clustered (example squamous cell carcinoma in situ); 3. serpiginous (example clear cell acanthoma); 4. linear (example pigmented squamous cell carcinoma in situ).*

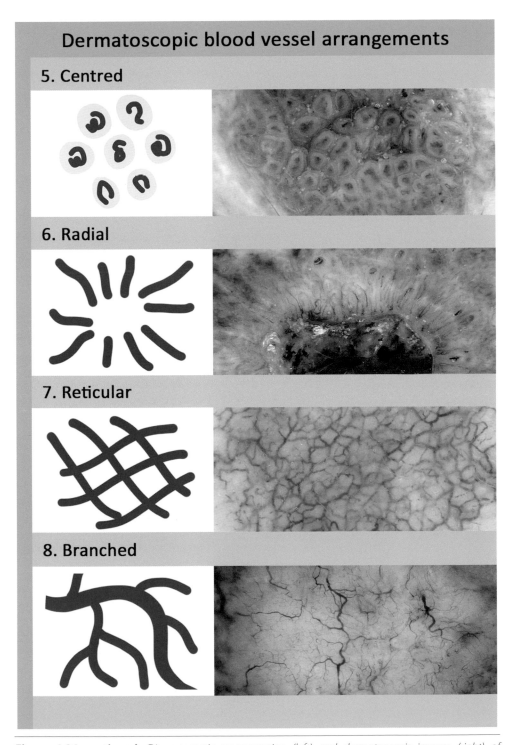

Dermatoscopic blood vessel arrangements

5. Centred

6. Radial

7. Reticular

8. Branched

Figure 4.34 continued: *Diagrammatic representation (left) and dermatoscopic images (right) of dermatoscopic blood vessel arrangements: 5. Centred (example seborrhoeic keratosis); 6. Radial (example squamous cell carcinoma); 7. Reticular (example telangiectasia on sun-damaged skin); 8. Branched (example basal cell carcinoma).*

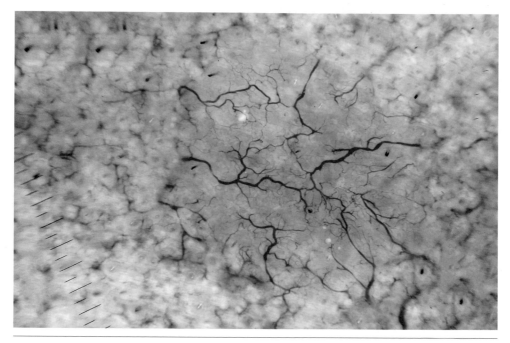

Figure 4.35: Branched serpentine vessels in a BCC are seen to blend seamlessly into the reticular pattern of vessels of the surrounding horizontal dermal plexus vessels which are visible through sun-damaged facial skin. The vessels of the BCC are seen more clearly and sharply because of the translucent stroma of the BCC.

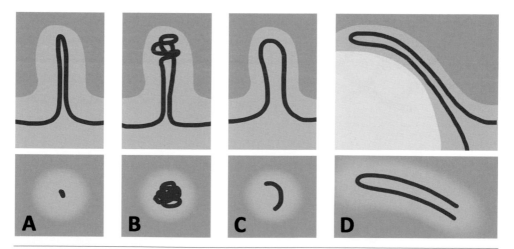

Figure 4.36: A diagrammatic representation of dermal papillary vessels (upper row) and corresponding dermatoscopic projections (lower row). A vessel in a flat lesion which enters the dermal papilla from below, ascends to the top and turns on itself sharply will appear as a dot (A), if it is convoluted it will appear as a coiled vessel (B). Once the lesion is raised the dermal papilla distorts laterally and if the papilla is wide it will project as a curved vessel (C), but if the papilla is not wide it will appear as a looped vessel (D).

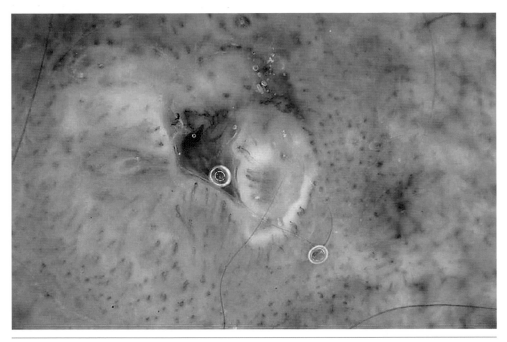

Figure 4.37: *Peripherally this lesion shows a pattern of coiled vessels consistent with squamous cell carcinoma in situ. Centrally the squamous cell carcinoma has become invasive and the dermal papillae vessels, being displaced sideways, appear as looped vessels.*

situ)[23]. This can be seen on dermatopathology to correlate with dermal papillae vessels in linear array which, in the case of dots which are pigmented, correlates with angiocentric melanin (*Figure 4.38*)[4].

In addition, we have observed that some angulated lines are a result of angiocentric melanin in relation to vessels of the horizontal dermal plexus (*Figure 4.39*). We propose two possible mechanisms for these examples

of angiocentric melanin in relation to both SCC *in situ* and melanoma, either separately or in combination. It has been shown that cutaneous blood vessels in blue naevus can phagocytose melanin[24] and maybe such phagocytosis also occurs in pSCC *in situ* and melanoma. Another possibility is that melanophages, having phagocytosed melanin, may then migrate towards lymphatic vessels in an angiocentric location.

 # 4.8 The cognition of dermatoscopy

"A method that cannot be taught is barely a method at all"[4].

Critics of algorithmic methods often state that in actual practice experts do not think with an algorithmic process. Of course, with experience and expertise most malignancies are recognised by a form of cognition which we call here 'rapid processing' which is in fact 'pattern recognition'. A clinician sees a lesion through the dermatoscope and, by

comparing it to a vast database of dermatoscopic 'memories' stored in the cerebral cortex, recognises it for what it is, in the same way that the clinician recognises the face of an acquaintance. The problem is that while facial recognition is a well-documented human practice, the application to disciplines like dermatoscopy is not automatic

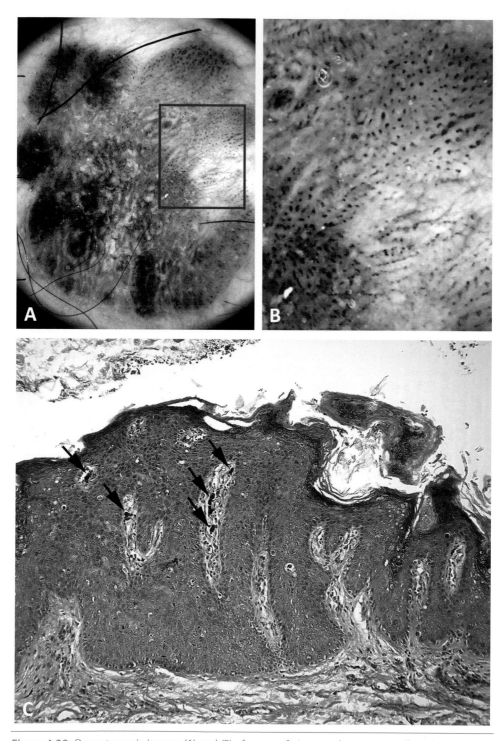

Figure 4.38: *Dermatoscopic images (A) and (B) of a case of pigmented squamous cell carcinoma* in situ *show red dots in linear array merging into lines of pigmented dots (boxed area in (A), enlarged in (B)). A photomicrograph (C) reveals the correlation of angiocentric melanin in the dermal papillae in proximity to papillary vessels (arrows).*

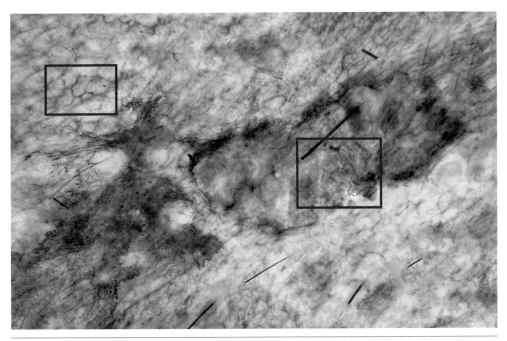

Figure 4.39: *Comparison of the angulated lines (boxed area right) shows a marked similarity to the morphology of vascular plexus vessels (boxed area left). This causes us to speculate that angiocentric melanin may underlie the morphology of angulated lines.*

and must be learned. Learning, without critical teaching, can lead to delusions of grandeur if the self-taught 'expert' assumes that what is not recognised does not exist. Malcolm Gladwell in his book *Outliers* asserts that to gain expertise in a new field, a time investment of approximately 10,000 hours is required[25]. A dermatologist who works for 8 hours 5 days a week and who examines every lesion with a dermatoscope might have his eye on the instrument for 2 hours a day. That is about 500 hours per year, reaching 10,000 hours in 20 years. Of course, a person who does nothing else apart from dermatoscopy, such as a technician working solely in that field, can arguably develop expertise a lot more rapidly. While expertise is being developed, algorithmic methods provide scaffolding on which accumulated education and experience can be organised and stored. After expertise is established these methods provide a systematic approach for the assessment of more difficult lesions so that they never become redundant in a universe such as ours, of infinite variation.

The algorithmic method of RPA is not for robots but rather for thoughtful students of science, a cohort which includes the readers of this book.

Finally, RPA is not set in stone. Every dermatoscopist is encouraged to adapt it to their own style, practice and experience and to share any innovations with others in the spirit of peer-review and adaptation.

References

1. Kittler H. Dermatoscopy: introduction of a new algorithmic method based on pattern analysis for diagnosis of pigmented skin lesions. *Dermatopathol Pract Concept,* 2007;13:3.

2. Kittler H, Riedl E, Rosendahl C, and Cameron

A. Dermatoscopy of unpigmented lesions of the skin: a new classification of vessel morphology based on pattern analysis. *Dermatopathol Pract Concept*, 2008;14:4.

3. Kittler H, Marghoob AA, Argenziano G, *et al.* Standardization of terminology in dermoscopy/dermatoscopy: results of the third consensus conference of the International Society of Dermoscopy. *J Am Acad Dermatol*, 2016;74:1093.

4. Kittler H, Rosendahl C, Cameron A, and Tschandl P. *Dermatoscopy,* 2nd Edition, 2016. Facultas.

5. Rosendahl C, Cameron A, Tschandl P, Bulinska A, Zalaudek I, and Kittler H. Prediction without pigment: a decision algorithm for non-pigmented skin malignancy. *Dermatol Pract Concept,* 2014;4:9.

6. Keir J. Dermatoscopic features of cutaneous non-facial non-acral lentiginous growth pattern melanomas. *Dermatol Pract Concept,* 2014;4(1):77.

7. http://greycircles.blogspot.com.au [accessed 5 Feb 2018].

8. Tschandl P, Rosendahl C, and Kittler H. Dermatoscopy of flat pigmented facial lesions. *J Eur Acad Dermatol Venereol*, 2015;29:120.

9. https://dermoscopedia.org [accessed 26 August 2022].

10. Argenziano G, Soyer HP, Chimenti S, *et al.* Dermoscopy of pigmented skin lesions: results of a consensus meeting via the internet. *J Am Acad Dermatol*, 2003;48:679.

11. Marghoob AA, and Braun R. Proposal for a revised 2-step algorithm for the classification of lesions of the skin using dermoscopy. *Arch Dermatol*, 2010;146:426.

12. Tschandl P, Rosendahl C, and Kittler H. Accuracy of the first step of the dermatoscopic 2-step algorithm for pigmented skin lesions. *Dermatol Pract Concept*, 2012;2:203.

13. Liebman TN, Rabinovitz HS, Balagula Y, Jaimes-Lopez N, and Marghoob AA. White shiny structures in melanoma and BCC. *Arch Dermatol*, 2012;148:146.

14. Peris K, Micantonio T, Piccolo D, and Concetta M. Dermoscopic features of actinic keratosis. *J Deutsch Dermatol Gesellsch*, 2007;5:970.

15. Rosendahl C, Cameron A, Argenziano G, Zalaudek I, Tschandl P, and Kittler H. Dermoscopy of squamous cell carcinoma and keratoacanthoma. *Arch Dermatol*, 2012;148:1386.

16. Berk DR, and Bayliss SJ. Milia: a review and classification. *J Am Acad Dermatol*, 2008;59:1050.

17. Bellucci C, Arginelli F, Bassoli S, Magnoni C, and Seidenari S. Dermoscopic yellow structures in basal cell carcinoma. *J Eur Acad Dermatol Venereol*, 2014;28:651.

18. Bryden AM, Dawe RS, and Fleming C. Dermatoscopic features of benign sebaceous proliferation. *Clin Exp Dermatol*, 2004;29:676.

19. Enei ML, Paschoal FM, Valdés G, and Valdés R. Basal cell carcinoma appearing in a facial nevus sebaceous of Jadassohn: dermoscopic features. *An Bras Dermatol*, 2012;87:640.

20. Jegou Penouil MH, Gourhant J-Y, Segretin C, Weedon D, and Rosendahl C. Non-choroidal yellow melanoma showing positive staining with Sudan Black consistent with the presence of lipofuscin: a case report. *Dermatol Pract Concept*, 2014;4:9.

21. Inskip M, James N, Magee J, and Rosendahl C. Pigmented primary cutaneous balloon cell melanoma demonstrating balloon cells in the dermoepidermal junction: a brief case report with dermatoscopy and histopathology. *Int J Dermatol*, 2016;55:e110.

22. Deutch CE. Browning in apples: exploring the biochemical basis of an easily-observable phenotype. *Biochem Mol Biol Educ*, 2018;46:76.

23. Cameron A, Rosendahl C, Tschandl P, Riedl E, and Kittler H. Dermatoscopy of pigmented Bowen's disease. *J Am Acad Dermatol*, 2010;62:597.

24. Sato S, and Kukita A. Electron microscopic study of melanin-phagocytosis by cutaneous vessels in cellular blue nevus. *J Invest Dermatol*, 1969;52:528.

25. Gladwell M. *Outliers: the story of success*, 2009. Penguin.

CHAPTER 5

The skin examination

5.1 The skin check consultation

This book is about dermatoscopy and its application to the diagnosis and management of skin malignancy. Every step in that pathway is critical to a favourable outcome, including the way in which the 'geographical landscape' on which skin cancers are found is explored.

One scenario is for the patient to present with a lesion of concern which the clinician examines and manages. Another situation, frequently relevant in general practice, is for the alert clinician to encounter and take notice of a skin lesion when examining the patient for another purpose altogether. While both of these are valid scenarios, this section presents a method of systematic examination for skin malignancy.

5.1.1 Who needs a full skin examination?

Any intervention which involves a cost, subsidised by taxpayer or insurance-payer contributions, should only be recommended when the potential cost/benefit ratio is reasonable. A skin examination is no exception and it is not only cost that is relevant but the availability of finite resources. Although anyone can get a skin malignancy, stratification of risk factors is appropriate in the assessment of which patients should be classified as being at high risk and therefore screened for skin cancer at regular intervals. In practice, we routinely offer a 6-monthly skin examination

to patients whose stratified risk factors give them a relative risk (RR), compared to the population as a whole, of 5 or higher, this being the recommendation according to the Australasian melanoma guidelines[1]. This includes patients with:

- a past history of melanoma (RR 10)
- a naevus count (any type) over 100 (RR 7)
- a previous history of NMSC or AK is borderline (RR 4), and we believe it is reasonable to see such patients again after 6 months but then every 12 months until a further NMSC or a melanoma is encountered
- multiple NMSCs, who can reasonably continue to have 6-monthly examinations.

Contrary to common belief, a family history of melanoma (RR 2) does not confer a high risk and the authors recommend examination at 12-monthly intervals if this is the only risk factor.

5.1.2 History taking

A consultation for skin cancer surveillance, like every other consultation, commences with appropriate history taking. The first time a patient attends for this purpose it may be appropriate to allocate extra time to elicit and record details of[1]:

- allergies
- regular medication
- family history
- previous history of medical and surgical conditions, including skin cancer

- lifestyle questions about occupational and recreational sun and other UV and radiation exposure
- information about geographic location in earlier life
- history of remembered episodes of sunburn.

The first inquiry at subsequent visits should be directed towards updating this data record with any new information. At both the initial and subsequent visits the patient should have an opportunity to indicate any current concerns, especially about new, changing or symptomatic lesions.

5.1.3 The skin examination

The skin examination is performed with an understanding that healthy skin is expected to display many benign lesions that must be recognised without undue delay to the examination process.

Benign lesions

There are 5 benign lesion types which include the vast majority of benign lesions encountered daily in routine practice[2]:
- naevus
- benign keratinocytic lesions (including freckles, solar lentigines and seborrhoeic keratoses, etc.)
- haemangioma
- dermatofibroma
- sebaceous gland hyperplasia.

These lesions will often be seen on the same patient and, although the dermatoscope will be applied to many of them, the diagnostic process employed will be pattern recognition, which is actually rapid processing of visual information.

Significant lesions

Similarly, the significant lesions, both benign and malignant, for the diagnosis and differential diagnosis of skin cancer can be conveniently classified as follows:
- Melanocytic: benign (naevus) and malignant (melanoma).
- Keratinocytic: benign (e.g. solar lentigo, seborrhoeic keratosis, LPLK, melanotic

macule and viral wart) and malignant SCC and BCC.
- Vascular/haematopoietic tumours: benign (e.g. haemangioma) and malignant (e.g. cutaneous lymphoma).
- Fibrous tumours: benign (e.g. DF) and malignant (e.g. dermatofibrosarcoma protuberans).
- Other: benign (e.g. benign sebaceous and adnexal tumours) and malignant (e.g. Merkel cell carcinoma; atypical fibroxanthoma, Kaposi sarcoma and various adnexal malignancies).

5.1.4 Clinical examination

Before considering the dermatoscopic algorithms, it is relevant to also look at what is actually done in the daily routine of clinical practice.

Clinical red flags

Clinical red flags represent the non-dermatoscopic features that may highlight a lesion as suspicious and therefore warranting formal algorithmic assessment. These features are such that they will either be known (patient concern) or be obvious (clinical pattern-breaker).
- **Patient concern or clinical evidence of change.** No lesion of patient concern should ever be dismissed without targeted examination including dermatoscopy[3]. Patients may be concerned because a seborrhoeic keratosis is large and black, because a haemangioma has apparently suddenly appeared or because a mole is perceived to have changed. Patient concern should automatically flag a lesion as suspicious and lead to an analytical assessment (*Figure 5.1*). Similarly, documented evidence of change at mature age, including deliberately monitored change, flags a lesion as suspicious therefore requiring focused dermatoscopic assessment.
- **Clinical pattern-breaker.** The same disorganised and uncontrolled behaviour of malignant tissue that causes dermatoscopic chaos often causes malignant lesions

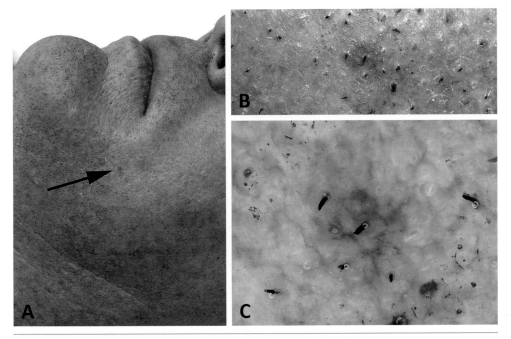

Figure 5.1: *Clinical (A), close-up (B) and dermatoscopic (C) images of a subtle pigmented skin lesion which was identified by a patient with a history of multiple melanomas as being present for only 6 weeks. Dermatoscopy revealed the clue to melanoma* in situ *of pigmented circles correlating with hair follicles in a lesion which did not have the unequivocal dermatoscopic morphology of a naevus (see Section 5.1.5)[4].*

to break the pattern of the surrounding skin clinically. Malignant lesions may arise randomly, have an irregular unexpected shape or colour, and eventually their unrestrained growth may make them larger than surrounding benign lesions. A lesion which breaks the pattern clinically should be flagged as suspicious and analysed dermatoscopically (see *Figure 5.2*)[2].

5.1.5 Dermatoscopic examination

Pattern recognition of common benign lesions

Although the clinician is ideally encouraged to apply the dermatoscope to all lesions on a patient, a detailed algorithmic analysis of every lesion is neither realistic nor necessary. The vast majority of skin lesions are benign and can be diagnosed dermatoscopically by pattern recognition (see *Section 4.8*)[5].

Benign lesions tend to have dermatoscopic biological symmetry and this symmetry occurs in the form of recognisable patterns, just as faces of different species of animals have recognisable patterns. We will recognise any dog's face by pattern recognition even though there are many different morphological varieties of dog faces.

In *Figure 5.3* there are six different images of animal faces. The first five are recognisable as 'normal' faces because even though they are not necessarily perfectly symmetrical they are biologically symmetrical and therefore recognisable. *They do not exhibit chaos.* The sixth image on the other hand is not biologically symmetrical. *It is chaotic* and therefore not as easily recognisable, which means that pattern analysis may need to be used to weigh clues to identify what it represents.

The common benign skin lesions we may see every day are also recognisable because

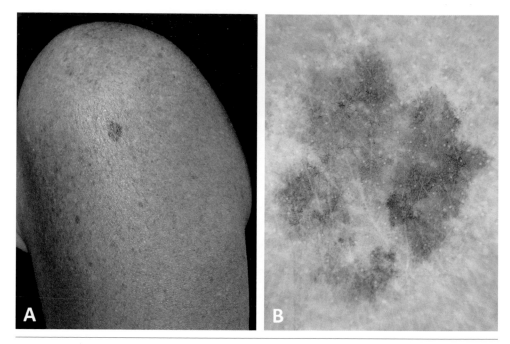

Figure 5.2: *Clinical (A) and dermatoscopic (B) images of a pigmented lesion which 'broke the pattern' on this patient's shoulder and which was noticed by the clinician while the patient was standing at the reception desk after consulting another doctor for an unrelated issue. The patient confirmed that it had only become apparent in the preceding 6 weeks; melanoma in situ.*

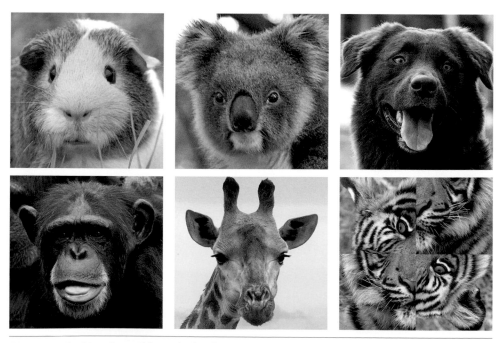

Figure 5.3: *In this collage of faces the first five are recognisable by pattern recognition because they are biologically symmetrical. The sixth exhibits biological asymmetry (chaos) and therefore may require analysis of the patterns present to achieve recognition.*

of characteristic biologically symmetrical patterns (*Figure 5.4*). Just as there are many different morphological varieties of dogs and fish, there are many different morphological types of naevi and of seborrhoeic keratoses. An experienced clinician will recognise them instantly through a dermatoscope as naevi or seborrhoeic keratoses and move to the next lesion. Becoming an expert at pattern recognition of common benign lesions requires just one thing – the deliberate examination of thousands of them with a dermatoscope.

5.1.6 A methodical approach to complete skin examination

This approach is used by both of the authors and offers a consistent methodical approach.

The patient undresses behind a curtain and sits on the edge of an adjustable couch wearing only underwear. No gown or sheet is routinely used but a sheet is available if the patient requests it. Make-up removal wipes and nail polish remover are available if required. The area over the couch is well illuminated with fluorescent lights (*Figure 5.5*).

The clinician is equipped with a dermatoscope, an LED torch and varieties of immersion fluid (*Figure 5.6*).

The method of examination employed by the authors is illustrated in *Figures 5.7–5.13*.

Equipment and workflow

Examination proceeds with the dermatoscope in the dominant hand of the clinician and a source of interface fluid in the other. This means that the illumination for the greater part of the examination will be provided by overhead fluorescent lights supplemented by the light source of the dermatoscope. This facilitates skin wetting and application of the dermatoscope to multiple lesions with a

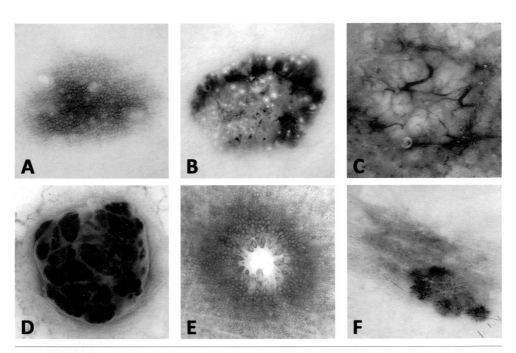

Figure 5.4: *To an experienced dermatoscopist the first five lesions in this collage are biologically symmetrical (no chaos) and will be diagnosed by pattern recognition as (A) naevus, (B) seborrhoeic keratosis, (C) sebaceous gland hyperplasia, (D) haemangioma, and (E) dermatofibroma. The last lesion (F) is asymmetrical and cannot be* recognised *as any of the common benign lesions, so pattern analysis is applied. It is disorganised (chaotic) with clues to malignancy (see* Chapter 6*); melanoma in situ.*

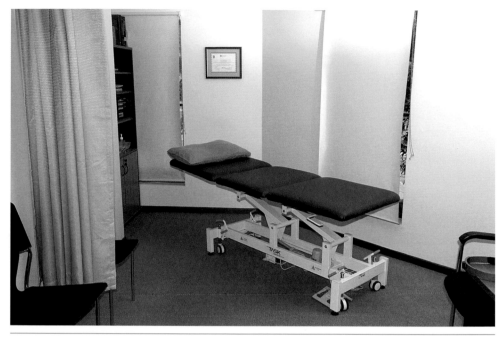

Figure 5.5: *The examination room contains an adjustable couch, set out from the wall, and which is brightly illuminated with fluorescent lights.*

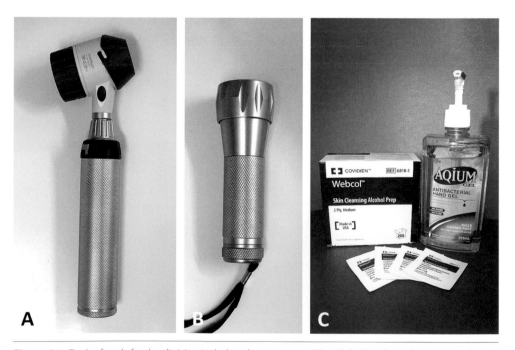

Figure 5.6: *Tools of trade for the clinician include a dermatoscope (A) with both polarised and non-polarised options, as well as an LED torch (B) and varieties of immersion fluid to facilitate fluid-immersion contact dermatoscopy (C).*

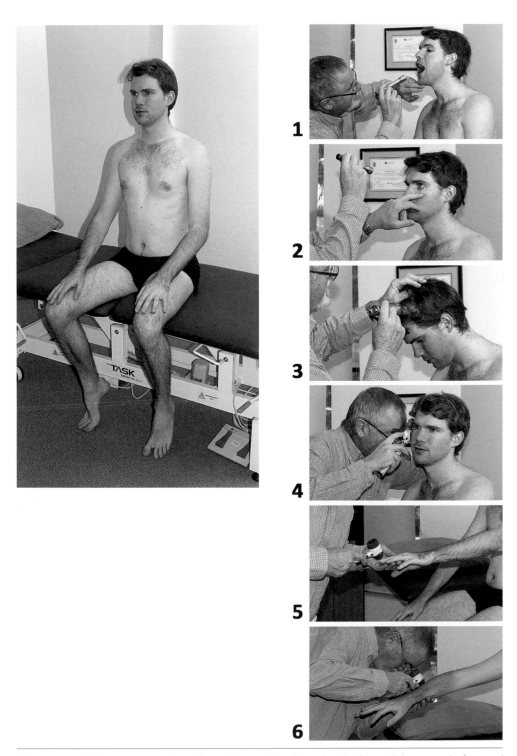

Figure 5.7: *With the patient seated and facing the examiner, the oral cavity, lips, eyelids, eyes, scalp, face, and upper limbs are examined in turn.*

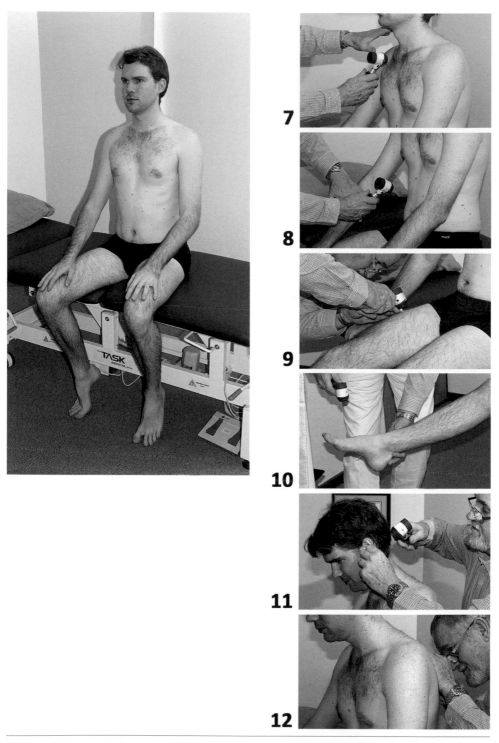

Figure 5.8: *The examination proceeds on the anterior torso and anterior lower limbs after which the clinician walks behind the patient and inspects the posterior scalp, posterior surface of the ears and the upper back. By using the dermatoscope as the light source for the clinical examination the clinician's eye is by necessity close to the patient's skin and application of the dermatoscope to lesions of interest is facilitated.*

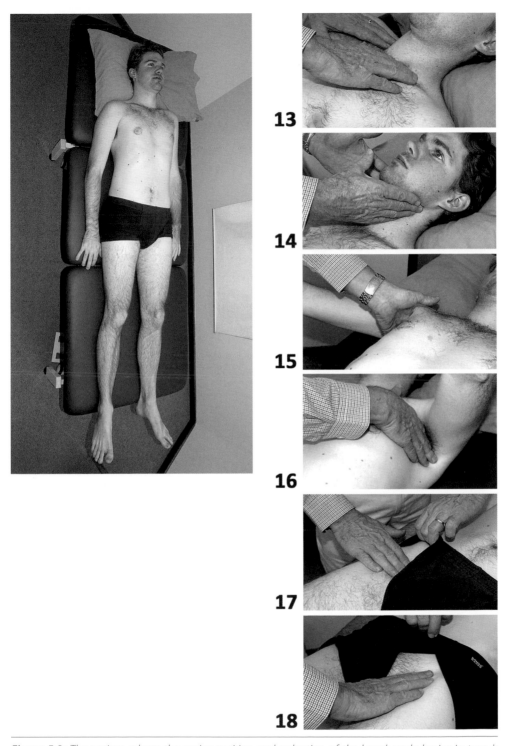

13

14

15

16

17

18

Figure 5.9: *The patient adopts the supine position and palpation of the lymph node basins in turn is performed first. This typically takes less than 30 seconds and the yield of relevant findings is significant.*

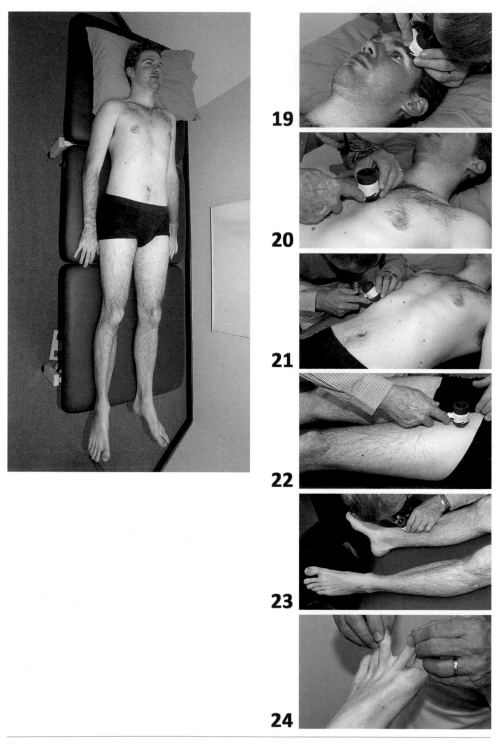

19

20

21

22

23

24

Figure 5.10: Next the anterior surface of the body is examined including the face, entire anterior torso, upper limbs and lower limbs including the nails and the interdigital skin. Underwear is retracted to expose the breasts in women and the pubic area in all patients. The genitalia are enquired about and inspected with permission in response to any concern.

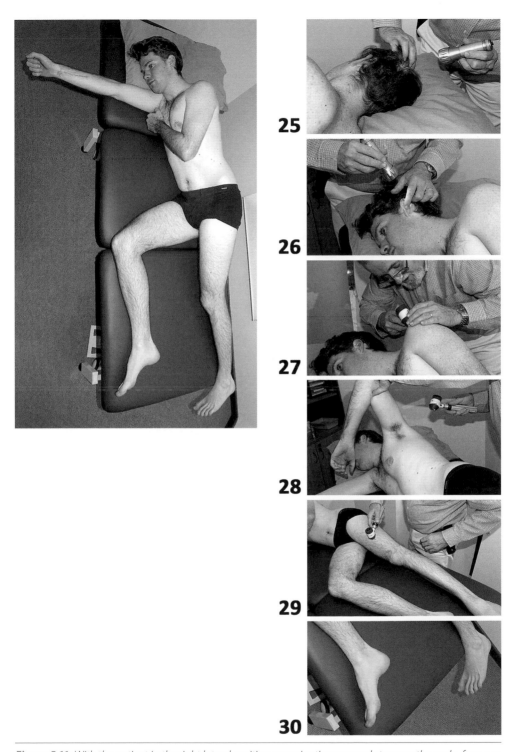

25

26

27

28

29

30

Figure 5.11: With the patient in the right lateral position, examination proceeds to cover the scalp, face, ear, neck, and torso as well as the exposed upper and lower limb surfaces, with the uppermost (left) limb retracted posteriorly.

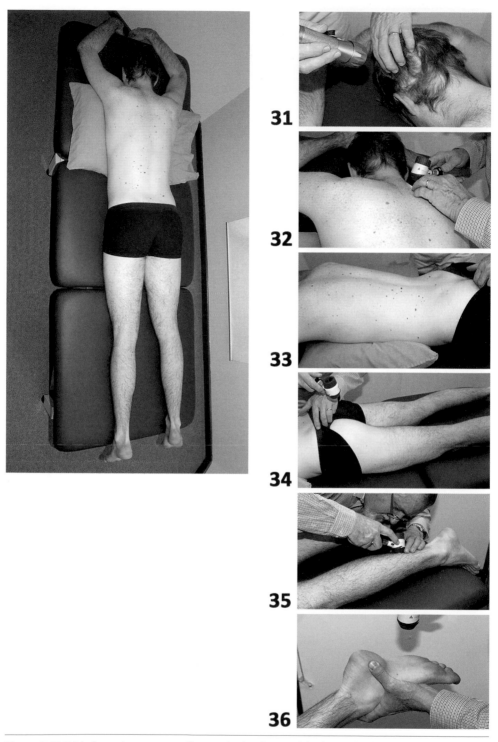

31

32

33

34

35

36

Figure 5.12: *With the patient prone, a pillow under the chest and the face in the breather hole in the couch, the entire posterior surface of the body is examined, commencing with the scalp and finishing with the soles of the feet. Underwear is retracted to facilitate the examination of each buttock in turn.*

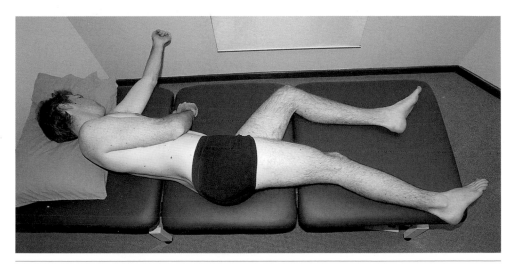

Figure 5.13: *Finally, with the patient in the left lateral position the entire right side is examined in the same manner as described for the left side (Figure 5.11).*

smooth workflow. It also brings the examiner's eyes into proximity with the patient's skin.

The initial examination is performed with the dermatoscope in polarised mode, routinely being done with contact dermatoscopy using interface fluid because the improved clarity makes small malignant lesions, particularly BCC, recognisable at a much earlier stage. Some clinicians prefer to start with non-contact polarised dermatoscopy, using a second dermatoscope when non-polarised information is required. Even when non-contact (polarised) dermatoscopy is used, the application of fluid to the lesion, as with an alcohol wipe, may greatly improve clarity, especially on sun-damaged, scaly skin. Others routinely use video dermatoscopy, viewing the lesion on a monitor screen, capturing images on demand and sharing the viewed images with the patient in real time. There is no single correct method. The important thing is that the clinician develops a method, becomes proficient with it and understands any limitations that may apply.

It is also important that a protocol is established and followed that includes an examination of all accessible skin and mucosal surfaces as well as the lymph node basins. The establishment of a consistent examination

protocol permits the examiner to focus on the skin rather than considering what to do next.

Examination of the oral cavity and lips

The examiner commences by inspecting the oral cavity and vermillion lips with a handheld LED light for illumination (see *Figure 5.7*). The most commonly observed abnormal pigmentation is amalgam tattoo from inadvertent amalgam implantation during dental intervention, which has a characteristic appearance with which the clinician should become familiar. Findings of interest include any unexpected pigmentation (*Figure 5.14*), interruption of mucosal integrity by white discoloration, or ulceration. The vermillion (non-hair-bearing) lips are carefully examined for any mucosal abnormality.

Examination of the eyes and eyelids

Next the eyelids are examined for any abnormality, with careful inspection of the eyelid margins for focal missing lashes which might accompany very early BCC, or for pigmented lesions suspicious for malignancy (*Figures 5.15* and *5.16*). Pigmentation of the sclera warrants careful assessment (*Figure 5.17*) and any irregularity of the iris should be noted.

The opportunity is taken when examining

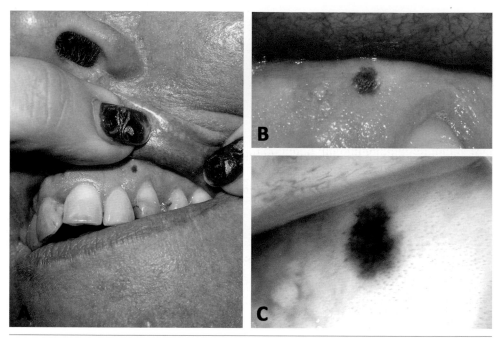

Figure 5.14: *Clinical (A), close-up (B) and dermatoscopic (C) images of a lesion on the gum which may need histological confirmation to exclude malignancy; melanotic macule.*

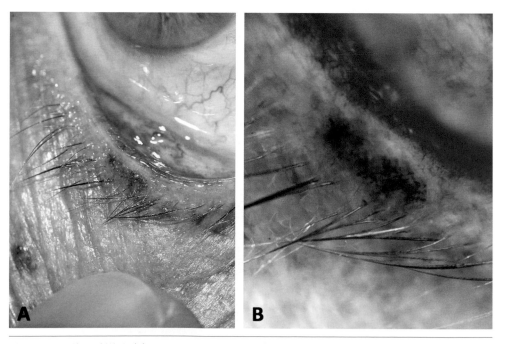

Figure 5.15: *Clinical (A) and dermatoscopic (B) images of a lesion discovered on the eyelid margin; melanotic macule.*

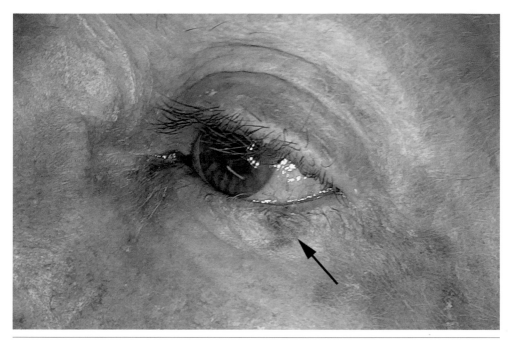

Figure 5.16: *A pigmented skin lesion is discovered on the lower eyelid; melanoma in situ.*

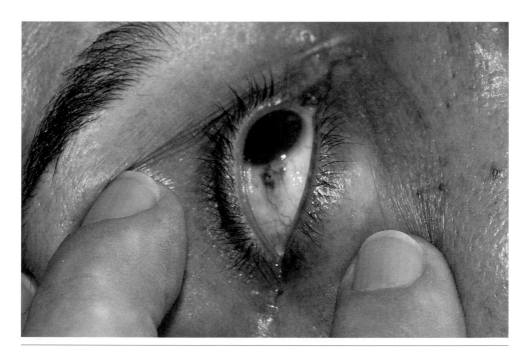

Figure 5.17: *A pigmented lesion is encountered on the lateral conjunctiva; melanoma in situ.*

the eyes to ask about routine optometry visits and to mention the relevance of requesting the optometrist to examine the inside of the eye for choroidal melanoma at the time of routine optometry assessment.

Examination of the face and scalp

Following an examination of the oral cavity, lips and eyes, the LED light is placed back in its scabbard on the examiner's belt. The dermatoscope is taken in the dominant hand and a spray bottle with 70% ethanol, or alternatively an alcohol wipe, is taken in the other hand and the anterior scalp and face are examined (*Figure 5.7*). When examining the face, contact dermatoscopy is used in polarised mode with interface fluid applied directly to the face-plate rather than being sprayed onto the skin, thus avoiding inadvertent spraying of the eyes. Alternatively, an alcohol wipe can be used.

The face is examined systematically with application of the dermatoscope to pigmented lesions as well as to other non-skin-coloured lesions, flat or raised, and to any raised lesions/skin indentations even if skin-coloured. The greatest likelihood of discovering a NMSC is on the head and neck, and there is a significant advantage in discovering it at a very early stage, particularly in that location, at which time it may only be identified by careful examination using contact dermatoscopy with fluid applied to the skin.

Examination of the upper limbs and the anterior surface of the body with the patient still seated

After the face, the upper limbs are examined with the patient still seated facing the clinician (*Figure 5.7*). Starting with the right hand the nails are inspected, each in turn, with the hand being rotated for a careful inspection of the thumbnail, this being the most common site of neoplasia of the nail apparatus. Then the palmar and dorsal surfaces of the hands and fingers and the interdigital spaces are examined, following which the forearms and arms are carefully examined, followed by a

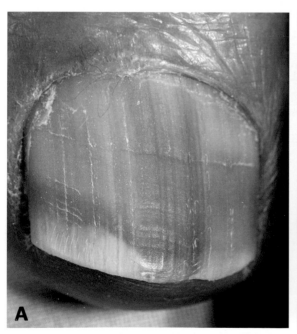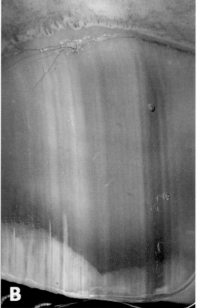

Figure 5.18: Close-up (A) and dermatoscopic (B) images. Examination of the toenails discovers longitudinal melanonychia with lines parallel chaotic on a hallux; melanoma in situ of the nail matrix.

scanning view of the front of the torso and lower limbs (*Figure 5.8*).

Examination of the back with the patient still seated

The clinician then walks to the back of the couch and, with the patient still seated, carefully examines the back of the neck, the top of the shoulders and the upper back (*Figure 5.8*).

Examination with the patient supine

Lymph node basins: the patient is then requested to lie down in the supine position and the lymph node basins (supraclavicular, posterior cervical, anterior cervical, submandibular, submental, axillary and inguinal) are each examined in turn (*Figure 5.9*). Disposable gloves may be worn during this part of the examination. Careful examination of the lymph node basins typically takes less than 30 seconds and surprising discoveries can be made (*Figure 5.19*).

Anterior surface of face, neck, torso and limbs: after the lymph node basins have been examined, the dermatoscope and spray bottle are again taken in hand while a systematic examination of the whole anterior surface of the body is repeated. This starts with the face, neck, upper limbs, anterior chest and abdomen and proceeds to the lower limbs, including feet, toes, interdigital spaces and toenails (*Figures 5.10 and 5.18*). With respect to female patients, each side of the bra is retracted in turn to permit inspection of the skin of the breasts. The same is done with underwear to permit inspection of the pubic area in men and women, this being a common location for congenital naevi. Genitalia are enquired about but not routinely examined, although there is no specific rationale for this apart from what the examiner is comfortable doing and the consent provided by the patient.

Left side of body including scalp under hair: the patient is then asked to roll onto

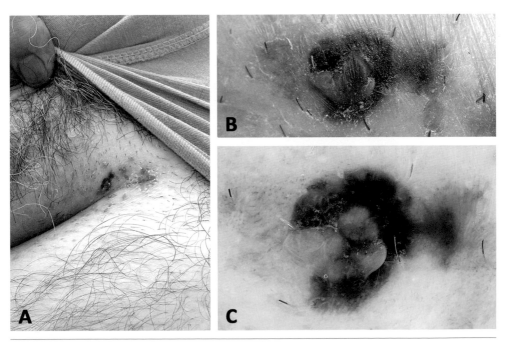

Figure 5.19: *Clinical (A), close-up (B) and dermatoscopic (C) images. Examination of the inguinal lymph node basins detected a palpable lesion. Retraction of the crural fold revealed an irregular pigmented skin lesion; invasive melanoma associated with a dermal naevus.*

the right side (*Figure 5.11*). The dermatoscope is returned to its scabbard then, with the aid of the LED torch, the left side of the scalp is carefully and systematically examined regardless of the presence or not of thick hair (*Figure 5.20*). Examination of the scalp in the presence of long thick hair is much easier when the patient is lying down because the hair stays in place when moved aside, in contrast to the situation if the patient is upright. Anecdotally, it appears quite common for patients to be instructed by examining clinicians to have their hairdresser check the scalp. Although this may conveniently permit the clinician to 'tick' that box, we believe that an instruction to delegate examination to an unqualified person is inappropriate, appearing to be in the interests of the doctor rather than the patient. Examination of skin under dense facial hair (a beard) is also greatly facilitated by a very bright LED light and, when necessary, this examination is included while the patient is in the supine, left lateral and right lateral positions (*Figures 5.10, 5.11* and *5.13*). After the scalp has been examined the dermatoscope

and spray bottle are again taken in hand while a systematic examination of the whole left side of the face, ear, neck and torso, as well as the exposed upper and lower limb surfaces, is performed, gently retracting underwear when appropriate. The most effective way to expose the skin of the medial thigh of the right lower limb is to gently retract the left (uppermost) limb posteriorly (*Figure 5.11*).

Examination with the patient prone
Following examination with the left side up, the patient is requested to roll into the prone position with the pillow placed under the chest and with the face in the breather hole in the couch (*Figure 5.12*).

Scalp under hair and posterior surface of torso and limbs: examination commences with the posterior scalp moving to the back of the neck and torso. Underwear is retracted as necessary to allow visualisation of each buttock in turn, proceeding to the posterior surface of the lower limbs and the plantar surfaces of the feet.

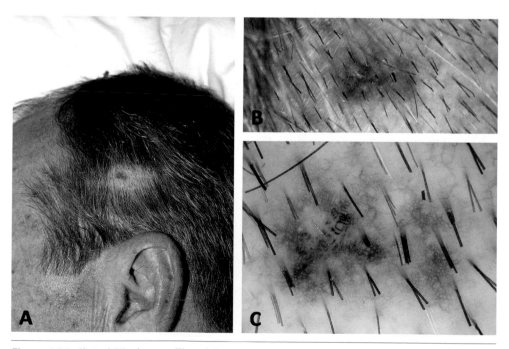

Figure 5.20: *Clinical (A), close-up (B) and dermatoscopic (C) images of a melanoma* in situ *which was concealed by hair. It is important to examine hair-covered scalp methodically.*

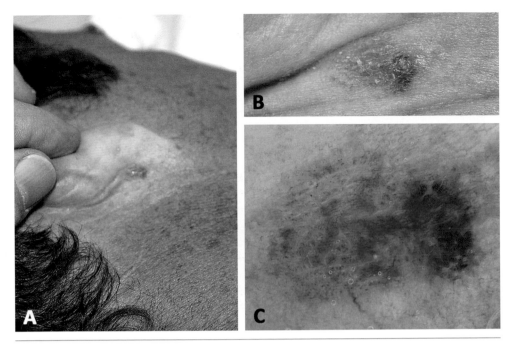

Figure 5.21: *Clinical (A), close-up (B) and dermatoscopic (C) images of a melanoma in the sulcus behind the right ear lobe. Retraction of the right ear was required to discover this lesion; melanoma* in situ *associated with a dermal naevus.*

Right side of body including scalp under hair: following examination in the prone position, the patient is asked to roll onto their left side and the right side of their body is finally examined in the same manner as described for the left (*Figures 5.13* and *5.21*).

One final question

The patient is then invited to sit up and before getting dressed is asked for a final time whether there are any specific lesions of concern that they think have been overlooked.

5.2 Photo-documentation

5.2.1 Workflow for photo-documentation

In our workflow, adhesive arrows are applied at the location of any lesions scheduled for monitoring or intervention (*Figure 5.22*). These are numbered consecutively and photo-documented starting when the patient is supine then before each successive postural shift (*Figure 5.22*). The method employed involves a separate worksheet for each examination with lesions numbered on a diagram of a mannequin (*Figure 5.23*). The patient's name,

written on the worksheet, is photographed prior to each series of images to facilitate organisation of images at the end of the day. Variations of this system exist with degrees of sophistication, reaching a pinnacle in certain video imaging systems. The method currently used by us has evolved and the use of high resolution dermatoscopes and cameras (*Figure 5.24*) has been useful in the context of collecting images for research and education purposes, but it is not necessarily the best method and may change as technology creates innovations in this field.

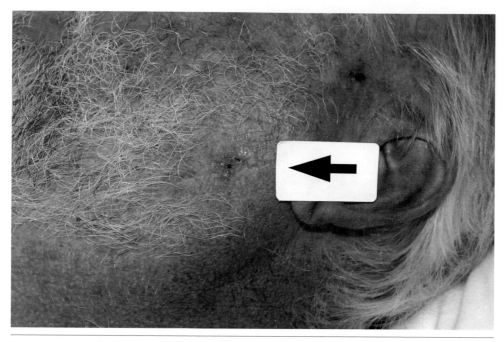

Figure 5.22: *An adhesive arrow has been applied to indicate a lesion of concern that has been encountered during a systematic skin examination. The adhesive sticker will be numbered and the number will correspond to that recorded on a spreadsheet for this examination (Figure 5.23).*

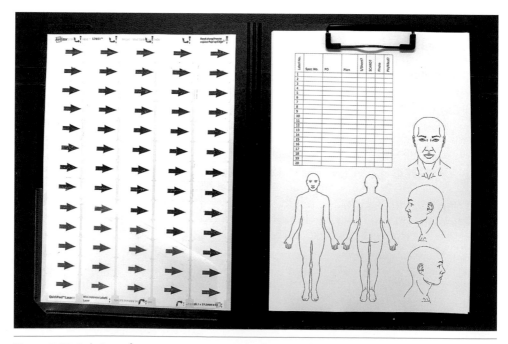

Figure 5.23: *As lesions of concern are encountered, adhesive stickers (left side of image) are applied to the skin. These are numbered and cross-referenced to a spreadsheet (right side of image). The patient's name, written on this spreadsheet, is photographed with each camera in turn prior to taking the various images of each lesion so that images can be filed correctly at the end of each day.*

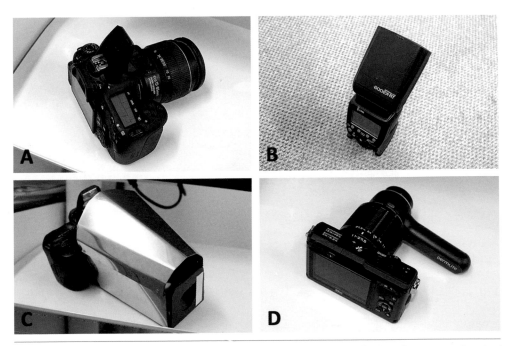

Figure 5.24: *Photographic equipment used by us includes (A) Canon EOS 60D for clinical images synchronised to a remote Canon 600EX-RT flash (B). Close-up images are taken with a Canon EOS 40D camera connected to a Canon macro lens EFS 60mm housed in a custom-made stainless steel flash concentrator apparatus (C) (not commercially available). A Nikon AW1 camera coupled magnetically to a DermLite DL4 dermatoscope (D) facilitates polarised and non-polarised dermatoscopic images.*

Digital dermatoscopic monitoring: a useful tool which is recommended in the Australasian guidelines for high-risk patients[1]. It can be used on flat lesions with a reticular or structureless dermatoscopic pattern when the diagnostic suspicion of melanoma is low, but present. Raised lesions should not be monitored because if a raised lesion is a melanoma it will already be invasive. Clod-pattern lesions should not be monitored because a clod-pattern melanoma has a predicted rapid growth rate[6].

Digital dermatoscopic monitoring can be used to *randomly* monitor lesions on high-risk patients and such monitoring needs a time lapse of approximately 12 months to identify the asymmetrical change of melanoma[7,8,9].

Digital dermatoscopic monitoring can also be used on selected lesions to confirm or exclude malignancy when the index of suspicion is higher, but when there is a desire to avoid unnecessary excision. In such cases short term monitoring (3 months) is advocated[8], but monitoring should continue for at least 12 months.

Total body photography: also recommended in the Australasian guidelines for high-risk patients[1]. The equipment and space required, as well as the need for a trained and expert photographer may be prohibitive for many practices; in such cases referral to an appropriate service provider may be an option. Although the cost may be a prohibitive factor, the option should be discussed with and offered to high-risk patients.

Generally, total body photography is used to establish a baseline of clinical images which can then be available at future consultations as a reference. In addition, it is common for a copy of the images to be provided to the patient, the patient being encouraged to self-examine periodically with the assistance of a partner, and to report any deviation from baseline.

Automated total body photography: this permits the procedure to be performed routinely after a lapse of time with subsequent comparison of images. This promises to facilitate the diagnosis of melanoma at a very early stage when dermatoscopic features of melanoma may not be recognisable (*Figures 5.28* and *5.29*)[9].

 ## 5.3   Patient safety: tracking specimens and self-audit

It is standard of care in surgical specialties to conduct self-audit of outcomes in the interests of validating evidence-based practice and optimising patient safety. Because in many places the management of skin cancer is not a regulated specialty, it has fallen upon practitioners of this craft to develop their own systems of self-audit. One such system is the Skin Cancer Audit Research Database (SCARD) system, developed in 2006 by Cliff Rosendahl and Tobias Wilson and made freely available

to all medical practitioners who manage skin cancer, regardless of their specialty or country of practice[10,11]. The SCARD system currently contains entries of over 1,000,000 specimens from over 1000 doctors. Participating doctors can monitor their own performance and generate reports on demand, evaluating their performance metrics for any time interval and comparing that to the metrics of the entire pool (*Figure 5.25*). Entries are colour-coded: yellow when scheduled, orange when

Specimens			
	New Lesions SCARD feedback	2212	
	Previously Biopsied Lesions	303	
	Total Lesions	2515	

Breakdown	Breakdown of all new lesions by HD	
	BCC (unspecified)	0
	BCC - Superficial	228
	BCC - Nodular/Solid	338
	BCC - Aggressive	121
	IEC/Bowens disease	335
	SCC	178
	Keratoacanthoma	40
	Merkel cell tumour	0
	Other malignant	9
	NMSC Metastasis	0
	Melanoma - in situ	75
	Melanoma - invasive	9
	Melanoma - invasive > 1mm	3
	Melanoma - metastasis	0
	Naevus - other	135
	Naevus - dysplastic/Clark	19
	Naevus - blue	1
	Naevus - Spitz/Reed	5
	Solar keratosis	99
	Solar lentigo	44
	Seborrhoeic keratosis	45
	Lichenoid keratosis (LPLK)	46
	Dermatofibroma	2
	Sebaceous gland hyperplasia	1
	Benign cyst	10
	Other - benign	111
	Histology Pending	272
	Percentage of new lesions tested which were malignant	71.75%
	Percentage of Definitively excised lesions that were malignant	77.14%
	Lesions tested to find one melanoma	3.64
	Percentage of lesions tested for NMSC which were NMSC	77.39%
	Ratio of New BCCs : New Melanomas	8:1

New Lesions SCARD feedback	748523	
Previously Biopsied Lesions	132060	
Total Lesions	880583	

Breakdown of all new lesions by HD	
BCC (unspecified)	34067
BCC - Superficial	67402
BCC - Nodular/Solid	95839
BCC - Aggressive	34058
IEC/Bowens disease	104963
SCC	75503
Keratoacanthoma	13669
Merkel cell tumour	66
Other malignant	957
NMSC Metastasis	34
Melanoma - in situ	13652
Melanoma - invasive	4950
Melanoma - invasive > 1mm	1096
Melanoma - metastasis	222
Naevus - other	40824
Naevus - dysplastic/Clark	30585
Naevus - blue	2470
Naevus - Spitz/Reed	1049
Solar keratosis	70864
Solar lentigo	10374
Seborrhoeic keratosis	40613
Lichenoid keratosis (LPLK)	14761
Dermatofibroma	5452
Sebaceous gland hyperplasia	1576
Benign cyst	11525
Other - benign	52909
Histology Pending	14144
Percentage of new lesions tested which were malignant	61.12%
Percentage of Definitively excised lesions that were malignant	77.40%
Lesions tested to find one melanoma	5.85
Percentage of lesions tested for NMSC which were NMSC	73.80%
Ratio of New BCCs : New Melanomas	12:1

Figure 5.25: SCARD report for one practitioner for 2017 compared to a report for the entire pool.

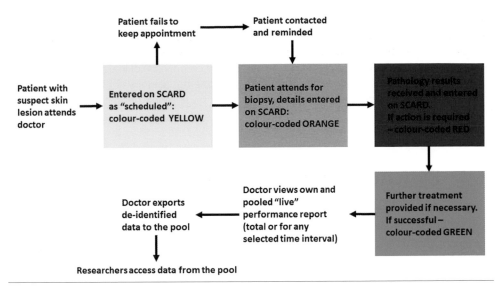

Figure 5.26: Flowchart demonstrating lesion tracking for the purpose of ensuring patient safety on the SCARD system.

awaiting histology, red when requiring action and green when completed, thus facilitating tracking for satisfactory completion of treat-

ment (*Figure 5.26*). To find out more about SCARD, including how to register, go to https://scard.co.

 The lives of lesions

Being a relatively new science, dermatoscopy has only become accessible to clinicians in the last 30 years. It is not surprising that dermatologists and primary care doctors, trained before dermatoscopy had been studied and validated, may still regard it as

an optional tool which at best can confirm a clinical impression or diagnosis. The idea that dermatoscopy can be used to diagnose lesions which are not clinically suspicious at all is a novel concept to many, and that belief can be reinforced by experience, due to the

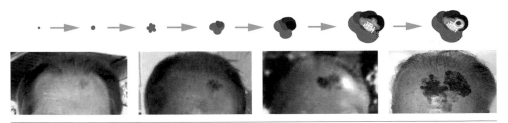

Figure 5.27: (Upper panel) The melanoma timeline: diagrammatic representation of the development of a melanoma from the juvenile stage, when it can only be detected by monitored change, to the childhood stage which can be diagnosed by dermatoscopy, to the mature stage of its life when it can be recognised clinically. (Lower panel) This large invasive melanoma (image far right), represents a lesion on the far right of the melanoma timeline, which can be diagnosed clinically, without dermatoscopy. By examining earlier opportunistic photographs it is possible to verify that this lesion has steadily grown and matured over at least 16 years, comparable to an infant growing and maturing into an adult. Lower images courtesy of Dr Ian McColl.

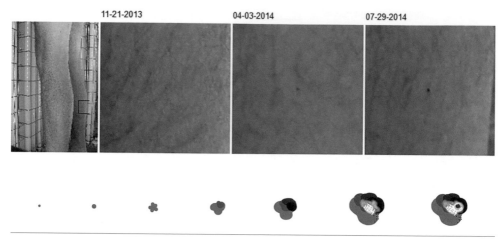

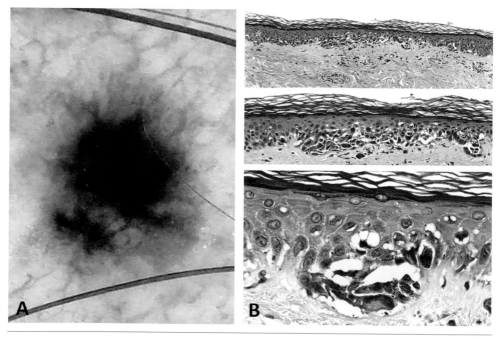

Figure 5.28: A lesion has been detected by automated interval photography, the image at the far right representing the lesion when it was first noted as a lesion of concern. Review of images taken 3 and 8 months earlier reveal that this lesion has appeared and grown over at least 8 months. Dermatoscopy and dermatopathology (see Figure 5.29) reveal that this lesion, still being on the extreme left of the diagrammatic melanoma timeline when it was noted as significant on 29 July 2014, is not a precursor lesion; melanoma in situ[9]. Reproduced from Aust J Dermatol, 2016;57:242 with permission.

Figure 5.29: Dermatoscopy (A) and dermatopathology (B) images of the 1.5mm diameter lesion shown in Figure 5.28 (at 29 July 2014). Dermatoscopically this lesion has minimal clues to malignancy and it would be reasonable to assume that the minute lesion present 8 months earlier would not have been recognisable as a melanoma dermatoscopically. There is no doubt, however, that the lesion excised, a lesion on the far left of the diagrammatic melanoma timeline, is dermatopathologically a melanoma[9]. Reproduced from Aust J Dermatol, 2016;57:242 with permission.

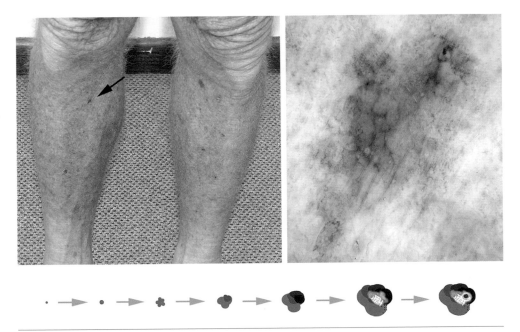

Figure 5.30: *Clinical image (left) of a lesion which was not clinically suspicious (arrow). All that was required for a diagnosis was the application of a dermatoscope revealing dermatoscopic chaos and angulated lines (right). Lesions at the centre of the melanoma timeline may be overlooked clinically but can be diagnosed if a dermatoscope is applied; melanoma in situ.*

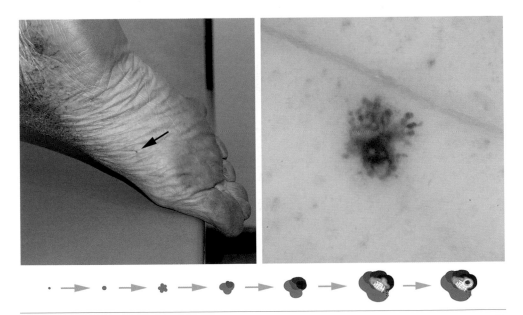

Figure 5.31: *Clinical image of a minute lesion (arrow left image) that was examined dermatoscopically (right image) by an astute dermatoscopist after a senior colleague had passed over it. Although very small it is not at the extreme left of the melanoma timeline because it has dermatoscopic chaos and the clue of lines radial (pseudopod type); melanoma invasive (Breslow thickness 0.6mm).*

assumption that what is not seen does not exist. In other words, a clinician examines a patient clinically, discovers worrying lesions, confirms those regarded as suspicious with dermatoscopy and proceeds with an inner glow of achievement, oblivious to lesions which were missed. It is only when the clinician accepts that every malignancy starts at a microscopic size, smaller than can be seen by the naked eye, that they appreciate that there is a size threshold below which he or she has failed to diagnose every malignancy (*Figures 5.27–5.31*). If the smallest melanoma one has diagnosed is 3mm in diameter then every melanoma smaller than that has been overlooked. In fact, very young (and therefore very small) melanomas will often lack diagnostic dermatoscopic clues and can only be suspected by the observation of change on monitoring, this being based on the assumption that malignant tissue changes continually.

Every systematic skin examination is a new journey of discovery. Like any voyage into the unknown it requires planning, functional equipment, meticulous execution and heightened awareness. Enjoy the experience!

References

1. Clinical Practice Guidelines for the Management of Melanoma in Australia and New Zealand. Cancer Council Australia and Australian Cancer Network, Sydney and New Zealand Guidelines Group, Wellington, 2008;17,18,30.

2. https://dermoscopedia.org [accessed 26 August 2022].

3. Bourne P, Rosendahl C, Keir J, and Cameron A. BLINCK—A diagnostic algorithm for skin cancer diagnosis combining clinical features with dermatoscopy findings. *Dermatol Pract Concept*, 2012;2(2):12.

4. Rosendahl C, Cameron A, Bulinska A, Harding-Smith D, and Weedon D. Embryology of a melanoma? A case report with speculation based on dermatoscopic and histologic evidence. *Dermatol Pract Concept*, 2012;2(4):8.

5. Kittler H, Rosendahl C, Cameron A, and Tschandl P. *Dermatoscopy*, 2nd Edition, 2016. Facultas.

6. Beer J, Xu L, Tschandl P, and Kittler H. Growth rate of melanoma *in vivo* and correlation with dermatoscopic and dermatopathologic findings. *Dermatol Pract Concept*, 2011;1(1):59.

7. Kittler H, Guitera P, Riedl E, *et al.* Identification of clinically featureless incipient melanoma using sequential dermoscopy imaging. *Arch Dermatol*, 2006;142:1113.

8. Altamura D, Avramidis M, and Menzies SW. Assessment of the optimal interval for and sensitivity of short-term sequential digital dermoscopy monitoring for the diagnosis of melanoma. *Arch Dermatol*, 2008;144:502.

9. Rosendahl CO, Drugge ED, Volpicelli ER, and Drugge RJ. Diagnosis of a minute melanoma assisted by automated multi-camera-array total body photography. *Aust J Dermatol*, 2016;57:242.

10. Rosendahl C, Hansen C, Cameron A, *et al.* Measuring performance in skin cancer practice: the SCARD initiative. *Int J Dermatol*, 2011;50:44.

11. Rosendahl C, Williams G, Eley D, *et al.* The impact of sub-specialization and dermatoscopy use on accuracy of melanoma diagnosis among primary care doctors in Australia. *J Am Acad Dermatol*, 2012;67:846.

CHAPTER 6

'Chaos and Clues' (Chaos, Clues and Exceptions): a decision algorithm for pigmented skin lesions

'Chaos and Clues'

Algorithmic methods are not intended for all skin lesions but rather for 'lesions of concern', which are lesions which cannot be given a confident benign diagnosis by dermatoscopic pattern recognition. With experience many benign lesions including naevi, benign keratinocytic lesions, dermatofibroma, haemangioma and sebaceous gland hyperplasia, will be diagnosed by pattern recognition. If that is not possible, or if there is some other cause for concern such as change at mature age, then the lesion must be managed as a 'lesion of concern'. Such a lesion, if pigmented, should be evaluated not only for 'chaos and clues', but also for 'exceptions'. To highlight that we suggest that the dermatoscopist consider 'Exceptions' as an integral part of 'Chaos and Clues': Chaos, Clues and Exceptions.

Revised pattern analysis (RPA) is designed to lead to a *provisional diagnosis* in a logical stepwise process. 'Chaos and Clues' is an algorithmic method which uses pattern analysis to guide the clinician in a stepwise process to the *decision* about whether (excision) biopsy is indicated.

The flowchart for the 'Chaos and Clues' algorithm is shown in *Figure 6.1*.

6.2 Chaos

Chaos is defined as the presence of dermatoscopic asymmetry of any, or all of, pattern, colour and border abruptness[1,2]. *This differs from asymmetry as assessed by the method described for RPA in that chaos of border abruptness is not included in that method*[3].

Any irregularity of the shape of a lesion is not relevant.

- Chaos of pattern requires that there be more than one pattern (a pattern covering a significant area of the lesion, arbitrarily defined as at least 20%), with the patterns being combined asymmetrically. If either of the highly specific defined clues: peripheral black clods, lines radial segmental, are present asymmetrically in a lesion, that

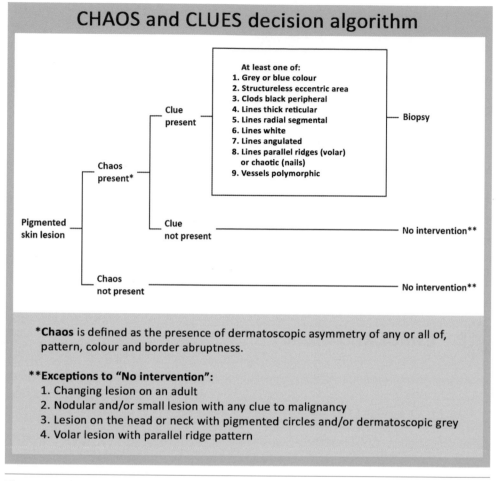

Figure 6.1: *Flowchart for the 'Chaos and Clues' algorithm. Pigmented lesions are first assessed for the presence of chaos (chaos being defined as the presence of dermatoscopic asymmetry of any, or all of, pattern, colour and border abruptness) and, if chaos is present, they are examined for any one or more of nine clues to malignancy. If a clue is present, an excision biopsy is considered. There are four exceptions for which excision biopsy is considered even for non-chaotic lesions.*

confers chaos even if the structure does not cover sufficient area to produce a pattern[1].

- Chaos of colour requires that there be more than one colour (light and dark brown being regarded as different colours if the transition between them is abrupt), with those colours being combined asymmetrically. There is no lower limit to the area required to be covered by a

colour to create asymmetry if that variation is obvious and abruptly demarcated[1].

- Chaos of border abruptness* is defined as significant and asymmetric variability in the abruptness of demarcation of the border of a lesion[1]. While border abruptness is also assessed in the ABCD method of dermatoscopy[4], this is given most significance in that method when the total border is abrupt. The ABCD method would there-

---

*Chaos of border abruptness was first recognised and described to us by Francis Drugge, the 12-year-old son of dermatologist Rhett Drugge (Stamford, Connecticut, USA).

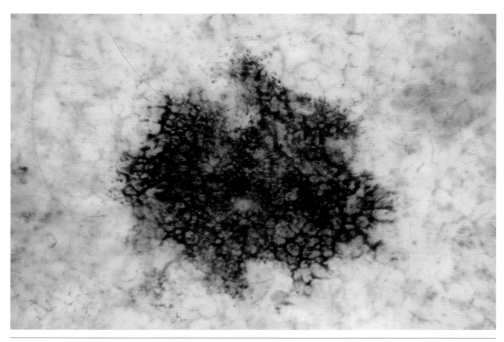

Figure 6.2: *Dermatoscopic image of an ink spot lentigo which exhibits an abrupt border over the total periphery which would give it a high score in the ABCD method of dermatoscopy. However, the lack of chaos of border abruptness is in fact a feature of benignancy in this lesion which also has a single pattern (lines branched) and a single colour (brown).*

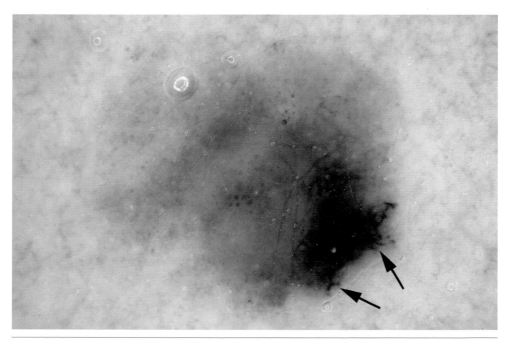

Figure 6.3: *Dermatoscopic image of a lesion which displays asymmetry of both pattern and colour. With an abrupt border at the lower right extremity of the image (arrows) and a gradual border elsewhere, it also has marked chaos of border abruptness; melanoma invasive.*

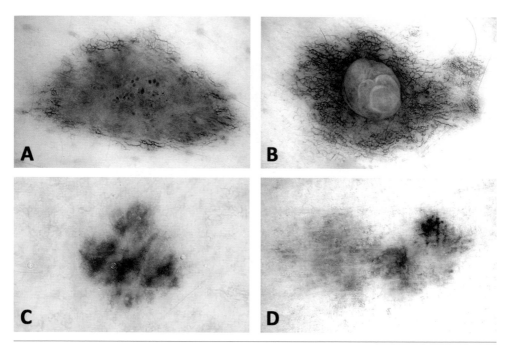

Figure 6.4: *Composite of dermatoscopic images of four lesions from the same patient showing only one (D) with chaos as defined. Only one of the three types of chaos is necessary to fulfil the definition but this lesion has chaos of pattern, colour and border abruptness; melanoma in situ. The other three lesions have been confirmed as benign (naevi) by stability over time.*

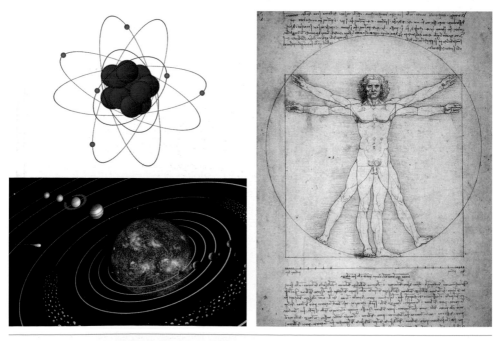

Figure 6.5: *The natural laws of physics and biology, including those defining electromagnetic and gravitational forces as well as those of biological feedback mechanisms, favour symmetry.*

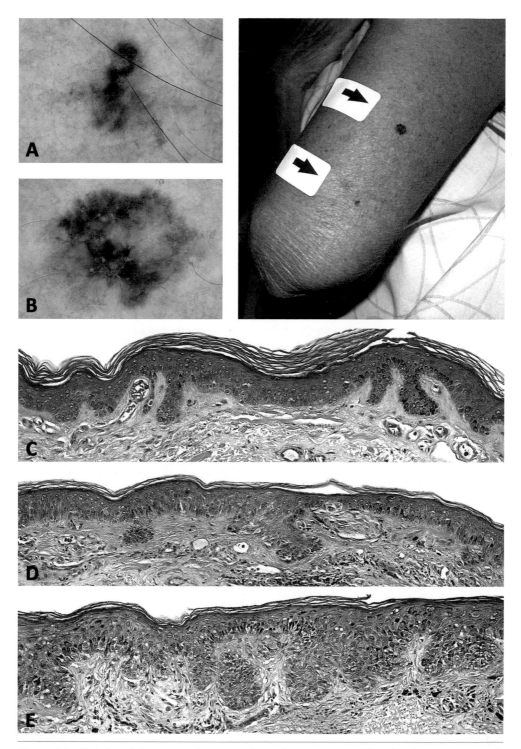

Figure 6.6: *Clinical and dermatoscopic images of a melanoma in situ (A) and melanoma invasive (B) are correlated with dermatopathological images. Histology of perilesional skin (C) has a relatively orderly architecture, with histological disorganisation increasing along with dermatoscopic chaos, moving from melanoma in situ (A, D) to invasive melanoma (B, E).*

fore allocate the highest score for border abruptness to an ink spot lentigo (*Figure 6.2*) or solar lentigo, and a lower score would be allocated for a lesion which has abruptness of only a portion of the border (*Figure 6.3*). In fact, abruptness of the total border is a feature of benignancy while chaos of border abruptness is more likely in a malignant lesion (see *Figures 6.2–6.4*).

By definition, if there is one pattern, one colour and no obvious variation of border abruptness there can be no chaos. While natural laws (gravity, electrical and magnetic fields, surface tension and feedback mechanisms) favour symmetry (*Figure 6.5*), malignant tissue defies natural laws and this is the basis for both dermatopathological and dermatoscopic chaos in malignant tissue (see *Figure 6.6*)[1].

6.3 Clues

6.3.1 Grey or blue colour

The clue of grey or blue colour, in a chaotic lesion, applies to both melanocytic and non-melanocytic malignancies.

Grey colour
Grey colour correlates with melanin in the superficial dermis and this can be in melanocytes, keratinocytes or as melanin incontinence in melanophages, which is frequently

the result of an immune attack even on lesions that remain confined to the epidermis. Grey colour is the most sensitive clue to malignancy and is seen in most *in situ* melanomas (*Figures 6.7* and *6.8*) in many pBCCs (*Figure 6.9*) and in some pSCCs (*Figure 6.10*)[5].

Grey colour due to melanin incontinence is also seen in benign lesions, including naevi and keratinocytic lesions which have undergone an immune attack with a degree of subsequent regression. Naevi are usually

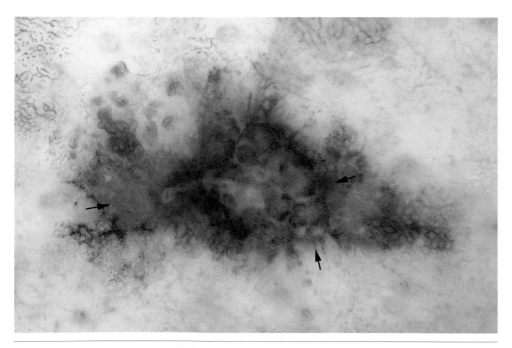

Figure 6.7: *Dermatoscopic image displaying grey colour in this* in situ *melanoma (arrows) contrasting with the background colour of brown – a colour invariably present in a pigmented (melanotic) melanocytic lesion.*

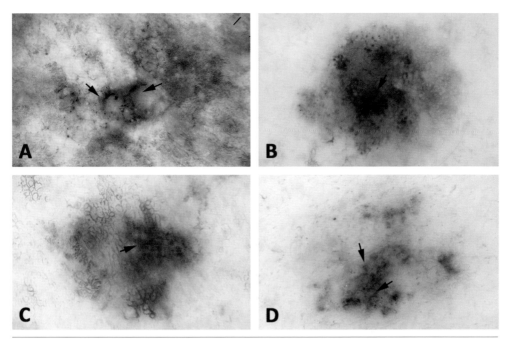

Figure 6.8: *Dermatoscopic images of four melanomas all exhibiting chaos and the clue of grey colour (arrows). (A) Melanoma invasive on the dorsum of the hand; (B) melanoma in situ on the arm; (C) melanoma in situ on the leg; (D) melanoma invasive on the leg.*

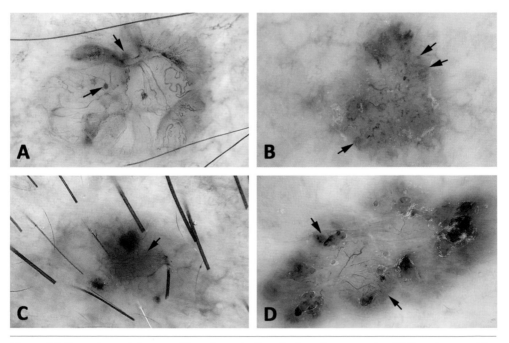

Figure 6.9: *Dermatoscopic images of four pigmented basal cell carcinomas each exhibiting chaos and the clue of grey colour, located on the: (A) back; (B) chest; (C) face; (D) back. A representative area of grey colour is indicated by arrows in each lesion.*

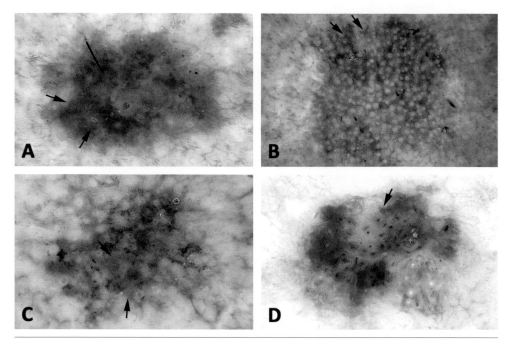

Figure 6.10: Dermatoscopic images of four pigmented squamous cell carcinomas in situ, each exhibiting chaos and the clue of grey colour, on the: (A) shoulder; (B) face (note white circles as a clue to invasion of adnexal openings); (C) face; (D) back (note pigment dots in linear arrangement as a highly specific clue for this diagnosis). A representative area of grey colour is indicated by arrows in each lesion.

recognisable by symmetry on pattern analysis, but LPLK may have chaotic grey colour leading to a need for excision biopsy and histological clarification. Grey colour is therefore a very sensitive clue to malignancy, but it has a relatively low specificity.

Blue colour

Blue colour correlates with pigment in the deep dermis, most commonly in nested melanocytes (*Figure 6.11*) or aggregates of BCC cells (*Figure 6.12*). Melanin can only be transported deep enough to cause dermatoscopic blue if it is within lesional cells that have moved to that location. Blue colour does occur in the benign lesions of blue naevus and combined naevus, but in a chaotic lesion it is a clue to the presence of melanin, associated with either melanocytes (in invasive pigmented melanoma) or keratinocytes (in pBCC or invasive pSCC), in the reticular dermis[1].

6.3.2 Structureless eccentric area

An eccentric structureless area must[1,6]:
- be eccentrically located
- have none of the basic structures (lines, circles and clods) predominating
- be a colour other than skin-coloured
- cover a sufficient portion of the lesion for it to form a pattern (at least 20%)
- be contrasted to a structured pattern or to a pattern of a distinctly different colour which is also within the lesion.

Eccentric structureless areas can have a variety of colours[1]:
- The chaotic behaviour of malignant melanocytes can produce black, brown, grey or blue.
- Increased blood flow from the high metabolic demand of tumour tissue can produce pink or red.
- Fibrosis after regression can produce white.

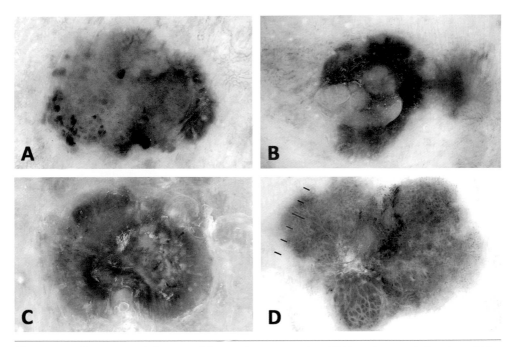

Figure 6.11: *Dermatoscopic images of four melanomas each exhibiting chaos and the clue of blue colour: (A) nodular melanoma on the leg; (B) melanoma invasive arising in a dermal naevus in the groin; (C) melanoma invasive on the forearm; (D) melanoma invasive on the abdomen.*

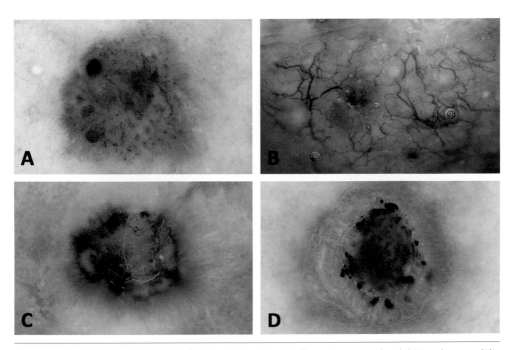

Figure 6.12: *Dermatoscopic images of four pigmented basal cell carcinomas each exhibiting chaos and the clue of blue colour located on the: (A) back; (B) ear; (C) wrist; (D) back.*

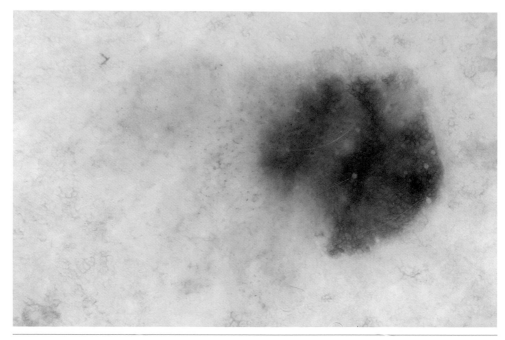

Figure 6.13: *An eccentric structureless (light brown) area extends to the left of a structured (lines reticular) area in this dermatoscopic image of an* in situ *melanoma.*

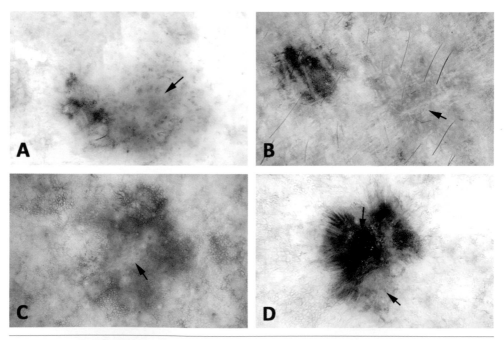

Figure 6.14: *Dermatoscopic images of four pigmented lesions each exhibiting chaos and the clue of an eccentric structureless area (arrows). (A) Pigmented basal cell carcinoma on the leg with a pattern of angulated lines lower left and an eccentric structureless pink area upper right; (B) a melanoma* in situ *on the back with an eccentric structureless pink area; (C) a melanoma invasive on the back with an eccentric structureless pink area; (D) a pigmented squamous cell carcinoma* in situ *on the back with a pattern of radial lines upper left, a structureless brown area centrally and an eccentric structureless area inferiorly (arrows).*

This clue applies to both melanocytic and non-melanocytic malignancies (*Figures 6.13* and *6.14*). If the eccentric structureless area includes the colour brown, it can be predicted that the melanin is present within an epidermis lacking a rete ridge pattern, otherwise a reticular network would be expected.

A skin-coloured structureless area, being the pattern of normal skin, has no diagnostic significance at all. Similarly, any interruption to a pigmented pattern caused by the presence of adnexal openings (hair follicles) has no diagnostic significance and should be regarded as an incidental interruption to whatever pattern might be present, rather than forming a pattern itself.

6.3.3 Clods black peripheral

These structures correlate with pigmented pagetoid melanocytes and nests of melanocytes carrying pigment to the outer layers of the epidermis in melanomas; this clue should therefore be specific to melanoma. Actually,

because minute clods (dots) are common in both pBCC and pSCC *in situ*, and because grey may be perceived as black, this clue can also be seen in those lesions. The reason for the designation that they be peripherally located is because black dots can be seen centrally in naevi which have been traumatised, correlating with pigment in ascending keratinocytes. Pagetoid spread can occur anywhere in a melanoma, so when black dots or clods are seen peripherally they are regarded as a clue to malignancy (*Figure 6.15*)[1,6].

6.3.4 Lines thick reticular

These are defined when the lines are at least as thick as the holes that they surround, and in melanocytic lesions they may correlate with rete ridges which are widened by pigment-laden malignant melanocytes[1,6]. They are a clue to malignancy in a chaotic lesion and will be focal rather than evenly widespread over the lesion (*Figure 6.16*). This clue is specific to melanoma because the presence of reticular

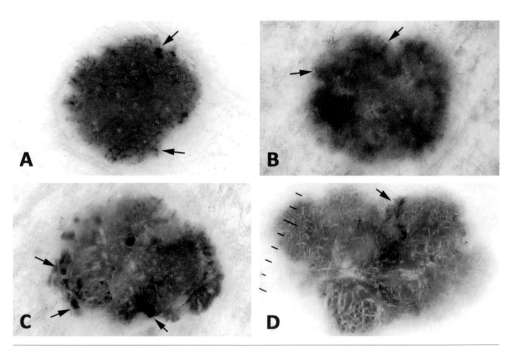

Figure 6.15: Dermatoscopic images of four pigmented lesions each exhibiting chaos and the clue of peripheral black clods (arrows). (A) Melanoma in situ *on the dorsal foot; (B) melanoma* in situ *on the back; (C) nodular melanoma on the calf; (D) melanoma invasive on the abdomen.*

lines effectively rules out the diagnosis of BCC or SCC. Thick reticular lines frequently occur in seborrhoeic keratoses due to acanthotic rete ridges (due to a proliferation of pigmented keratinocytes), but they will be widespread in that context and other clues to seborrhoeic keratosis are expected to be present.

The term 'thick lines reticular' differs from 'atypical network' because, unlike the latter, it can be precisely defined.

6.3.5 Lines radial segmental

Lines radial segmental are clues to malignancy, being found in all three pigmented malignancies[1,6]. In melanocytic lesions these structures correlate with fascicles of pigmented melanocytes extending from the periphery of a lesion and they signify growth. In melanomas they are expected to be distributed asymmetrically, and to extend from reticular lines, clods or structureless areas of equivalently dense pigmentation to the radial lines (see *Figures 6.17–6.19*)[1].

This can sometimes distinguish them from the radial lines seen in BCCs, which invariably converge and may (but not always) project from hypopigmented structureless areas (*Figures 6.20–6.21*).

Lines radial segmental are also seen in pSCC *in situ* in which they are usually created by dots in a linear arrangement (*Figure 6.22*)[7]. As with all clues to malignancy, lines radial segmental may also be found in benign lesions, most commonly as an unexpected finding in solar lentigo.

6.3.6 Lines white

To be defined as white, lines must be whiter than normal surrounding skin and they may be polarising-specific (polarising-specific blue lines have the same significance[1]) or, alternatively, white lines that are seen with both modalities[1,6].

Polarising-specific white lines are:
- bright white lines seen only with polarised dermatoscopy
- orientated perpendicularly to each other and not crossing

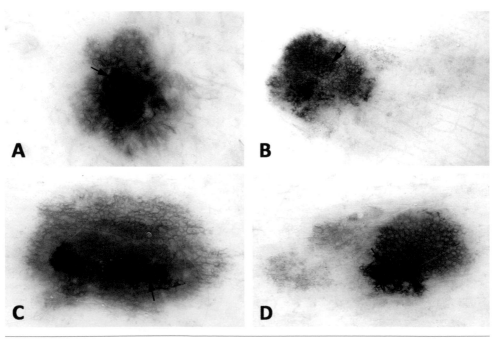

Figure 6.16: *Dermatoscopic images of four pigmented lesions (all are melanoma in situ) each exhibiting chaos and the clue of thick reticular lines (arrows). They are located on the: (A) abdomen, (B) knee and (C, D) back.*

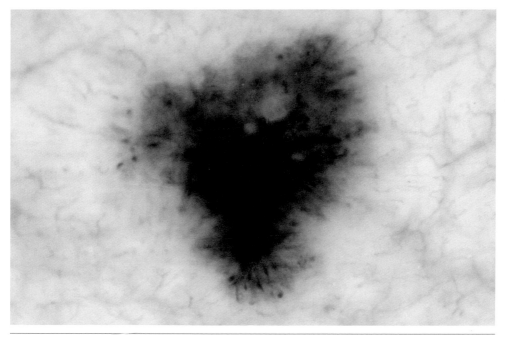

Figure 6.17: *Dermatoscopic lines radial segmental, in a melanoma in situ, extend from pigmented structures as dark as or darker than the radial lines.*

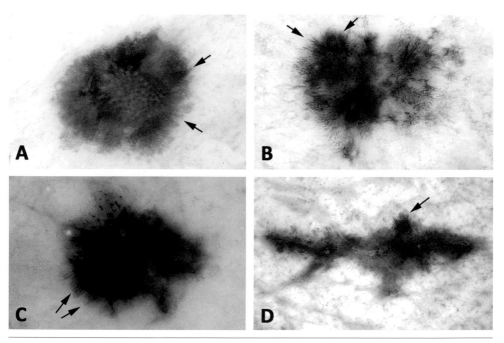

Figure 6.18: *Dermatoscopic images of four pigmented lesions each exhibiting chaos and the clue of lines radial segmental (arrows). (A) Melanoma in situ on the forearm; (B) melanoma in situ on the shoulder; (C) melanoma in situ on the back; (D) melanoma invasive on the posterior neck.*

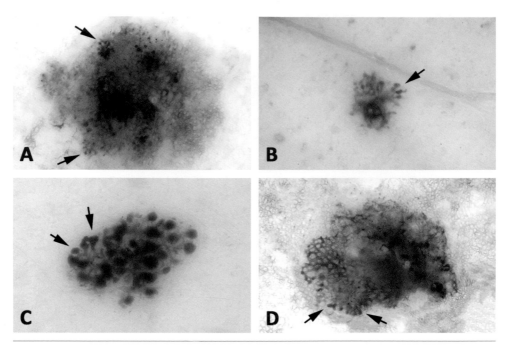

Figure 6.19: *Dermatoscopic images of four melanomas, each with chaos and segmental lines radial (pseudopod type) (arrows).*

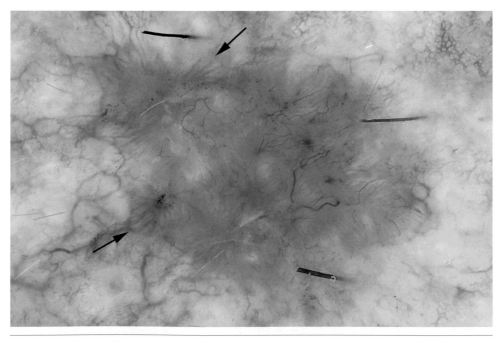

Figure 6.20: *In this dermatoscopic image of a pigmented basal cell carcinoma, the radial lines are morphologically very specific to basal cell carcinoma in that they converge and also extend from a non-pigmented part of the lesion (arrows).*

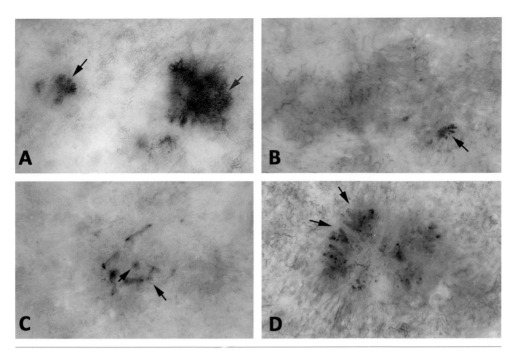

Figure 6.21: *Dermatoscopic images of four pigmented basal cell carcinomas each exhibiting chaos and the clue of lines radial segmental (black arrows) on the: (A) back with lines radial segmental on the pigmented portion on the left but lines reticular on the right (red arrow) – an extremely rare finding in basal cell carcinoma; (B) shoulder; (C) back; (D) neck. Note that in (B–D) the radial lines converge and also extend from hypopigmented areas.*

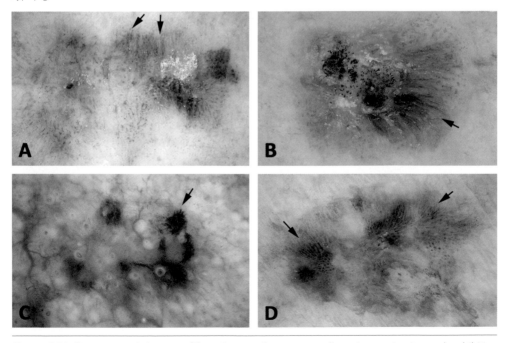

Figure 6.22: *Dermatoscopic images of four pigmented squamous cell carcinomas in situ, each exhibiting chaos and the clue of lines radial segmental (arrows) on the: (A) leg; (B) back; (C) face; (D) back. In (A, B and D) the radial lines are seen to be formed by dots in linear arrangement.*

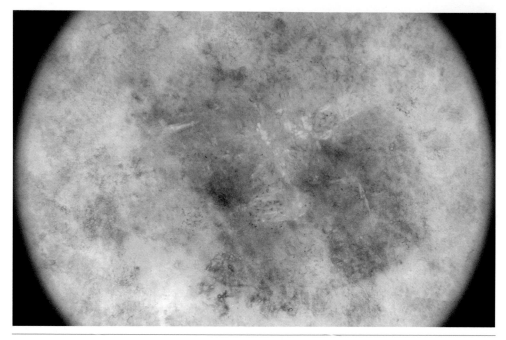

Figure 6.23: *Polarised dermatoscopy of this melanoma* in situ *displays white lines which are seen to be in a perpendicularly orientated arrangement.*

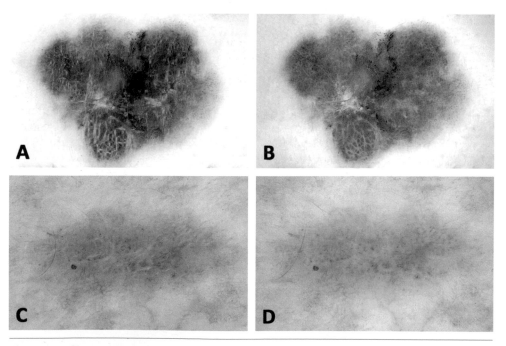

Figure 6.24: *Dermatoscopic images of two melanomas taken with polarised (A, C) and non-polarised (B, D) dermatoscopy. The invasive melanoma (upper images) exhibits polarising-specific white and blue lines (A), some of which also correlate with non-polarising-specific white/blue lines (B). The* in situ *melanoma (lower images) shows polarising-specific white lines (C) as the only clue to malignancy. Although there may be some skin-coloured lines in the non-polarised image (D), there are no white lines.*

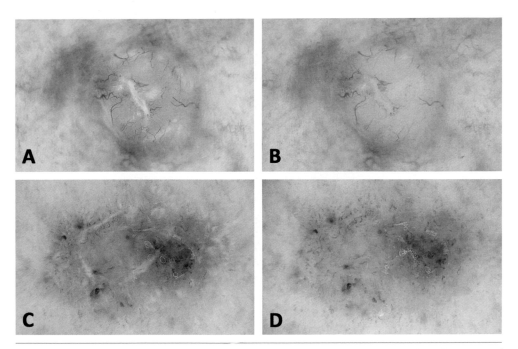

Figure 6.25: Dermatoscopic images of two basal cell carcinomas taken with polarised (A, C) and non-polarised (B, D) dermatoscopy. Polarising-specific white lines, orientated at right angles to each other but not crossing (A, C) are seen to disappear in non-polarising mode (B, D).

- commonly seen in BCC, melanoma, DF and Spitz naevus.

Although polarising-specific white lines are only seen with polarising dermatoscopy (see *Figures 6.23* and *6.24A,C*), they may sometimes correlate with reticular white lines seen with non-polarised dermatoscopy (*Figure 6.24B*). Polarising-specific white lines are commonly seen in BCC (pigmented or non-pigmented) (*Figure 6.25*) and they are not unusual in melanoma (pigmented or non-pigmented) (*Figures 6.23* and *6.24*). They are only rarely seen in pSCC *in situ*. They are also commonly seen in both DF and Spitz naevus, but their presence is not expected in any other type of naevus (unless traumatised) nor in seborrhoeic keratosis[3].

6.3.7 Lines angulated

Angulated lines are straight lines, not reticular or branched, meeting at angles of 90° or more, but not crossing. This definition includes pigment interfaces between darkly and lightly pigmented areas. Angulated lines may join to enclose a polygon[8]. This clue, in a chaotic lesion, is a valuable clue to melanoma (*Figures 6.26* and *6.27A,B,D*), but may also rarely be seen in pBCC (*Figure 6.27C*)[1].

6.3.8 Lines parallel on the ridges (volar) or lines parallel chaotic on the nails

These melanoma-specific clues are the only ones that are site-dependent, applying on volar skin (palms and soles; see *Figure 6.44*), or on the nail apparatus due to lesions in the nail matrix (*Figure 6.28*)[9]. It is important to remember that the longer a volar or nail matrix melanoma remains untreated the more likely it is to develop any of the other clues to malignancy. Melanoma may also arise in a volar (acral) naevus in which case any of the other eight clues will override a benign parallel furrow pattern which may be present (see *Figure 6.29*).

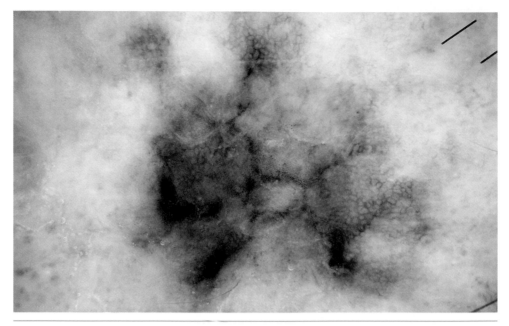

Figure 6.26: *Angulated lines form both complete and incomplete polygons in this dermatoscopic image of a melanoma* in situ.

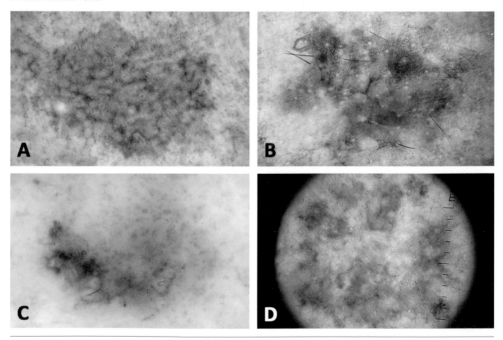

Figure 6.27: *Dermatoscopic images of four lesions with the clue to malignancy of angulated lines. (A) Melanoma* in situ *on the face which is non-chaotic, but it does not have the clear morphology of any benign lesion and it has the exception of pigmented circles (see* Section 6.4); (B) melanoma in situ *on the forearm; (C) pigmented basal cell carcinoma on the thigh; (D) melanoma* in situ *on the back.*

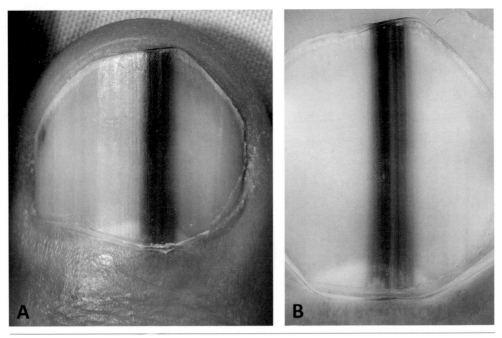

Figure 6.28: *Clinical (A) and dermatoscopic (B) images of pigmentation of the nail plate due to a nail matrix melanoma exhibiting lines parallel chaotic (varying in width, interval and colour)[9].*

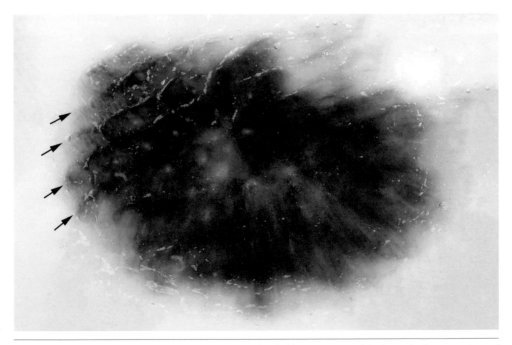

Figure 6.29: *In this dermatoscopic image, the clue of radial lines segmental (right and inferior portions of the image) overrides the clue of lines parallel in a furrow pattern (arrows). This is a melanoma arising in a volar (acral) naevus. Note that in the benign furrow pattern there is pigment over the ridges but the lines (as assessed at the edges) lie in the furrows. Image courtesy Dr Agata Bulinska.*

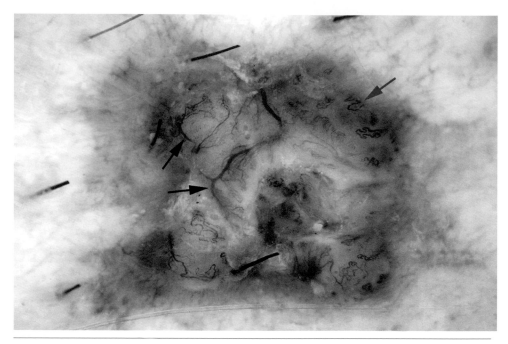

Figure 6.30: *This basal cell carcinoma displays dermatoscopic linear polymorphous vessels, branched serpentine (black arrows) and looped (one example – blue arrow).*

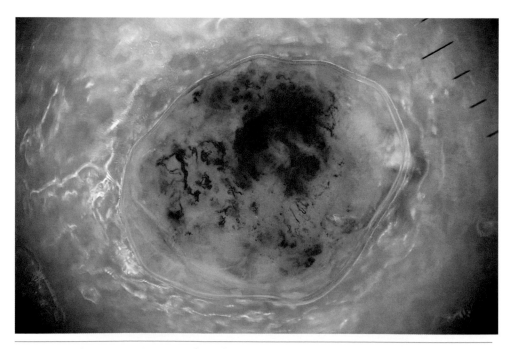

Figure 6.31: *Dermatoscopic image of an ulcerated (non-pigmented) BCC with polymorphous vessels, including some dots.*

6.3.9 Vessels polymorphic

A pattern of polymorphous vessels is a clue to both melanoma and pBCC, but not to pSCC *in situ* which is expected to have a monomorphous pattern of coiled vessels. A pBCC often has a monomorphous pattern of serpentine or serpentine-branched vessels, but it may have a pattern of polymorphous linear vessels (see *Figure 6.30*).

A pattern of dot vessels is not expected in pBCC but ulceration, commonly present in BCC, and associated keratinisation may produce polymorphous vessels including looped vessels in radial arrangement surrounding ulceration and even dot vessels (*Figure 6.31*)[1].

In melanomas, polymorphous vessels may include various types of linear vessels in raised portions, and a pattern of dot vessels, as well as any pattern of linear vessels in macular portions. Generally, other clues apart from polymorphous vessels (pigment clues and/or white lines) are expected in a melanoma and the vessel clues are then useful in differentiating melanoma from pBCC and pSCC *in situ* (see *Figures 6.32* and *6.33*).

It must be remembered that benign lesions such as seborrhoeic keratoses and dermal naevi may have polymorphous vessels, but such lesions, having the unequivocal pattern-recognition morphology of their benign diagnosis, should not be lesions of concern (see *Section 5.1.5*).

SCC *in situ* (pigmented or non-pigmented) is expected to have a monomorphous pattern of coiled vessels which may resolve as dots depending on visual acuity and magnification (*Figure 6.34*)[7].

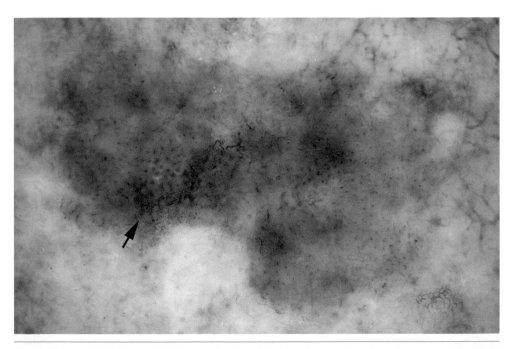

Figure 6.32: *In this dermatoscopic image chaos and the clue of grey colour (arrow) point to malignancy. A pattern of serpentine vessels centrally, combined with a vast pattern of dot vessels is consistent only with melanoma; melanoma invasive*[1].

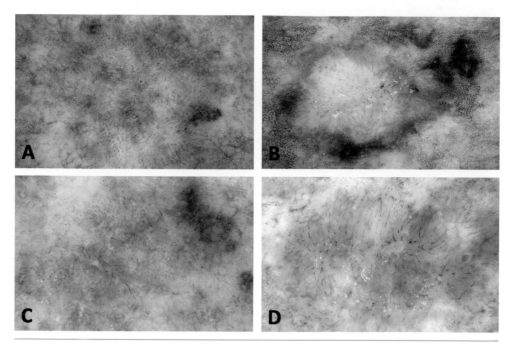

Figure 6.33: *Dermatoscopic images of four lesions with various degrees of pigmentation, each exhibiting chaos and the clue of polymorphous vessels including a pattern of dot vessels. All are invasive melanomas, as is often the case by the time lightly pigmented melanomas are diagnosed, and all are located on the back.*

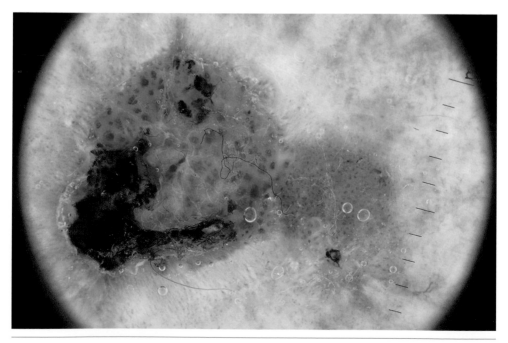

Figure 6.34: *A (non-pigmented) SCC* in situ *displays a dermatoscopic pattern of coiled vessels on the left side of this image while on the right side the vessels resolve as dots. There is also adherent fibre as a dermatoscopic clue to evident ulceration.*

6.4 Exceptions

'Chaos and Clues' was tested on a consecutive series of pigmented lesions (all of which had been excised on suspicion of malignancy), the majority of melanomas in the series being *in situ*. The algorithm was found to have a diagnostic sensitivity of 90.6% (BCC 98.5%, SCC 86.5%, melanoma 79.3%), with a specificity of 62.7% for the diagnosis of malignancy, any type[5]. In an attempt to move the sensitivity closer to 100%, the following sections describe which exceptions are included, to *consider* lesions for biopsy, even if not chaotic[1].

6.4.1 Any changing lesion on an adult

This includes any lesion with a history of change, lesions with monitored change (*Figure 6.35*) and lesions with dermatoscopic clues to change, such as the presence of peripheral clods (see *Figures 6.36–6.38*) or peripheral radial lines[1]. The presence of peripheral clods must be considered in the context of the age

of the patient. Peripheral clods in an otherwise unremarkable lesion, with the morphology of a naevus, is consistent with the diagnosis of a growing naevus on a patient under the age of 30, but not over the age of 50 (*Figure 6.39*). In between these ages the clues must be weighed and discretion exercised; if doubt remains then excision biopsy is prudent (*Figure 6.37*)[1]. In such a situation, examination of other lesions on the patient for context can be useful.

6.4.2 A nodular or small lesion which has any of the clues to malignancy

We define small, arbitrarily, as less than 6mm in diameter[1], this being the size cited in the clinical ABCD method for the diagnosis of melanoma[10]. The 3mm diameter nodular melanoma shown in *Figure 6.38* on the flank of a 60-year-old woman was arguably symmetrical, but it did not have the morphology of any

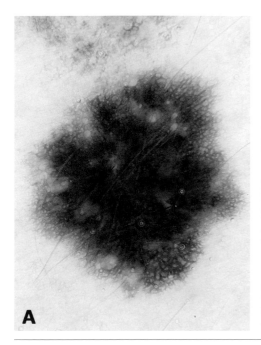 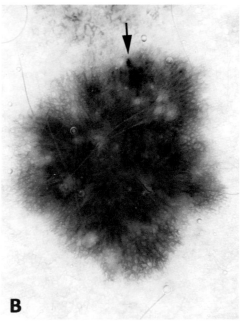

A   **B**

Figure 6.35: A pigmented skin lesion (A) has been dermatoscopically monitored over 6 months (B). The structural change of the appearance of a small cluster of peripheral black dots (arrow) led to excisional biopsy; melanoma in situ *arising in a naevus.*

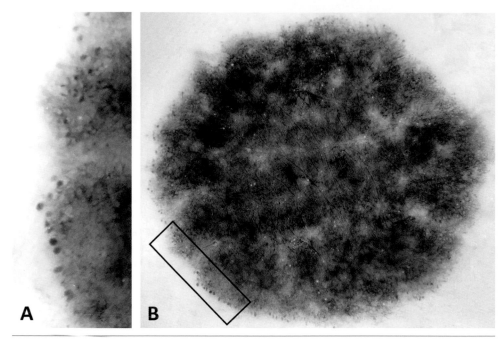

Figure 6.36: *A large lesion on the abdomen of a 70-year-old man is symmetrical, but the dermatoscopic clue to growth of peripheral clods is not expected at mature age. The left border of the image (boxed in (B)) is enlarged in (A) showing the peripheral clods clearly: melanoma invasive.*

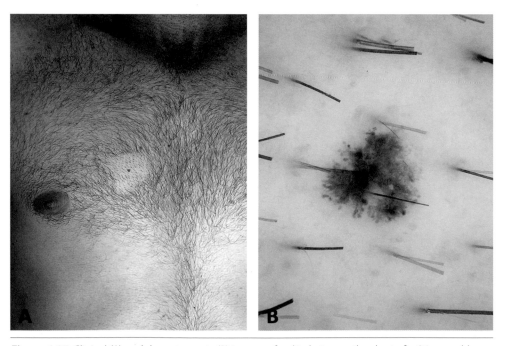

Figure 6.37: *Clinical (A) and dermatoscopic (B) images of a skin lesion on the chest of a 34-year-old man displaying only borderline asymmetry, but peripheral clods indicated that the lesion was growing. Under the age of 30 growth is expected, but at the age of 34 the lesion was assessed in context with other naevi on the patient. No others were found to have clues to growth. Excision biopsy revealed it to be a melanoma in situ.*

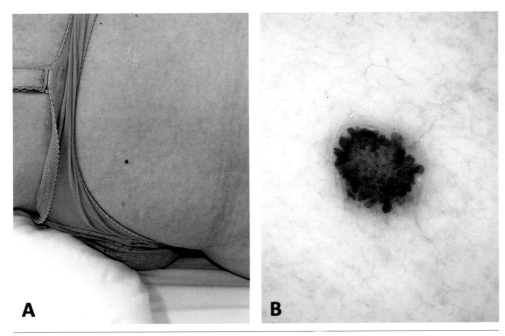

Figure 6.38: *This pigmented skin lesion on the flank of a 60-year-old woman (A) was only 3mm in diameter and it was raised. Although it had dermatoscopic structural symmetry (B) it could not be recognised as a known benign lesion and there were two relevant exceptions: first, there was the dermatoscopic clue to change of peripheral clods and, secondly, it was both small and nodular with the clue of grey structures; nodular melanoma (Breslow thickness 0.9mm)[11].*

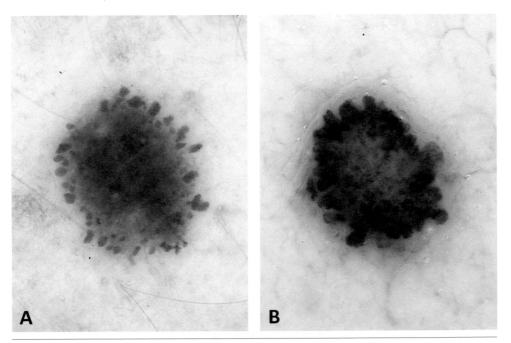

Figure 6.39: *Two lesions both with the dermatoscopic clue to change of peripheral clods. The lesion on the left was a growing naevus on the back of an adolescent (not excised). The lesion on the right was on the back of a 60-year-old woman (from Figure 6.38) and it was excised: nodular melanoma 3mm in diameter with a Breslow thickness of 0.9mm[11]. Note that the melanoma, although arguably symmetrical, has a disorganised structure compared to the naevus, consistent with the chaotic behaviour of malignant tissue.*

of the five common benign lesions (see *Section 5.1.5*) and, in addition to peripheral clods as a dermatoscopic clue to change, it had the clue of grey colour (*Figures 6.38* and *6.39B*)[11].

*This particular exception should only be applied with respect to **small** lesions if there is an additional significant cause for concern.* Many naevi have grey colour or even patterns that could be interpreted as angulated lines, but if they are non-chaotic and a uniform gradual border supports the diagnosis of naevus, there being no historical information to cause concern, a biopsy may not be indicated (see *Figure 6.40*)[1].

DF is frequently a small nodular lesion which often has central polarising-specific white lines, but if the diagnosis of DF can be made confidently by historical, clinical and dermatoscopic criteria, excision biopsy is not necessary (see *Figure 6.41*)[1].

6.4.3 Any lesion on the head or neck with pigmented circles and/or any dermatoscopic grey

This clue acknowledges the fact that young melanomas at these locations, possibly related to a physical barrier effect of numerous follicles, may be symmetrical (*Figure 6.42A,B,C*). They may also be asymmetrical (*Figures 6.42D* and *6.43*). A study of flat pigmented facial lesions found that the presence of any grey structures in the series examined had sensitivity and specificity for melanoma of 95.8% and 30.5%, respectively, while grey circles had a sensitivity of 54.2% and a specificity of 83.3%[12]. Unpublished data from the same study showed that pigmented circles (any colour) were similar to grey circles with a sensitivity and specificity for melanoma of 70.83% and 76.9%, respectively.

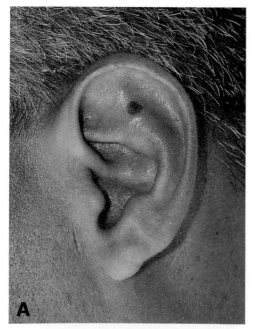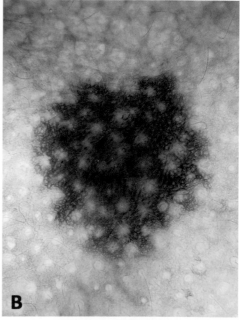

Figure 6.40: A 4mm diameter pigmented skin lesion on the ear of an adult man (A) is both a small lesion with a clue (dermatoscopic grey) (B) and also a lesion on the head and neck with dermatoscopic grey. However, a lesion which has the unequivocal morphology of a naevus (symmetry and a gradual border over the total periphery), as well as historical stability, does not need to be excised[1]. Note that there is not a pattern of pigmented circles in this lesion – it has a pattern of reticular lines interrupted by follicular openings.

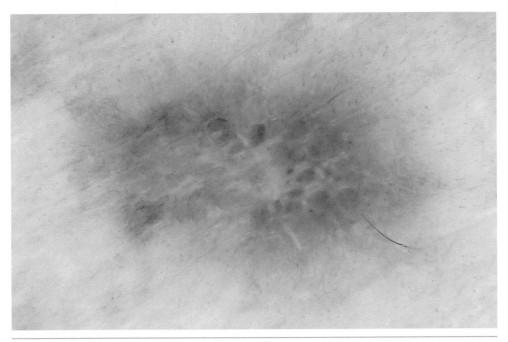

Figure 6.41: *Dermatoscopic image of a small nodular lesion with the clue to malignancy of polarising-specific white lines. It has the morphology of a DF with symmetry of pattern and colour and a central white area and, being historically stable, it does not require excision.*

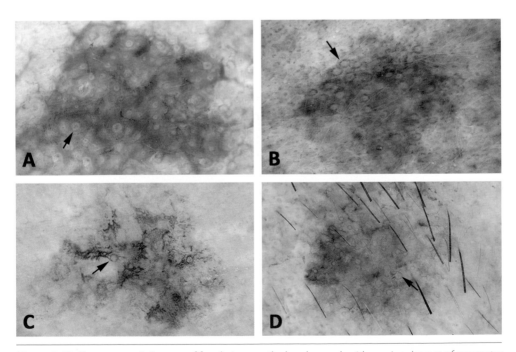

Figure 6.42: *Dermatoscopic images of four lesions on the head or neck with varying degrees of symmetry and all exhibiting the clue of pigmented circles (arrows indicate representative pigmented circles). Chaos of border abruptness precludes the unequivocal diagnosis of any known benign lesion. (A) Nasal side wall; (B) ear lobe; (C) neck; (D) eyebrow: all are melanoma in situ.*

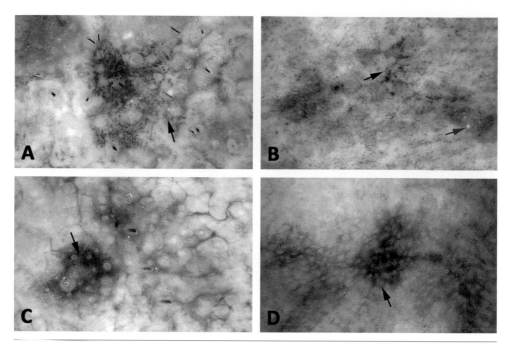

Figure 6.43: *Dermatoscopic images of four lesions on the head or neck with varying degrees of symmetry and all exhibiting the clue of grey colour (black arrows). Chaos of border abruptness precludes the unequivocal diagnosis of any known benign lesion. (A) Cheek; (B) neck (note shiny white dots due to collision seborrhoeic keratosis (blue arrow)); (C) cheek; (D) ear lobe; all are melanoma* in situ.

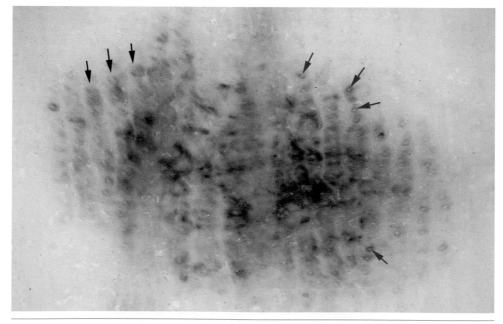

Figure 6.44: *This symmetrical (with respect to pattern, colour and border abruptness) pigmented skin lesion on the sole of a 55-year-old woman's foot has a dermatoscopic pattern of lines parallel. Although pigment is present on both dermatoglyphic ridges and furrows, the pattern of lines, best assessed at the edges of the lesion, is a parallel pattern located on the broad ridges (black arrows) rather than the narrow furrows. Pigmented circles marking the centre of the ridges correlate with pigmented malignant melanocytes in the eccrine ducts (blue arrows).*

As with the exception of a small or nodular lesion with any clue to malignancy, this particular exception should only be applied if there is an additional significant cause for concern. If a lesion has the unequivocal morphology of a naevus (*Figure 6.40*) or solar lentigo and a history of stability, it should not require (excision) biopsy[1].

6.4.4 Any lesion on volar skin (palms or soles) with a parallel ridge pattern

This clue acknowledges the fact that young melanomas at these locations may be symmetrical (*Figure 6.44*)[1].

6.5 Excluding unequivocal seborrhoeic keratoses from biopsy

If a lesion is assessed as chaotic and one or more clues to malignancy are present, consideration of (excisional) biopsy is appropriate. The specificity of 'Chaos and Clues' can be increased without sacrificing sensitivity if unequivocal seborrhoeic keratoses can be diagnosed by pattern analysis and excluded from biopsy[1,6]. Although such exclu-

sion is appropriate before the deployment of 'Chaos and Clues', we will consider it in detail here. Seborrhoeic keratoses are frequently asymmetrical and may also have dermatoscopic grey colour, peripheral black clods and even thick reticular lines, however, if they have unequivocal dermatoscopic clues to seborrhoeic keratosis then biopsy is not necessary

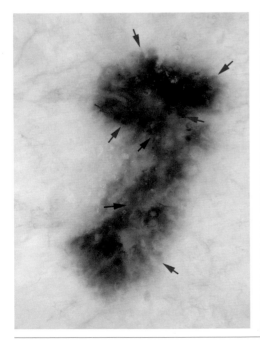
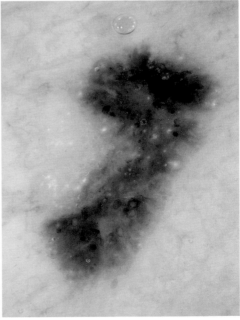

Figure 6.45: *Dermatoscopic images of a pigmented skin lesion. The polarised image (A) shows a chaotic lesion with the clues to malignancy of grey colour (black arrows), segmental radial lines (blue arrows) and some peripheral black clods (red arrows). Non-polarised dermatoscopy (B) reveals multiple white clods and this, along with the well-defined border over the total periphery and a rough surface texture, enabled a confident diagnosis of seborrhoeic keratosis.*

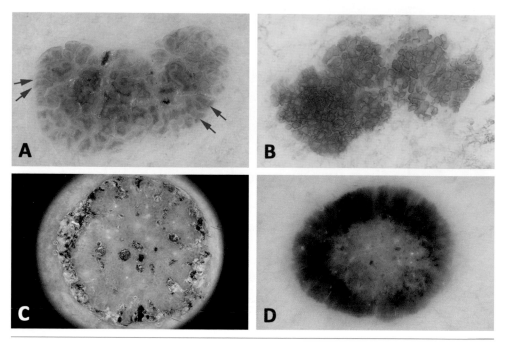

Figure 6.46: *Dermatoscopic images of four lesions which have unequivocal features of seborrhoeic keratosis by pattern analysis, all having a sharply demarcated border over the total periphery as well as: (A) thick curved lines (blue arrows); (B) pigmented circles (not related to follicles); (C) multiple orange and white clods; (D) white clods and circumferential radial lines.*

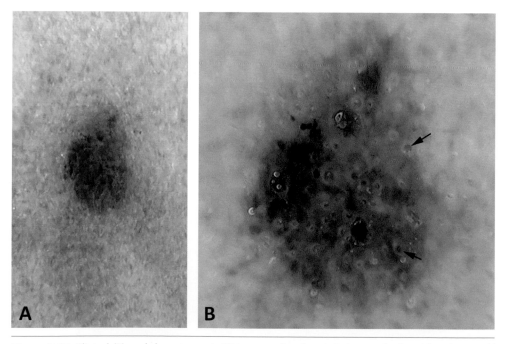

Figure 6.47: *Clinical (A) and dermatoscopic (B) images of a chaotic lesion on the face of a 52-year-old man which is considered for biopsy due to the clue of blue colour. While blue colour can be seen in some seborrhoeic keratoses and there are orange clods in this lesion (arrows) the lack of a sharply demarcated border over the total periphery precludes the diagnosis of seborrhoeic keratosis: melanoma invasive.*

(*Figure 6.45*). The dermatoscopic clues should include at least one of: multiple orange and white clods or thick curved lines, as well as, in every case, a uniformly abrupt border over the total periphery (*Figure 6.46*)[1]. If a lesion is chaotic and has clues to malignancy and there is any doubt about the diagnosis of seborrhoeic keratosis, an adequate biopsy should be performed (*Figure 6.47*).

'Chaos and Clues' is not a method designed for robots and it should not be regarded as an ultimate method, set in stone. It has been designed as a useful tool, avoiding tedious mathematical calculations, unburdened by a language of innumerable poorly defined metaphorical terms carrying preconceived diagnostic implications, and it is suitable for seamless integration into routine practice. Individuals are encouraged to use it as a framework on which to organise their accumulated experience as they individualise the method for their own style and practice.

References

1. https://dermoscopedia.org [accessed 26 August 2022].

2. Fomiatti J, Clark S, and Rosendahl C. Dermatoscopic chaos of border-abruptness led to diagnosis of a minute melanoma. *Aust J Dermatol*, 2019; in press (DOI 10.1111/ajd.12841).

3. Kittler H, Rosendahl C, Cameron A, and Tschandl P. *Dermatoscopy*, 2nd Edition, 2016. Facultas.

4. Nachbar F, Stolz W, Merkle T, *et al*. The ABCD rule of dermatoscopy. *J Am Acad Dermatol*, 1994;30:551.

5. Rosendahl C, Tschandl P, Cameron A, and Kittler H. Diagnostic accuracy of dermatoscopy for melanocytic and nonmelanocytic pigmented lesions. *J Am Acad Dermatol*, 2011;64:1068.

6. Rosendahl C, Cameron A, McColl I, and Wilkinson D. Dermatoscopy in routine practice – "Chaos and Clues." *Aust Fam Physician*, 2012;41:482.

7. Cameron A, Rosendahl C, Tschandl P, Riedl E, and Kittler H. Dermatoscopy of pigmented Bowen's disease. *J Am Acad Dermatol*, 2010;62:597.

8. Keir J. Dermatoscopic features of cutaneous non-facial non-acral lentiginous growth pattern melanomas. *Dermatol Pract Concept*, 2014;4(1):77.

9. Rosendahl C, Cameron A, Wilkinson D, Belt P, Williamson R, and Weedon D. Nail matrix melanoma: consecutive cases in a general practice. *Dermatol Pract Concept*, 2012;2(2):13.

10. Friedman RJ, Rigel DS, and Kopf AW. Early detection of malignant melanoma: the role of the physician examination and self-examination of the skin. *CA Cancer J Clin*, 1985;35:130.

11. Rosendahl C, Hishon M, Cameron A, Barksdale S, Weedon D, and Kittler H. Nodular melanoma: five consecutive cases in a general practice with polarized and non-polarized dermatoscopy and dermatopathology. *Dermatol Pract Concept*, 2014;4(2):15.

12. Tschandl P, Rosendahl C, and Kittler H. Dermatoscopy of flat pigmented facial lesions. *J Eur Acad Dermatol Venereol*, 2015;29:120.

CHAPTER 7

'Prediction without Pigment': a decision algorithm for non-pigmented skin lesions

7.1 'Prediction without Pigment'

For the purpose of this method non-pigmented lesions are defined as being amelanotic: lesions without evidence of melanin pigmentation. There must be no brown or grey colour. Black, purple or blue colour, when present, must be apparently due to blood rather than melanin; this is usually the case if they are otherwise associated with red colour only, with no brown[1].

Melanomas in particular may be hypopigmented, in which case it is not always possible to determine whether pigment is due to background or collision lesions. Such lesions will often be regarded as non-pigmented for the purpose of assessment until the histological diagnosis is determined, after which they will be classified as hypopigmented melanoma.

Most benign non-pigmented lesions, as for pigmented lesions, can rapidly and accurately be diagnosed clinically and dermatoscopically by pattern recognition, into one of five groups (see *Section 5.1.3*):

- naevus
- benign keratinocytic lesion (e.g. wart, seborrhoeic keratosis)
- haemangioma
- dermatofibroma
- sebaceous gland hyperplasia.

Benign cyst can be added to this list for non-pigmented lesions[2].

For such lesions algorithmic analysis is usually not needed.

It should also be remembered that there are clinical situations which take priority over algorithmic assessment. In particular, any elevated, firm and continuously growing (EFG) lesion, whether pigmented or non-pigmented, should be excised, primarily to confirm or exclude nodular melanoma[3,4].

The short version of 'Prediction without Pigment' is a *decision* algorithm (*Figure 7.1*). This short version, analogous to 'Chaos and Clues' for pigmented skin lesions[5] (see *Chapter 6*), is not primarily a method to lead to a specific diagnosis but is designed to lead the clinician in a stepwise process to a decision about the need to perform an excision biopsy[1]. This chapter will elaborate on this short version which is recommended as a starting point for students of dermatoscopy because of its balance of simplicity and efficacy, making it ideal for seamless integration with routine practice.

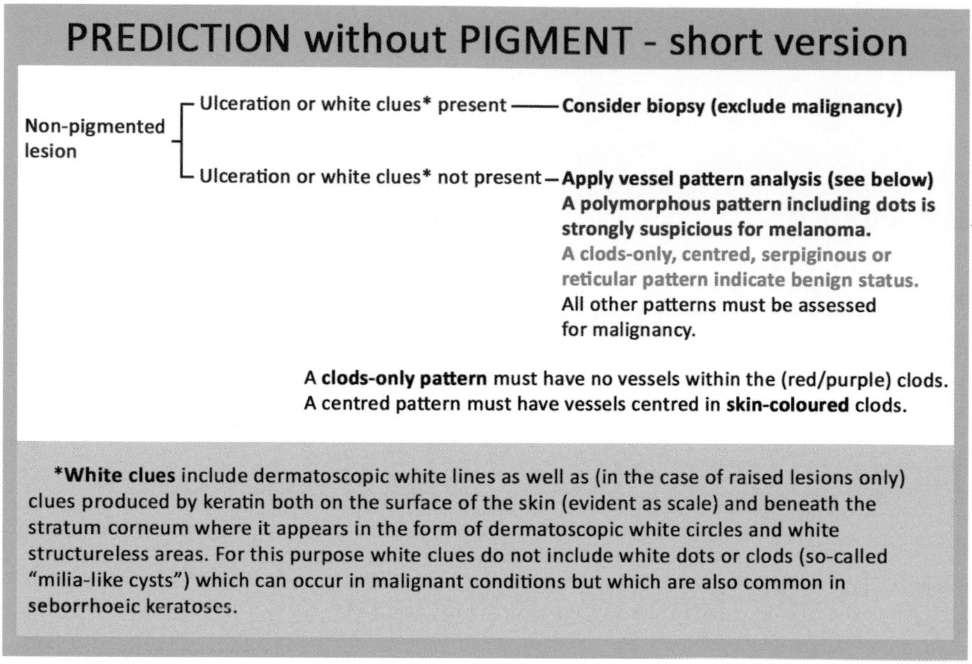

PREDICTION without PIGMENT - short version

Non-pigmented lesion
- Ulceration or white clues* present —— **Consider biopsy (exclude malignancy)**
- Ulceration or white clues* not present — **Apply vessel pattern analysis (see below)**
  A polymorphous pattern including dots is strongly suspicious for melanoma.
  A clods-only, centred, serpiginous or reticular pattern indicate benign status.
  All other patterns must be assessed for malignancy.

A **clods-only pattern** must have no vessels within the (red/purple) clods.
A **centred pattern** must have vessels centred in **skin-coloured** clods.

*White clues include dermatoscopic white lines as well as (in the case of raised lesions only) clues produced by keratin both on the surface of the skin (evident as scale) and beneath the stratum corneum where it appears in the form of dermatoscopic white circles and white structureless areas. For this purpose white clues do not include white dots or clods (so-called "milia-like cysts") which can occur in malignant conditions but which are also common in seborrhoeic keratoses.

Figure 7.1: *Flowchart for 'Prediction without Pigment' decision algorithm – short version.*

The full version of 'Prediction without Pigment' involves application of RPA to proceed to a *provisional* diagnosis (*Figure 7.2*), on the basis of considering all of the clues which are observed[1,2].

7.1.1 Prioritisation of clues in 'Prediction without Pigment'

Structures pigmented by melanin provide valuable patterns and clues for the assessment of pigmented lesions and, when such structures are present and are unequivocally part of the lesion even focally, the lesion should generally be evaluated as a pigmented lesion[3]. When such structures are absent the process is more challenging. Because of this it helps to use all available information, both clinical and dermatoscopic, when examining such lesions[2].

While ulceration is not a strong clue to a specific diagnosis, in the absence of trauma or a specific infective or vascular disorder, it is a good clue to malignancy, in particular to the most common skin malignancy, basal cell carcinoma (BCC)[3].

Ulceration: the presence of ulceration, often best determined clinically, is given first priority in the 'Prediction without Pigment' decision algorithm.

White lines: it is known that the presence of white lines seen with either polarised or non-polarised dermatoscopy, a clue to malignancy in the assessment of pigmented lesions[5], is also a useful clue in the non-pigmented variants of those same lesions, and for this reason it is prioritised after ulceration.

Keratin clues: a study has shown that with respect to the evaluation of *raised* non-pigmented lesions, the keratin clues of surface keratin, white structureless areas and white circles are more robust than vessel clues[6], and therefore they are given priority over them. Because one of the purposes of dermatoscopy is to render keratin invisible, surface keratin is often best displayed clinically, but in raised lesions it is generally also seen dermatoscopically, particularly if immersion fluid is not used. The clues of white structureless areas and white circles are dermatoscopic clues.

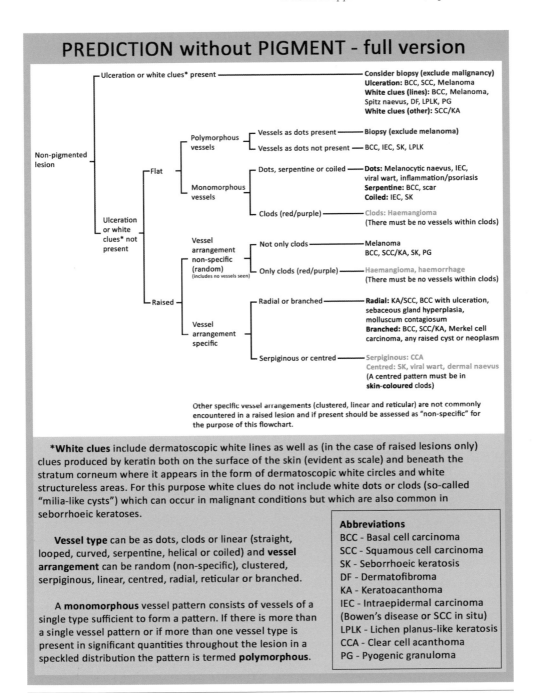

PREDICTION without PIGMENT - full version

Non-pigmented lesion

— **Ulceration or white clues* present** —— **Consider biopsy (exclude malignancy)**
Ulceration: BCC, SCC, Melanoma
White clues (lines): BCC, Melanoma, Spitz naevus, DF, LPLK, PG
White clues (other): SCC/KA

Ulceration or white clues* not present

Flat

Polymorphous vessels
— Vessels as dots present —— **Biopsy (exclude melanoma)**
— Vessels as dots not present —— BCC, IEC, SK, LPLK

Monomorphous vessels
— Dots, serpentine or coiled —— **Dots:** Melanocytic naevus, IEC, viral wart, inflammation/psoriasis
Serpentine: BCC, scar
Coiled: IEC, SK
— Clods (red/purple) —— Clods: Haemangioma
(There must be no vessels within clods)

Raised

Vessel arrangement non-specific (random) (includes no vessels seen)
— Not only clods —— Melanoma
BCC, SCC/KA, SK, PG
— Only clods (red/purple) —— Haemangioma, haemorrhage
(There must be no vessels within clods)

Vessel arrangement specific
— Radial or branched —— **Radial:** KA/SCC, BCC with ulceration, sebaceous gland hyperplasia, molluscum contagiosum
Branched: BCC, SCC/KA, Merkel cell carcinoma, any raised cyst or neoplasm
— Serpiginous or centred —— Serpiginous: CCA
Centred: SK, viral wart, dermal naevus
(A centred pattern must be in **skin-coloured** clods)

Other specific vessel arrangements (clustered, linear and reticular) are not commonly encountered in a raised lesion and if present should be assessed as "non-specific" for the purpose of this flowchart.

*White clues include dermatoscopic white lines as well as (in the case of raised lesions only) clues produced by keratin both on the surface of the skin (evident as scale) and beneath the stratum corneum where it appears in the form of dermatoscopic white circles and white structureless areas. For this purpose white clues do not include white dots or clods (so-called "milia-like cysts") which can occur in malignant conditions but which are also common in seborrhoeic keratoses.

Vessel type can be as dots, clods or linear (straight, looped, curved, serpentine, helical or coiled) and **vessel arrangement** can be random (non-specific), clustered, serpiginous, linear, centred, radial, reticular or branched.

A **monomorphous** vessel pattern consists of vessels of a single type sufficient to form a pattern. If there is more than a single vessel pattern or if more than one vessel type is present in significant quantities throughout the lesion in a speckled distribution the pattern is termed **polymorphous**.

Abbreviations
BCC - Basal cell carcinoma
SCC - Squamous cell carcinoma
SK - Seborrhoeic keratosis
DF - Dermatofibroma
KA - Keratoacanthoma
IEC - Intraepidermal carcinoma (Bowen's disease or SCC in situ)
LPLK - Lichen planus-like keratosis
CCA - Clear cell acanthoma
PG - Pyogenic granuloma

Figure 7.2: *Flowchart for specific diagnosis of non-pigmented lesions by RPA – full version.*

Vessel pattern analysis: finally, for a non-pigmented lesion which cannot be diagnosed clinically or by dermatoscopic pattern recognition, and in which no ulceration or white clues are detected, vessel pattern analysis must be performed[1].

7.2 'Prediction without Pigment': short version

7.2.1 Step 1: is there ulceration?

As stated above, the first step in evaluating a non-pigmented lesion in the 'Prediction without Pigment' algorithm is to determine whether it is ulcerated (*Figures 7.3–7.6*). Considering that the dermatoscope is generally applied to non-pigmented lesions of concern for which the diagnosis is not obvious, ulceration caused by significant trauma or by a specific infectious or vascular disorder should not be a confounding factor. If ulceration is observed with the naked eye, that only increases the appropriateness of dermatoscopic examination, because if the lesion is malignant additional dermatoscopic clues can be expected to add weight to the suspicion of malignancy, as well as providing evidence for the precise diagnosis. Dermatoscopy may actually make ulceration more difficult to appreciate because the application of immersion fluid, or even the use of polar-

ised light with non-contact dermatoscopy, may render the optical features of ulceration invisible. There is, however, a dermatoscopic clue to ulceration which may frequently be observed, even in cases of micro-ulceration which is not apparent clinically, and that is the presence of adherent fibre (*Figures 7.6* and *7.7*)[1,3]. Ulceration results in a serum exudate which may trap clothing fibre or other environmental or intrinsic matter, including hair, and the observation of such material may be a clue to ulceration which may not have been otherwise apparent[2].

It should also be remembered that ulceration can have secondary effects including the promotion of angioneogenesis; unexpected vessel morphology, including a polymorphous vessel pattern, may result (see *Figure 7.8*). In some cases keratinisation may also occur, leading to features such as surface keratin (*Figure 7.9*) or white circles, normally expected in SCC[6] but not BCC.

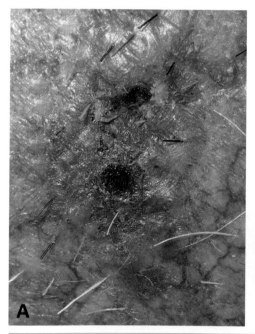
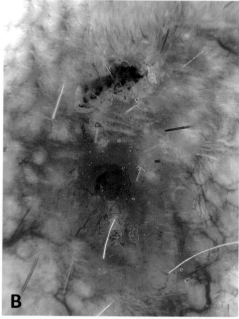

Figure 7.3: *Although ulceration is clearly evident clinically (A) and attracted attention to this subtle non-pigmented lesion, it requires dermatoscopy (B) to appreciate the additional clues to the diagnosis of basal cell carcinoma. These include polarising-specific white lines and fine serpentine vessels.*

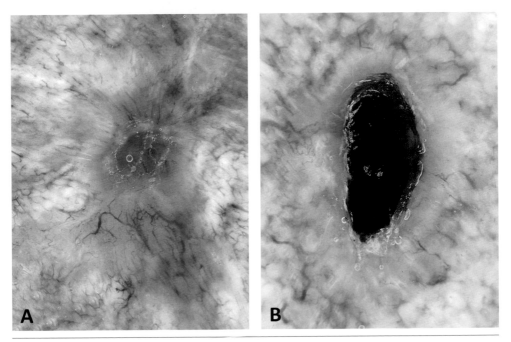

Figure 7.4: *The variety of dermatoscopic presentations of ulceration is illustrated by an orange clod due to serum exudate in (A) and a black clod due to a blood clot in (B), both lesions being examples of basal cell carcinoma.*

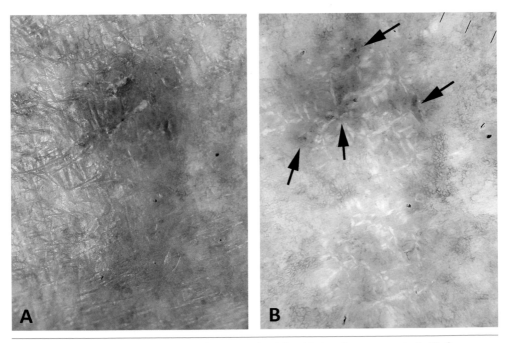

Figure 7.5: *A clinical image (A) displays ulceration of a defined lesion. Dermatoscopically (B), fine orange clods (arrows) correlate with the areas of micro-ulceration and very prominent polarising-specific white lines provide an additional clue to the specific diagnosis of basal cell carcinoma.*

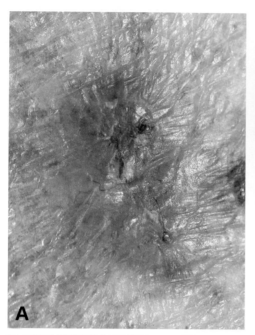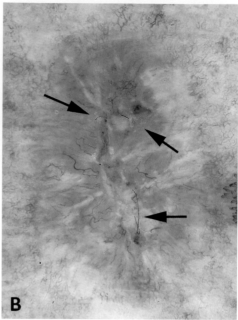

Figure 7.6: *Clinical (A) and dermatoscopic (B) images of a defined ulcerated lesion. Orange clouds as a dermatoscopic clue to micro-ulceration are supplemented by the presence of adherent fibres (arrows); basal cell carcinoma.*

7.2.2 Step 2: are there 'white clues'?

'White clues' are defined as:
- White lines in *any* non-pigmented lesion[3].
- Keratin clues in *raised* non-pigmented lesions of:
  - surface keratin (clinical or dermatoscopic)
  - white structureless areas (dermatoscopic)
  - white circles (dermatoscopic).

As for pigmented lesions, the clue of white lines may be seen with non-polarising and/or polarising dermatoscopy and to be classified as white lines they must be whiter than the perilesional skin.

Polarising-specific white lines, which are straight, orientated perpendicularly to each other, not crossing and frequently shifting as the dermatoscope is rotated, are the white lines most frequently seen in non-pigmented lesions, and are a valuable clue particularly to

BCC (see *Figures 7.10* and *7.11*). They can also be seen (uncommonly) in SCC *in situ* and LPLK, and correlation with vessel morphology may be necessary when attempting to predict a specific diagnosis. Differentiation from the other benign lesions where this clue may be seen, DF and Spitz naevus, is less often a concern when pigment is absent. Apart from DF, the distinction is not critical because there is a strong argument that Spitz naevi should probably be excised regardless of the age of the patient[7,8], because differentiation from spitzoid melanoma cannot be made with confidence without histological confirmation, and even that may be equivocal. Similarly, polarising-specific white lines may be seen in amelanotic melanoma (see *Figure 7.12*), where vessel clues can often, but not always, be used to distinguish BCC from melanoma, where a polymorphous pattern including patterns of dot vessels is a frequent feature of melanoma but not of BCC[1].

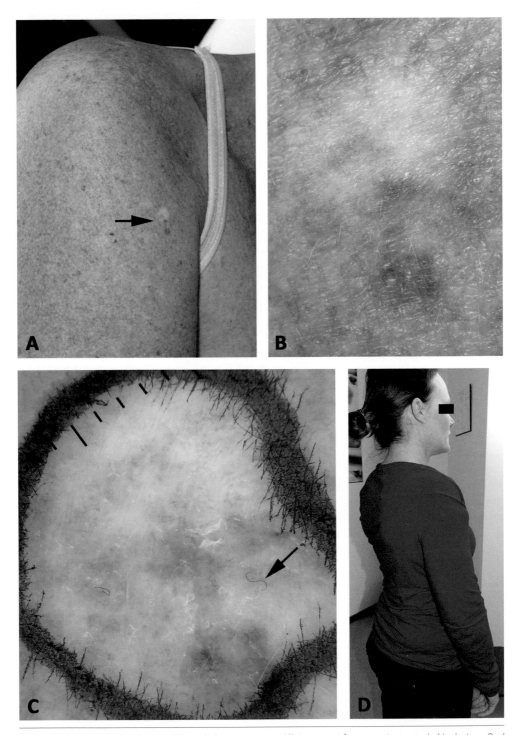

Figure 7.7: *Clinical (A), close-up (B) and dermatoscopic (C) images of a non-pigmented skin lesion. Red adherent fibre (arrow in C) is seen as a dermatoscopic clue to micro-ulceration of a subtle basal cell carcinoma (arrow in A) which lacks any other clue to ulceration. See also the second red fibre at the left inferior extremity. The source of the red fibre is evident in the image of the dressed patient (D). Image reproduced with permission.*

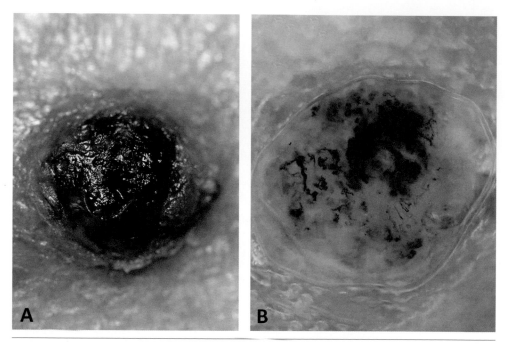

Figure 7.8: *Polymorphous vessels including dots, clods, and linear straight, linear curved, linear looped and linear serpentine vessels, in a dermatoscopic image (B) of a broadly ulcerated basal cell carcinoma (close-up image (A)).*

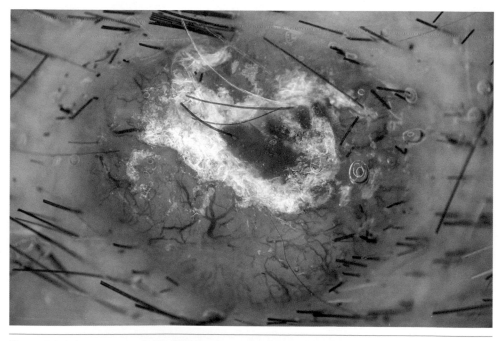

Figure 7.9: *A dermatoscopic image displaying secondary keratinisation in an ulcerated basal cell carcinoma.*

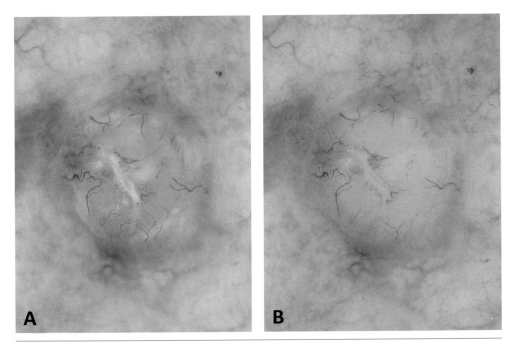

Figure 7.10: *Polarising-specific white lines, straight and perpendicularly orientated are a striking dermatoscopic feature only seen with polarised dermatoscopy (A). A monomorphous pattern of branched serpentine vessels as well as the characteristic translucent stroma, appreciated best in the polarised image (A) which casts the vessels into sharp focus, are supporting evidence that this is a basal cell carcinoma. A non-polarised dermatoscopic image is also shown (B).*

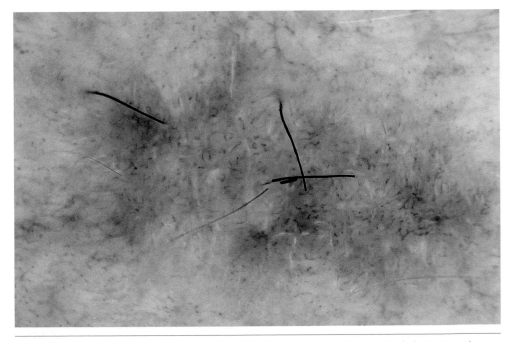

Figure 7.11: *Dermatoscopic polarising-specific white lines, straight and perpendicularly orientated, are a very evident clue in this basal cell carcinoma.*

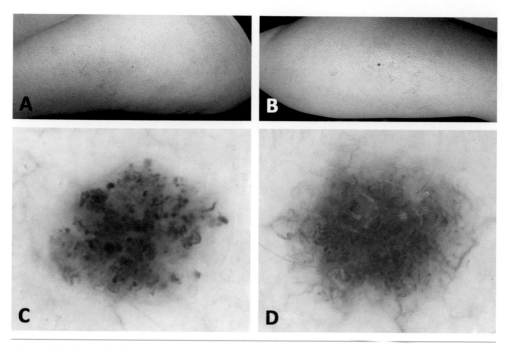

Figure 7.12: *Clinical (A, B) and dermatoscopic (C, D) images of two lesions on the same 30-year-old woman. On the left thigh (A, C) is a lesion with the dermatoscopic pattern recognition features of a haemangioma (clods-only pattern with a few linear variants as commonly seen with very small haemangiomas). The lesion on the right thigh (B, D) does not have the pattern recognition morphology of any of the common benign groups so is analysed carefully. Polarising-specific white lines are clearly visible and take priority over vessels (there are none of the four benign vessel patterns anyway) leading to excision biopsy; amelanotic melanoma, Breslow thickness 0.8mm.*

The keratin clues of surface keratin (*Figures 7.13–7.15*), white structureless areas (*Figures 7.13* and *7.15*) and white circles (*Figures 7.16–7.19*) are only applicable to *raised* non-pigmented lesions with respect to predicting malignancy. A raised lesion is defined as a lesion which is visible or palpably raised, other than due to surface keratin, or a lesion which has the dermatoscopic clue to a raised lesion of looped vessels[3]. Actinic keratoses may have surface keratin and/or white circles but such lesions, not being raised and therefore not being predicted to harbour invasive malignancy, may be suitable for non-surgical treatment without biopsy. Similarly, the keratin clue of a white structureless area does not apply in a flat *keratinising* lesion, because white structureless areas in

SCC/KA correspond to significant acanthosis of highly keratinised keratinocytes[3] and if this is present the lesion will not be flat.

While the presence of any of the three keratin clues in a raised non-pigmented lesion should lead to consideration of biopsy on suspicion of SCC/KA, the clue of white circles is regarded as the most useful clue. White circles were found to be 87% specific for SCC/KA in the consecutive test series examined, while nearly half (44%) of SCC/KA in that series displayed dermatoscopic white circles[6]. In the experience of the authors, dermatoscopic white circles have frequently enabled the confident prediction of the diagnosis of very small SCC where that diagnosis would not have been possible for such small lesions prior to that clue being described (*Figure 7.18*).

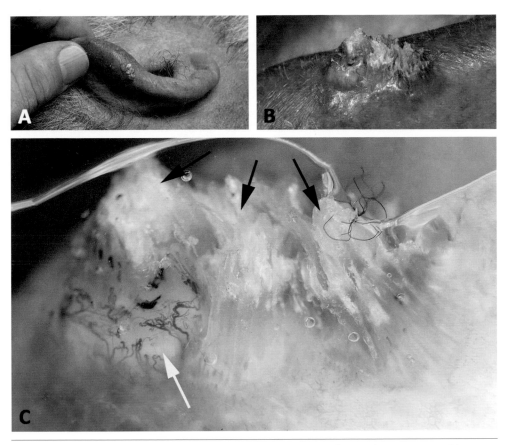

Figure 7.13: *Clinical (A), close-up (B) and dermatoscopic (C) images of a raised non-pigmented lesion on the ear. Surface keratin (black arrows) and a white structureless area (yellow arrow) are clues to malignancy; squamous cell carcinoma.*

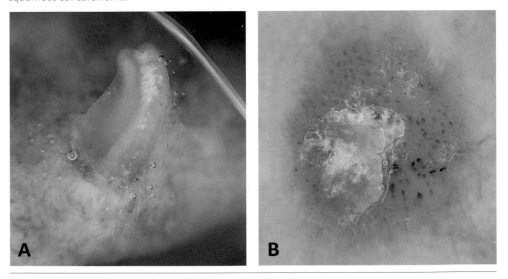

Figure 7.14: *Surface keratin is seen in dermatoscopic images of two non-pigmented lesions: (A) a keratin horn on an invasive squamous cell carcinoma; (B) a monomorphous pattern of coiled vessels is a clue to the specific diagnosis of squamous cell carcinoma in situ.*

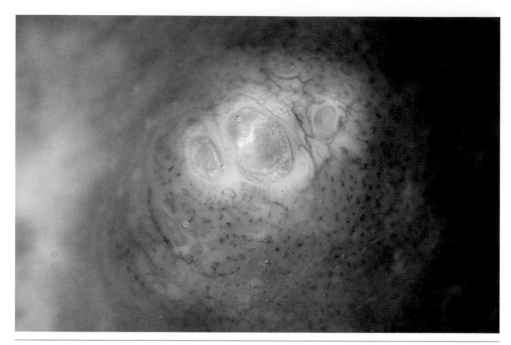

Figure 7.15: *Dermatoscopic image of a raised lesion with surface keratin over a white structureless area. Note the polymorphous vessel pattern including serpentine and coiled/dot vessels. The white keratin clues take priority over vessel clues and point to the correct diagnosis in this case; invasive squamous cell carcinoma.*

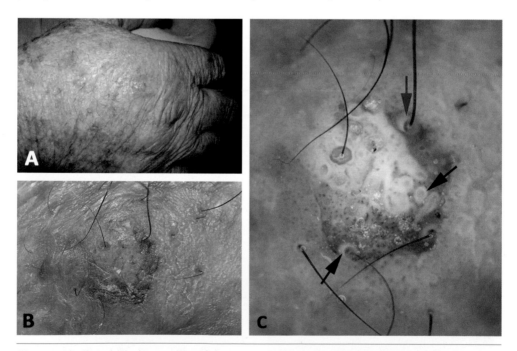

Figure 7.16: *Clinical (A), close-up (B) and dermatoscopic (C) images of a raised non-pigmented lesion on the hand of a 75-year-old man. There are several dermatoscopic white circles (black arrows). A red arrow points to an obliquely orientated structure with a white cylinder surrounding a hair shaft – this displays the dermatoscopic correlate of invasion of a hair follicle by highly keratinised malignant keratinocytes.*

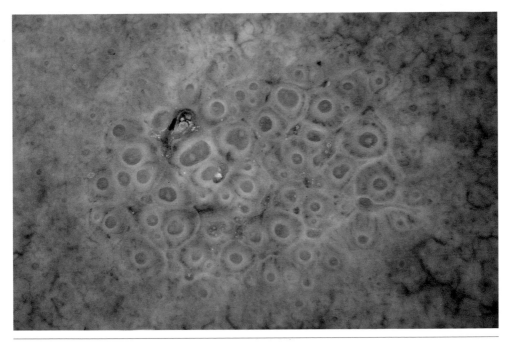

Figure 7.17: *A dermatoscopic pattern of white circles in a squamous cell carcinoma on the scalp of a 48-year-old man.*

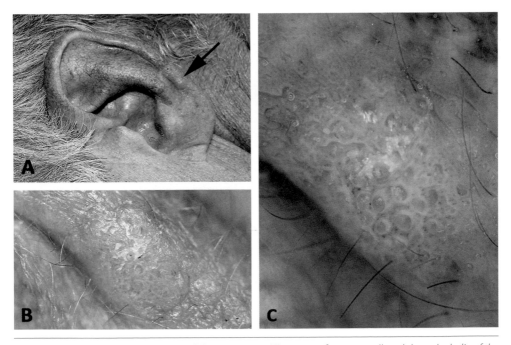

Figure 7.18: *Clinical (A), close-up (B) and dermatoscopic (C) images of a very small nodule on the helix of the ear which is confidently diagnosed as a squamous cell carcinoma due to the compelling dermatoscopic clue of white circles.*

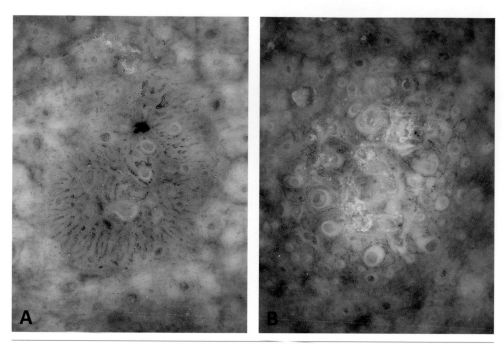

Figure 7.19: *Two examples of squamous cell carcinoma with dermatoscopic white circles which can be thin (A) or thick (B).*

7.2.3 Step 3: is the vessel pattern consistent with malignancy?

It is only when a non-pigmented lesion of concern has neither ulceration nor white clues that analysis of vessel patterns is necessary[3]. In fact, if either of those priority clues are present then, as a general rule, vessels should be considered as additional clues to a specific diagnosis rather than being relied on to avoid biopsy. However, if a non-pigmented lesion is not ulcerated and has no white lines, nor in the case of a raised lesion any keratin clues, vessel pattern analysis is the only remaining assessment possible and should proceed in the following manner.

There are four monomorphous vessel patterns which are consistent with a benign diagnosis when seen in a non-pigmented skin lesion[3].

A pattern of (red and/or purple) clods-only: this is consistent with the diagnosis of haemangioma in an apparently stable lesion

(see *Figure 7.20*)[3]. Normally, haemangiomas are diagnosed with confidence clinically and the dermatoscopist is encouraged to look at thousands of such lesions to become familiar with their distinctive but protean morphology. While it has been regarded as a rule that a clods-only pattern excludes lesions with any linear vessels, it is not at all uncommon to see haemangiomas with linear vessels peripherally as well as clods (see *Figure 7.12C*); indeed, this is almost universal with very small haemangiomas. Clinical correlation is required in the evaluation of such lesions. If there is some additional cause for concern, such as reported recent change, then biopsy may be indicated regardless of dermatoscopic findings and, in such a situation, the presence of any linear vessels would increase the index of suspicion. Certainly, any apparent haemangioma with any vessels seen *within* the red or purple clods should be excised[1]. Another frequent finding in haemangiomas is the presence of fibrous septa between the clods, projecting as white lines (*Figure*

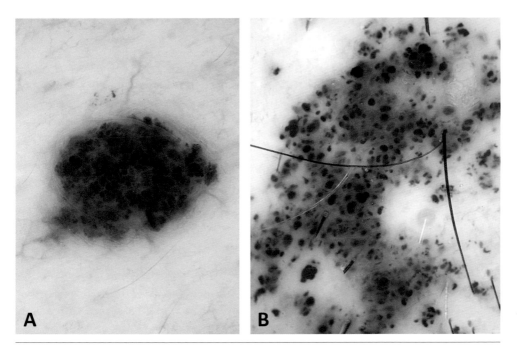

Figure 7.20: Two examples of a clods-only pattern in haemangiomas.

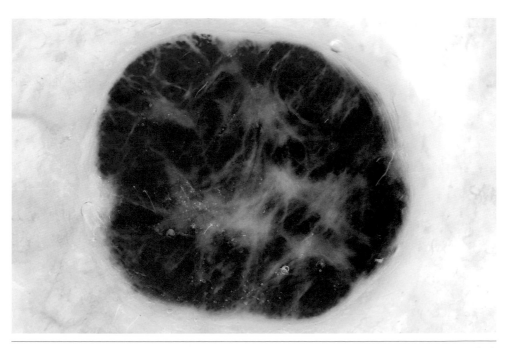

Figure 7.21: Dermatoscopic image of a haemangioma with fibrous septa projecting as white lines, which separate red clods.

7.21). The deliberate examination of multiple haemangiomas, when multiplicity supports benignancy, will permit the dermatoscopist to become familiar with this appearance.

A pattern of centred vessels-only: this is consistent with a benign diagnosis of verruca, congenital naevus or seborrhoeic keratosis in an apparently stable lesion (*Figure 7.22*)[3]. A centred vessel pattern is defined as the presence of vessels (any type) centred in *skin-coloured clods*; it cannot be applied if the clods are red because such a background colour can be seen in some nodular melanomas with vessels centred in red clods (*Figure 7.23*)[1]. Note that the presence of white lines (see *Figure 7.23*), also seen in some nodular melanomas, takes priority over vessel analysis and, if seen in association with an otherwise apparent centred vessel pattern, should lead to excision even if there is a monomorphous pattern of centred vessels. A background red colour can be falsely rendered as skin-coloured if undue pressure is exerted on the dermatoscope footplate. In such a situation, observation of red colour on clinical examination

should override observation of skin-colour on dermatoscopy and the diagnosis of a centred pattern should not be made.

A pattern of serpiginous vessels-only: in a stable lesion this is consistent with the diagnosis of clear cell acanthoma with no differential diagnosis (*Figure 7.24*)[3].

A pattern of reticular vessels-only: in a stable lesion this predictably corresponds to a benign diagnosis, with this pattern commonly seen in isolated patches on sun-damaged skin (*Figure 7.25*) as well as in the form of mastocytosis known as telangiectasia macularis perstans[3].

All other vessel patterns in lesions of concern should be assessed with a view to biopsy *(see Figures 7.26–7.30).*

While any polymorphous pattern of vessels can be a clue to malignancy, it should be remembered that benign lesions such as seborrhoeic keratoses and most dermal naevi can also have polymorphous (linear) vessels. The dermatoscopist is encouraged to look at

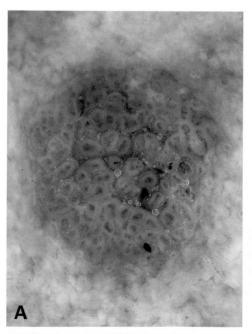
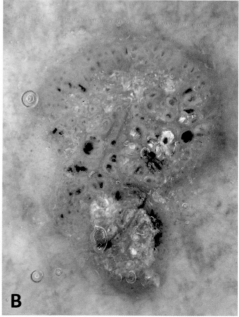

Figure 7.22: A centred vascular pattern in dermatoscopic images of two examples of seborrhoeic keratosis.

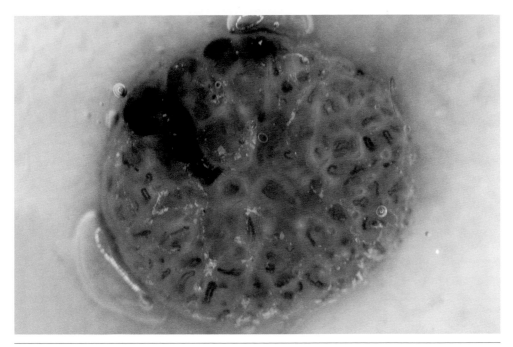

Figure 7.23: *Dermatoscopic image of a lesion in which vessels are mostly centred in non-pigmented clods. The unequivocal white lines take priority over the vessels and mandate biopsy; nodular melanoma, Breslow thickness 2.5mm. While white lines may separate the clods in a haemangioma, the white lines in this lesion do not have the morphology of septa as seen in Figure 7.21. Image reproduced from* Dermatol Pract Concept, *2014;4(1):91 with permission from the authors.*

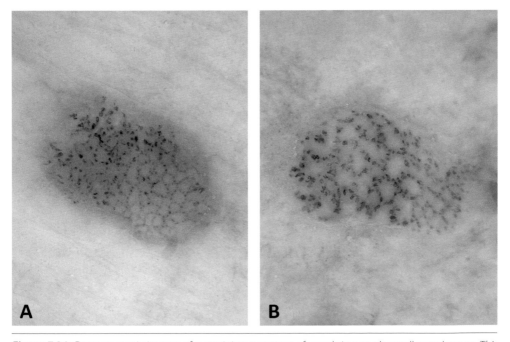

Figure 7.24: *Dermatoscopic images of a serpiginous pattern of vessels in two clear cell acanthomas. This very distinctive pattern is known as a 'string of pearls' pattern in metaphorical terminology.*

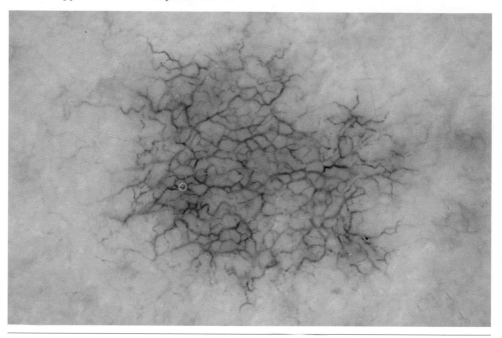

Figure 7.25: *Dermatoscopic image of a reticular vessel pattern on sun-damaged skin, also known as a telangiectasia (not excised). What is seen here are the vessels of the dermal vascular plexus made visible by solar-induced atrophy of the overlying dermis.*

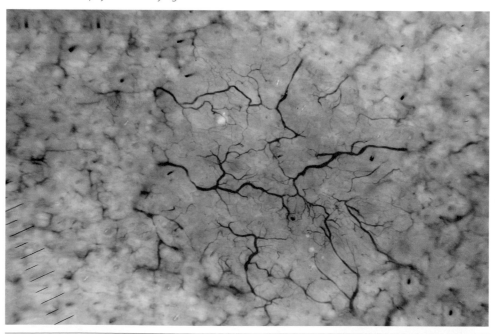

Figure 7.26: *Dermatoscopic image of a non-pigmented lesion on the cheek of a 62-year-old man which shows no evidence of ulceration or white clues (white clods/dots are not regarded as white clues in the 'Prediction without Pigment' algorithm because they are commonly encountered in benign lesions). None of the four benign vessel patterns are present and, in the context of a discrete lesion, a pattern of branched serpentine vessels, thrown into sharp relief by translucent stroma, is most consistent with a diagnosis of basal cell carcinoma. Note that the serpentine branched vessels are not unique to the lesion, blending seamlessly with the perilesional dermal vascular plexus.*

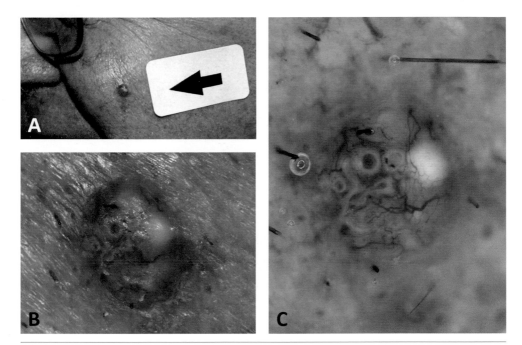

Figure 7.27: *A nodular lesion on the cheek of a 68-year-old man (A, B) has dermatoscopic serpentine branched vessels (C) which might be considered consistent with a diagnosis of basal cell carcinoma. Applying the 'Prediction without Pigment' algorithm, there is neither ulceration nor white lines, but there are white circles and a white structureless area. These clues have priority over vessel clues leading to the correct diagnosis of squamous cell carcinoma.*

thousands of obviously benign examples of these lesions in situations where their multiplicity is compelling evidence of their benignity, to become familiar with their distinctive but protean vessel morphology.

Any polymorphous vessel pattern which includes a pattern of dots in addition to any pattern of linear vessels raises suspicion for melanoma (see *Figures 7.28–7.30*)[3]. This assumes again that the lesion is not an unequivocal seborrhoeic keratosis or dermal naevus, because scattered linear and dot vessels are not uncommon in such lesions. It is assumed that vessel analysis is being applied to a discrete lesion that does not have compelling criteria of any common benign entity. Also, a few dot vessels in a lesion with predominantly linear vessels does not constitute a pattern of dot vessels. The pattern of dot vessels in a melanoma will usually, but not always, appear as a separate pattern of

vessels rather than speckled in between linear vessels. Dot vessels are only expected in the macular part of a melanoma because they actually represent prominent dermal papillae vessels projecting vertically from the dermal vascular plexus towards the epidermis. Once a melanoma becomes invasive the normal organised morphology of the dermal papillae becomes distorted with lateral displacement, meaning that dermal papillae vessels will project as linear vessels of various types[3]. Linear vessels, either laterally displaced dermal papillae vessels, dilated dermal plexus vessels (usually serpentine) or polymorphous linear vessels (looped, curved, serpentine, helical or coiled) can be seen in both macular and raised portions of a melanoma. A melanoma may also have a polymorphous pattern of linear vessels without a pattern of dots in which case the different vessel types are likely to be combined in a random arrangement.

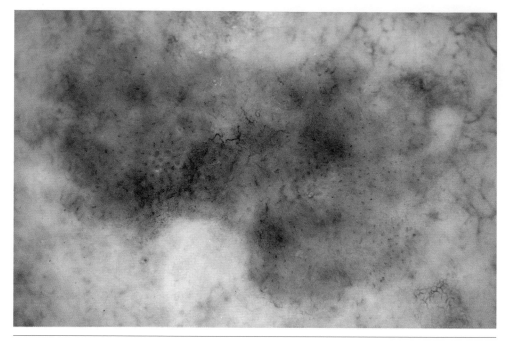

Figure 7.28: *Dermatoscopic image of a hypopigmented melanoma with a polymorphous vascular pattern including linear serpentine vessels (centrally) and a vast pattern of dot vessels (peripherally).*

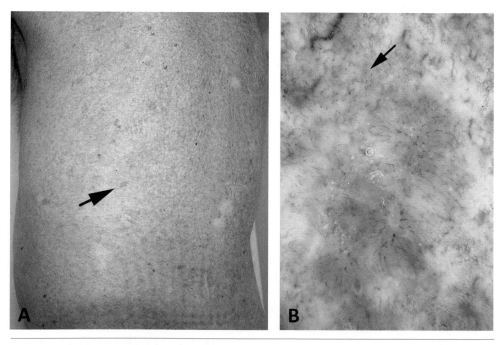

Figure 7.29: *A non-pigmented lesion (arrow in A) was treated by curettage and cautery on suspicion of basal cell carcinoma. Fortunately, because the diagnosis of basal cell carcinoma was not made with absolute certainty a shave biopsy 1mm thick was performed first, and a histological diagnosis of invasive melanoma (Breslow thickness 0.3mm) was made. In retrospect, as well as a dermatoscopic (B) pattern of linear serpentine vessels, there is a cluster of dot vessels at the upper extremity of the image (arrow).*

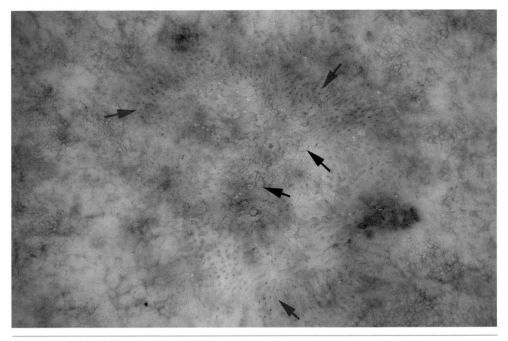

Figure 7.30: Dermatoscopic image of a hypopigmented melanoma with a polymorphous vascular pattern including patterns of linear (black arrows) and dot vessels (blue arrows).

7.3 Conclusion

As with 'Chaos and Clues', 'Prediction without Pigment' should not be regarded as an ultimate method set in stone. It has been designed as a useful diagnostic tool, suitable for seamless integration into routine practice. We encourage colleagues to use it as a framework on which to organise their accumulated experience and to adapt and individualise the method for their own style and practice.

References

1. Rosendahl C, Cameron A, Tschandl P, Bulinska A, Zalaudek I, and Kittler H. Prediction without pigment: a decision algorithm for non-pigmented skin malignancy. *Dermatol Pract Concept*, 2014;4(1):9.

2. Kittler H, Rosendahl C, Cameron A, and Tschandl P. *Dermatoscopy*, 2nd Edition, 2016. Facultas.

3. https://dermoscopedia.org [accessed 26 August 2022].

4. Chamberlain AJ, Fritschi L, and Kelly JW. Nodular melanoma: patients' perceptions of presenting features and implications for earlier detection. *J Am Acad Dermatol*, 2003;48:694.

5. Rosendahl C, Cameron A, McColl I, and Wilkinson D. Dermatoscopy in routine practice – "Chaos and Clues." *Aust Fam Physician*, 2012;41:482.

6. Rosendahl C, Cameron A, Argenziano G, Zalaudek I, Tschandl P, and Kittler H. Dermoscopy of squamous cell carcinoma and keratoacanthoma. *Arch Dermatol*, 2012;148:1386.

7. Gelbard SN, Tripp JM, Marghoob AA, *et al*. Management of Spitz nevi: a survey of dermatologists in the United States. *J Am Acad Dermatol*, 2002;47:224.

8. Weedon D. *Weedon's Skin Pathology,* 3rd Edition, 2002. Churchill Livingstone.

CHAPTER 8

Pattern analysis

8.1 Revised pattern analysis – a diagnostic algorithm

Algorithmic methods are useful when clinical assessment or pattern recognition does not provide a confident diagnosis. Most naevi, seborrhoeic keratoses, warts, haemangiomas and DFs will be recognised clinically. While the authors encourage the dermatoscopic assessment of as many lesions as possible, even obviously benign ones, they also know and acknowledge what happens in clinical practice.

- Dermatoscopic pattern analysis was first introduced in 1987: it was applied only to pigmented skin lesions[1]. We will refer to that published version as 'classic pattern analysis' to distinguish it from the generic process of 'pattern analysis'.
- Revised pattern analysis (RPA) was introduced 20 years later by Kittler in 2007: Kittler expanded the method to include all skin lesions, including those that were not pigmented by melanin[2,3].
- 'Chaos and Clues'[4] and 'Prediction without Pigment'[5] are decision algorithms based on RPA: they are designed to guide the clinician in a stepwise process, not necessarily to a specific diagnosis, but rather to a decision as to whether excision biopsy is appropriate.
- The next step is the application of pattern analysis to make a specific diagnosis: this is the ultimate goal of dermatoscopy and that process of pattern analysis is

presented here in the form of a simplified and practical method. With experience, the process of pattern analysis becomes rapid and merges into the process of pattern recognition so that most lesions, both benign and malignant, are recognised without measurable cognition, in the same way that one recognises the face of an acquaintance. Facial recognition is innate human behaviour but pattern recognition of skin lesions must be learned. We believe that learning is best achieved by a method which is reproducible and teachable. In other words, a method that cannot be taught is barely a method at all[6].

- Kittler presented RPA in the form of a flowchart[7] on which patterns, colours and clues were in turn analysed to lead logically in a stepwise fashion to either a provisional diagnosis or a limited number of options for that diagnosis[6]. Patterns were organised into a hierarchical order of specificity: lines (reticular, branched, angulated, parallel, radial and curved), pseudopods, circles, clods, dots and structureless. This could be applied to lesions with a single pattern and, in the case of lesions with more than one pattern, the pattern which appeared first in the above list was regarded as the primary pattern, the lesion being assessed based on the options according to that pattern.

- The stepwise process presented in these flowcharts permits assessment of lesions in a logical progression starting with an assessment of the patterns, colours and finally the clues. Patterns and colours are assessed as if from a distance, actually avoiding attention to subtle details, and when that assessment discovers biological symmetry the likelihood of malignancy is very low. On the other hand, the discovery of patterns and/or colours combined *asymmetrically* raises the possibility of malignancy and should lead to a careful examination for clues that may or may not support that suspicion.

An aide-memoire for revised pattern analysis of pigmented skin lesions

In practice we have found that with respect to pigmented skin lesions, including lesions containing white structures (whiter than surrounding skin), a simple aide-memoire can guide the clinician rapidly to a very limited differential diagnosis based on pattern, which can then be sorted according to specific clues to the defined alternatives.

The vast majority of skin lesions which will be encountered, pigmented and non-pigmented, both benign and malignant, fall into one of six categories:

1. Melanocytic.
2. Benign keratinocytic.
3. Basal cell carcinoma (BCC).
4. Squamous cell neoplasia (including squamous cell carcinoma (SCC), SCC *in situ* and actinic keratosis (AK)).
5. Dermatofibroma (DF).
6. Other; this group includes pigmented lesions not in the first five categories, including some lesions pigmented other than by melanin, such as haemangiomas.

It greatly simplifies the diagnostic process if each of these categories is considered each time a lesion which requires analysis is assessed. Not only is the consideration of six categories manageable, it also ensures that all likely options are considered.

Based on the flowchart for RPA it is possible to predict which of these categories are relevant to a pigmented lesion simply by identifying that lesion's pattern or primary pattern: a specific provisional diagnosis, or limited range of options, can then be predicted by weighing the clues which may be present.

This simplified approach is presented as an aide-memoire for RPA (*Figure 8.1*). Instructions for applying this method are as follows:

- Select the *first* pattern seen in the order shown on the left-hand side.
- The differential diagnosis will be as shown for *that pattern* regardless of other patterns.
- A pattern should cover a significant portion of the lesion (approximately 20% or more) to rate as a pattern rather than a clue.

Considering that the groups 'DF' and 'Other' do not generally provide a diagnostic challenge, the application of RPA can concentrate primarily on the use of clues to establish a provisional diagnosis of lesions in the first four categories defined in the RPA aide-memoire: melanocytic lesions, benign keratinocytic lesions, BCC, and SCC (including AK and SCC *in situ*).

Of relevance it should be noted that no pattern excludes the possible diagnosis of melanoma.

The reader is reminded before proceeding further that deployment of this method of pattern analysis is an optional further step after application of the decision algorithms presented in *Chapter 6* (Chaos and Clues) and *Chapter 7* (Prediction without Pigment) and because of that it is not critical with respect to *management* decisions.

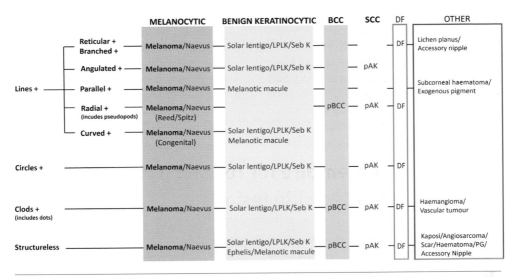

Figure 8.1: *An aide-memoire based on RPA to provide a manageable list of diagnostic categories. A lesion is examined for patterns and the first pattern encountered in the order shown above is the primary pattern. The differential diagnosis will be limited to the categories populated for that primary pattern. The '+' indicates that other patterns may or may not be present; the possible diagnostic options will be the same either way. Abbreviations: DF (dermatofibroma); LPLK (lichen planus-like keratosis); pAK (pigmented actinic keratosis including pigmented squamous cell carcinoma in situ); pBCC (pigmented basal cell carcinoma); PG (pyogenic granuloma); SCC (squamous cell carcinoma); Seb K (seborrhoeic keratosis).*

8.3 Applying the aide-memoire in practice

8.3.1 A pattern or primary pattern of lines

A pattern, or primary pattern of lines reticular or branched

Lines reticular and branched are very similar and while the presence of branched lines can be a useful clue to ink spot lentigo, as patterns the two will be considered together.

A lesion with one pattern, lines reticular/branched, or a lesion with more than one pattern but with a primary pattern of lines reticular/branched, and which is not lichen planus, an accessory nipple or DF, will be limited to only two categories (*Figures 8.2–8.4*):

- **melanocytic**
- **benign keratinocytic.**

These differential options are further sorted according to specific clues as detailed below and also in Sections 9.1, 9.2 *and* 9.4.

This means that for such a lesion the range of diagnostic options is limited to **melanoma, naevus and benign keratinocytic lesions**[6].

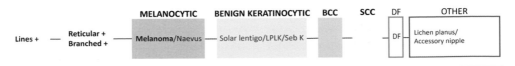

Figure 8.2: *Aide-memoire for a pattern, or primary pattern of lines reticular or branched.*

The other categories (BCC and SCC) are effectively excluded by any lesional reticular lines either pigmented or white[6].

As well as for pigmented reticular lines, this aide-memoire is applicable to a primary pattern of white (whiter than perilesional skin) reticular lines, which is a rare but compelling pattern highly specific for melanoma (*Figure 8.3B*). In contrast, polarising-specific white lines, being straight lines, orientated perpendicularly to each other, not crossing, and which may shift on rotation of the dermatoscope, are regarded as a clue rather than a pattern in RPA.

Melanocytic lesions

Melanoma: this should be suspected in a lesion with a single or primary pattern of reticular lines if asymmetry is present, as well as at least one clue to melanoma (*Figure 8.3*)[4].

The nine clues to malignancy were defined in *Chapter 6* and, while they point to generic pigmented malignancy in the 'Chaos and Clues' algorithm, they all apply to melanoma:
1. Grey or blue colour
2. Structureless eccentric area
3. Clods black peripheral
4. Lines thick reticular
5. Lines radial segmental
6. Lines white
7. Lines angulated
8. Lines parallel ridges (volar) or chaotic (nails)
9. Vessels polymorphic.

Melanoma should also be suspected and excluded even in non-chaotic lesions, on the basis of the four exceptions presented in the 'Chaos and Clues' method including:
1. New or changing lesions on adults.
2. Small or nodular lesions with any of the nine defined clues to melanoma.

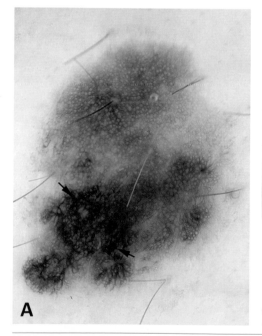
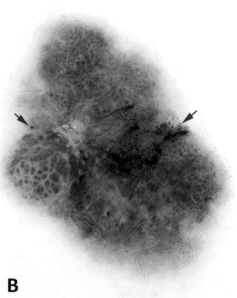

A

B

Figure 8.3: *Dermatoscopic images of two pigmented skin lesions, one with one pattern (pigmented) lines reticular (A) and the other with a primary pattern of (white) lines reticular (B). Additional clues to the specific correct diagnosis of melanoma in each case include: in (A) grey structures (blue arrow) and focal thick lines reticular (black arrows); in (B) grey structures, an eccentric structureless (grey) area (blue arrow) and peripheral black dots (red arrows).*

3. Lesions on the head and neck with pigmented circles or dermatoscopic grey.
4. Parallel ridge pattern (volar skin).

As clarified in *Chapter 6* the presence of an exception does not automatically mandate the need for excision biopsy. For example, many solar lentigines on the face will have pigmented circles, but if the other morphological features expected in solar lentigo (e. g. sharply demarcated scalloped border, regular short curved lines) are present then biopsy is not necessarily indicated[8]. Similarly, many congenital naevi on the face will have dermatoscopic grey centrally but if symmetry, a gradual border over the total periphery, and historical stability confirm the diagnosis of naevus, excision biopsy is not appropriate.

Naevus: the dermatoscopic features of the various categories of melanocytic naevi are described in detail in *Section 9.2*.

Benign keratinocytic lesions

The majority of benign keratinocytic lesions, including solar lentigo and ink-spot lentigo, melanotic macule, seborrhoeic keratosis and LPLK can confidently be distinguished from melanoma and naevus based on clinical and/or dermatoscopic morphology.

Solar lentigines: with one pattern, lines reticular (thin or thick), lines curved or a structureless pattern, solar lentigines are expected to have one colour, brown, and an abrupt border over the total periphery which is commonly scalloped in parts. Any shades of brown are expected to have a gradual transition[8].

The ink spot lentigo variant: has a distinct morphology with a single colour (black or dark brown) and a pattern of reticular, or more often branched, lines ending very abruptly and 'broken off' at the periphery (*Figure 8.4A*).

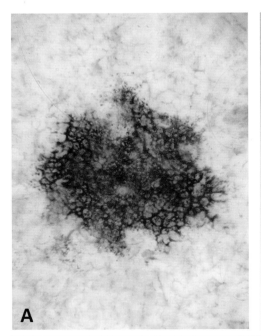 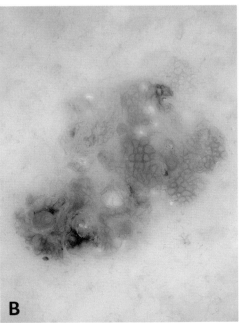

A **B**

Figure 8.4: Dermatoscopic images of two pigmented skin lesions. In (A) there is one pattern of lines branched, sharply cut-off at the periphery and one colour, brown, consistent with an ink spot lentigo. In (B) there is more than one pattern with a primary pattern of lines reticular. Orange and white clods combined with a sharply demarcated border are clues to the specific diagnosis of seborrhoeic keratosis.

Melanotic macules: with the exception of some melanotic macules of the lip, melanotic macules (e.g. of the genitalia and nail matrix) are not expected to have a reticular pattern but rather a lines curved or structureless pattern.

Seborrhoeic keratosis: if a reticular solar lentigo becomes acanthotic it then becomes raised and this is one form of transition from solar lentigo to seborrhoeic keratosis. The morphology will be similar to solar lentigo but additional clues to seborrhoeic keratosis may appear, including thicker curved lines and white dots and clods. Seborrhoeic keratoses with multicomponent patterns, including a primary pattern of lines reticular (*Figure 8.4B*) are not uncommon. Frequently they are asymmetrical and may have clues to malignancy including grey colour, thick lines reticular, peripheral black clods/dots and even segmental radial lines. Such lesions may require careful assessment because it is possible for melanoma to arise in collision with seborrhoeic keratosis or for parts

of a melanoma to mimic seborrhoeic keratosis. If there are clues to malignancy, multiple seborrhoeic keratosis criteria should be present for a benign diagnosis to be made. These may include multiple orange and white clods, thick curved lines and an abrupt border over the total periphery. The authors regard the feature of the total abrupt border to be critical if a diagnosis of seborrhoeic keratosis is to be made in such a situation. If that is not present the lesion should be considered for excision biopsy.

Lichen planus-like keratosis: this is a diagnosis made by the pathologist when a lesion has undergone immune regression. The original lesion is often a solar lentigo or seborrhoeic keratosis and LPLK frequently display portions of the precursor lesion. Another clue to the precursor lesion can be the 'skeletal morphology' of that lesion revealed by the pattern of grey dots correlating with residual melanin in melanophages. For a detailed description of the morphology of LPLK see *Section 9.4.3*.

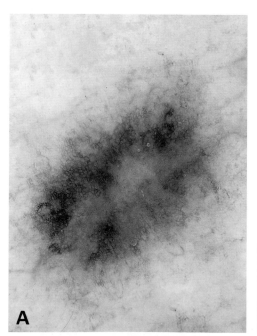 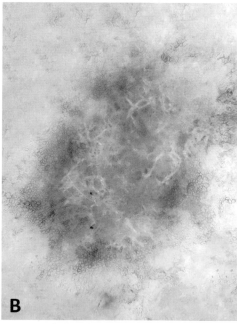

Figure 8.5: Dermatoscopic images of two pigmented skin lesions, both of which have a primary pattern of lines reticular. The peripheral arrangement of the reticular lines combined with a paler central structureless area (A) and central white lines (B) are consistent with a diagnosis of dermatofibroma in both cases.

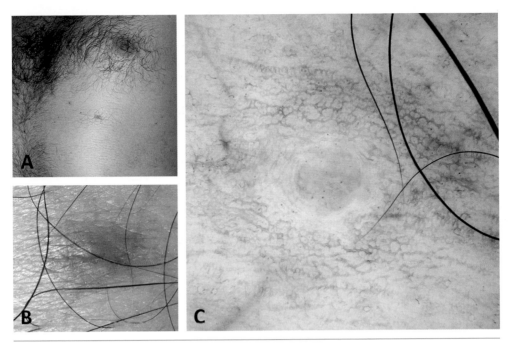

Figure 8.6: *Clinical (A), close-up (B) and dermatoscopic (C) images of a pigmented skin lesion with a primary pattern of lines reticular surrounding a central structureless area. It is located in the anatomical 'milk line'; accessory nipple.*

Dermatofibroma

While a DF cannot have a single pattern of reticular lines, it commonly presents with a central hypopigmented structureless area and a pattern of lines reticular (or circles or clods) peripherally (*Figure 8.5*). For a detailed description of the morphology of DF see *Section 9.6*.

Other

An accessory nipple can also have a primary pattern of lines reticular with a central structureless pattern, but the anatomical context should prevent confusion (*Figure 8.6*).

A pattern or primary pattern of lines angulated

A lesion with one pattern, lines angulated, or a lesion with more than one pattern but with a primary pattern of lines angulated will be limited to the following categories (*Figures 8.7–8.9* and *4.7F*):

* **melanocytic**
* **benign keratinocytic**
* **pigmented AK/SCC** *in situ.*

These differential options are further sorted according to specific clues as detailed below and also in Sections 9.1–9.4.

Melanocytic

Melanoma: a lesion which has one pattern of angulated lines with chaos of colour, or which has a primary pattern of angulated lines combined asymmetrically with another pattern, should be excised on suspicion of malignancy, most likely melanoma[8]. While

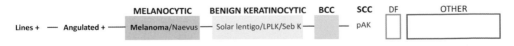

Figure 8.7: *Aide-memoire for a pattern, or primary pattern of lines angulated.*

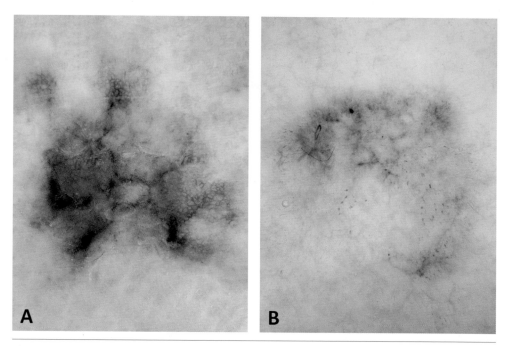

Figure 8.8: *Dermatoscopic images of two pigmented lesions each with a pattern of lines angulated. The lesion shown in (A) arguably has a pattern of lines angulated-only, with the reticular lines scattered throughout the lesion not actually covering 20% of the lesion in any specific location; melanoma in situ. The lesion shown in (B) has a primary pattern of lines angulated combined with a structureless pattern; basal cell carcinoma. Because this is an extremely rare pattern in basal cell carcinoma it is not included in the aide-memoire – an incorrect prediction of melanoma will not impact the decision to biopsy.*

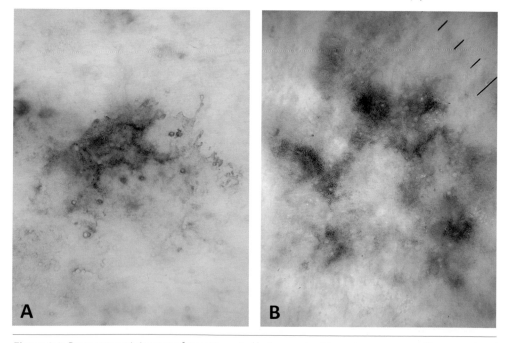

Figure 8.9: *Dermatoscopic images of two pigmented lesions each with a primary pattern of lines angulated combined with a structureless pattern: (A) solar lentigo, (B) seborrhoeic keratosis. Both lesions were excised on suspicion of malignancy.*

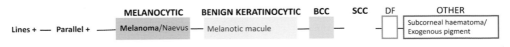

		MELANOCYTIC	BENIGN KERATINOCYTIC	BCC	SCC	DF	OTHER

Lines + —— Parallel + —— **Melanoma/Naevus** — Melanotic macule —— [ ] — [Subcorneal haematoma/ Exogenous pigment]

Figure 8.10: *Aide-memoire for a pattern or primary pattern of lines parallel on volar skin or nail apparatus.*

---

angulated lines may cover enough of a lesion to form a pattern it is extremely rare to see it as the only pattern on a lesion (*Figure 8.8A*).

Naevus: it is extremely uncommon to see a pattern of lines angulated in a naevus, and although symmetry and a uniform gradual border would favour that diagnosis, the index of suspicion should be very high for melanoma.

Benign keratinocytic

The clue of angulated lines, which may form complete or incomplete polygons[9], is occasionally seen in solar lentigo or seborrhoeic keratosis (*Figure 8.9*)[6].

Pigmented AK/SCC in situ

The pattern or clue of angulated lines may be seen in pAK/SCC *in situ* (*Figure 4.7F*). It may also very rarely be seen in BCC (*Figure 8.8B*) and although we have not included BCC in the aide-memoire for this pattern, this is not critical because if a BCC is mistaken for a melanoma it will be excised.

A pattern or primary pattern of lines parallel (volar skin)

A lesion on volar skin with one pattern, lines parallel, or with more than one pattern but with a primary pattern of lines parallel and which is pigmented by melanin will be restricted to the following categories (*Figures 8.10, 8.11A* and *8.12A*)[6]:

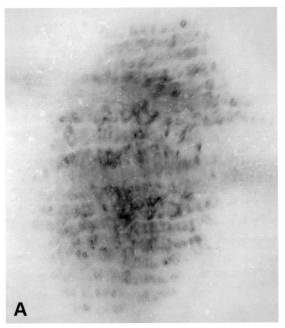

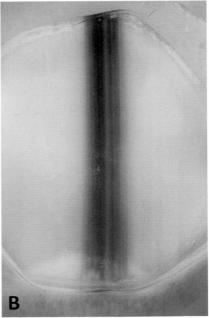

Figure 8.11: *Dermatoscopic images of two pigmented lesions. (A) A lesion on volar (plantar) skin with a pattern of lines parallel (on the broad dermatoglyphic ridges) peripherally, combined symmetrically with a structureless pattern centrally; melanoma in situ. (B) A nail plate (thumb) with lines parallel chaotic (varying in width interval and colour); melanoma in situ of the nail matrix.*

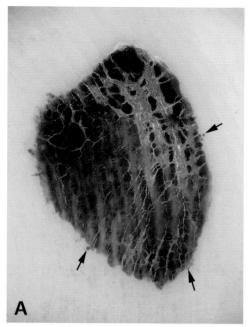 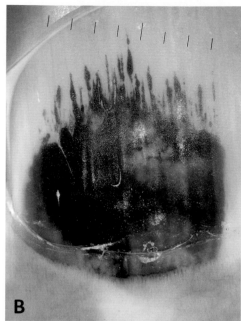

Figure 8.12: Dermatoscopic images of two pigmented lesions. (A) Lines parallel on the dermatoglyphic ridges of volar (plantar) skin; corneal haemorrhage. Arrows indicate the clue of satellite clods. (B) A primary pattern of lines radial segmental combined asymmetrically with a structureless pattern beneath a nail plate; subungual haematoma. The pigment in each case is haem, mimicking melanin.

- **melanocytic**
- **benign keratinocytic**
- **other.**

These differential options are further sorted according to specific clues as detailed below and also in Sections 9.1, 9.2 and 9.4.

Volar skin

Lines parallel on volar skin most commonly correlate with the dermatoglyphic furrows or ridges. A crossing pattern as a pattern of lines parallel on volar skin, with lines crossing both ridges and furrows should be resolved by tilting the dermatoscope each way at right angles to the direction of the lines, until the pattern resolves into either a furrow or ridge pattern.

Melanocytic

Melanoma: a solo pattern of lines parallel on volar skin in which the lines, pigmented by melanin, are located on the dermatoglyphic ridges, is a clue to volar melanoma (*Figure*

8.11A) but can also rarely be seen with any type of volar (acral) naevus. Clues to naevus include onset in youth combined with long term stability, but the index of suspicion should be high with any parallel ridge pattern on volar skin; evidence of onset at mature age and/or of change should lead to consideration of an appropriate biopsy. Of course, very large size or variations in pigment density in poorly defined lesions may be additional clues to melanoma. It should be remembered that melanomas in these locations may be very lightly pigmented but with small areas of subtle ridge-pattern pigmentation.

A lesion with a primary pattern of lines parallel in the furrows combined asymmetrically with any other pattern should raise suspicion for melanoma arising in a naevus and a careful search for clues to malignancy is warranted (see *Figure 6.29*).

Naevus: a solo pattern of lines parallel on volar skin in the dermatoglyphic furrows and pigmented by melanin is consistent with the diagnosis of volar (acral) naevus.

A primary pattern of lines parallel, in the furrows, combined with another pattern, may be consistent with a diagnosis of naevus if the lesion is concentrically symmetrical and there are no clues to melanoma. But, if the lesion is asymmetrical and there are any of the described clues to melanoma then, as mentioned in the previous section, the possibility of melanoma arising in association with a naevus must be considered.

Very rarely pSCC *in situ* **(pigmented Bowen's disease):** may be associated with a chaotic pattern of lines parallel on volar skin[6].

Other

Parallel patterns on volar skin can be caused by pigments other than melanin:

- **Blood:** a pattern of lines parallel on volar skin, pigmented by blood products, is due to intracorneal haemorrhage, a common additional clue being the presence of satellite clods (*Figure 8.12A*).
- **Exogenous pigment:** including that caused by silver nitrate treatment to warts can also result in a ridge pattern[6].

Nail apparatus

A lesion on the nail plate with one pattern, lines parallel, and which is pigmented by melanin will be restricted to the following categories:

- **melanocytic**
- **benign keratinocytic.**

A solo pattern of lines parallel on the nail plate, extending from the proximal nail fold or lunula to the free edge of the nail plate is known variously as longitudinal melanonychia or melanonychia striata[6]. It is consistent with a process in the germinal nail matrix which is transferring melanin to the stratum corneum and therefore into the developing nail plate.

Melanocytic

Melanoma: if the onset is in adulthood and the lines are chaotic (varying in width interval and colour) with change over time the diagnosis is consistent only with melanoma (*Figure 8.11B*).

While pigmentation of adjacent soft tissue (Hutchinson's sign) is an additional clue to melanoma of the nail matrix it can also be seen in benign conditions including congenital naevus and trauma. Micro-Hutchinson's sign (pigmentation of the nail cuticle) is a reliable clue to melanoma (see *Figure 9.12*).

As a general rule, any longitudinal melanonychia of a single nail, with onset after puberty, and with progression, should be considered for biopsy.

Naevus: if the onset is in childhood and the lines are regular in width, interval and colour, with stability over time, then the predicted diagnosis is congenital naevus of the nail matrix. Acquired naevi are not expected in the nail matrix.

Benign keratinocytic

Melanotic macule: may occasionally produce a pattern of lines parallel on the nail plate (usually the pigmentation will be structureless) but it will be expected to occur on multiple nails, this being compelling evidence against a diagnosis of melanoma.

Other causes of apparent nail pigmentation (blood, trauma, some drugs and pSCC *in situ*) are expected to cause structureless, often grey, pigmentation of the nail plate rather than lines parallel.

Subungual haematoma may initially extend distally from the proximal nail fold and typically has lines radial at the distal edge, which does not necessarily extend to the

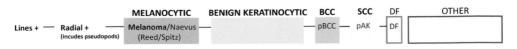

Figure 8.13: Aide-memoire for a pattern, or primary pattern of lines radial.

free edge of the nail plate (*Figure 8.12B*). As it clears proximally, convex morphology will be evident at the proximal border.

A pattern or primary pattern of lines radial

A lesion with one pattern, lines radial, or a lesion with more than one pattern but with a primary pattern of lines radial: will be limited to the following categories (*Figures 8.13–8.17*):

- **melanocytic**
- **BCC**
- **SCC**
- **DF.**

These differential options are further sorted according to specific clues as detailed below and also in Sections 9.1, 9.2, 9.3, 9.5 and 9.6.

The pattern of lines radial always occurs in combination with another pattern (*Figures 8.14–8.17*)[6].

For radial lines to cover a sufficient area to rate as a pattern they would generally need to be circumferential.

Focal or segmental radial lines will generally rate as a clue rather than a pattern but will be discussed here. If the lesion is asymmetrical then the radial lines must be segmental and this is a clue to malignancy, either melanoma, pBCC or pSCC *in situ* (*Figures 8.15A and 8.16*)[4].

Melanocytic

Melanoma and naevus: the radial lines will be connected to either lines reticular, a pigmented structureless area, or to pigmented clods as heavily pigmented as the radial lines (*Figure 8.14 and 8.15*)[8].

Naevus: if an otherwise symmetrical lesion with circumferential radial lines has a centre that is structureless and brown, black or grey,

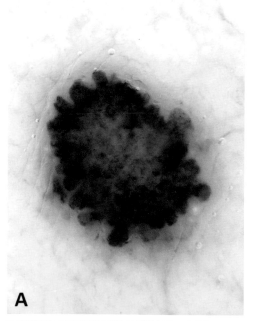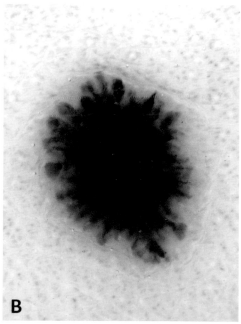

Figure 8.14: Dermatoscopic images of two arguably symmetrical pigmented lesions each with a circumferential pattern of lines radial (including pseudopod type) or alternatively they may reasonably be described as peripheral clods. In such a situation the pattern can be regarded as a single pattern indicating peripheral growth and the provisional diagnosis depends heavily on the context. (A) This lesion with arguably symmetrical but internally disorganised morphology, on a 60-year-old, is consistent with melanocytic malignancy; nodular melanoma diameter 3mm and Breslow thickness 0.9mm. (B) This symmetrical lesion on an 8-year-old is predictably benign; Reed naevus.

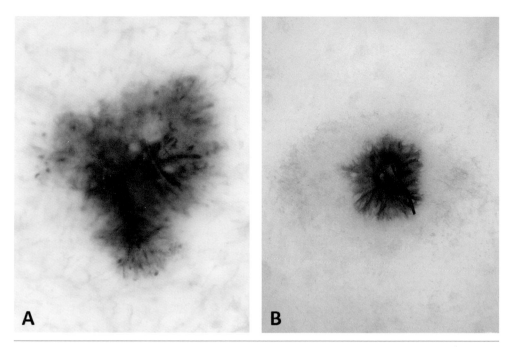

Figure 8.15: *Dermatoscopic images of two pigmented lesions both with a primary pattern of lines radial combined with a structureless pattern. (A) A chaotic lesion with lines radial segmental; melanoma in situ; (B) a symmetrical lesion; recurrent naevus.*

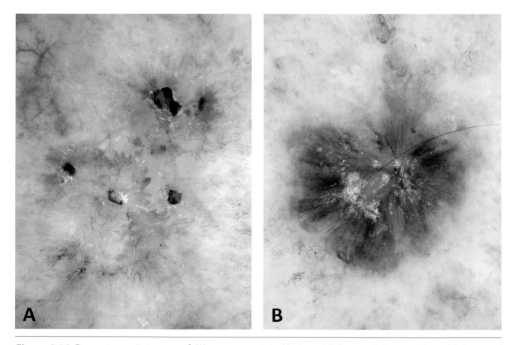

Figure 8.16: *Dermatoscopic images of: (A) an asymmetrical lesion with lines radial converging which extend from hypopigmented areas; BCC; and (B) an arguably symmetrical lesion with lines radial peripheral formed partly at least of dots in linear arrangement, combined with a central structureless area and surface scale; pigmented squamous cell carcinoma in situ.*

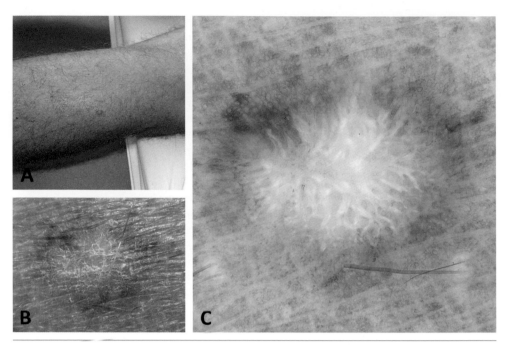

Figure 8.17: Clinical (A), close-up (B) and dermatoscopy (C) images of a pigmented lesion with a primary pattern of lines reticular peripherally combined symmetrically with a central pattern of white lines radial surrounding in turn a white structureless centre; dermatofibroma.

or alternatively with a pattern of dark clods (with the radial lines being of a similar colour), that favours a diagnosis of Reed naevus (*Figure 8.14B*) or recurrent naevus (*Figure 8.15B*).

Basal cell carcinoma
In pBCC the radial lines at the periphery will be segmental rather than circumferential and are expected to converge (*Figure 8.16A*), and this convergence may or may not be to a central clod, dot or line. Radial lines, converging to a central point within a lesion rather than at the periphery, are highly specific for BCC[10]. Also in BCC, in contrast to melanoma, the radial lines may project from a hypopigmented area (*Figure 8.16A*)[8].

Squamous cell carcinoma
In pigmented Bowen's disease (pSCC *in situ*) radial lines peripheral segmental are usually composed of dots in linear arrangement (*Figure 8.16B*)[11].

Dermatofibroma
A stable symmetrical lesion with a pattern of radial lines (pigmented or white) surrounding a structureless pale centre will predictably be a DF (*Figure 8.17*).

A pattern or primary pattern of lines radial with a terminal clod (lines radial – pseudopod type)
A lesion with more than one pattern but with a primary pattern of lines radial (pseudopod type) will be limited to a single category (*Figure 8.14*):
- **melanocytic.**

The specific diagnosis is further sorted according to specific clues as detailed below and also in Sections 9.1 and 9.2.

Melanocytic
A lesion with a pattern of lines radial (pseudopod type) will always have this pattern in combination with another

pattern and its diagnosis is restricted to the melanocytic category only (*Figure 8.14*)[6]. While lines radial (pseudopod type) have been described in seborrhoeic keratosis that entity is not expected to have that as a pattern.

Melanoma: a primary pattern of lines radial (pseudopod type) circumferential will occur in combination with a central pattern which may be structureless (*Figure 8.14A*) or have a pattern of clods (*Figure 8.14B*). In all cases after puberty the differential diagnosis of such a lesion includes melanoma (*Figure 8.14A*) and Reed, or rarely, Spitz naevus.

Although dermatoscopic descriptions should be independent of factors such as age, such factors are relevant to treatment decisions. After puberty all such lesions, whether symmetrical or not, should be excised to exclude spitzoid melanoma[12].

Lines radial (pseudopod type) which are segmental will be unlikely to cover a large enough area to rate as a pattern and will therefore be relevant as a clue to malignancy, specifically melanoma.

Naevus: before puberty, a darkly pigmented symmetrical lesion with the morphology of circumferential lines radial (pseudopod type) can reliably be predicted to be a Reed naevus (*Figure 8.14B*).

A pattern or primary pattern of lines curved

A lesion with one pattern, lines curved, or a lesion with more than one pattern but with a primary pattern of lines curved will be limited to the following categories (*Figures 8.18–8.20*)[6]:

- **melanocytic**
- **benign keratinocytic.**

These differential options are further sorted according to specific clues as detailed below and also in Sections 9.1, 9.2 *and* 9.4.

A skin lesion with one pattern, lines curved, which has one colour, brown, can be a naevus, solar lentigo, or a seborrhoeic keratosis. A lesion with more than one pattern including a primary pattern of lines curved can in addition have a differential diagnosis of melanoma.

A primary pattern of lines curved, combined with a secondary pattern, can be combined with any of the other non-linear patterns and if it has only one colour, brown, is also likely to be a solar lentigo or a seborrhoeic keratosis whether symmetrical or not. If any other colours of melanin are present a careful search for clues to melanoma is necessary before making a diagnosis of either seborrhoeic keratosis or LPLK.

Melanocytic

Melanoma: expected to have dermatoscopic chaos (often including chaos of border abruptness) as well as one or more clues to malignancy (see *Section 6.3*).

Naevus: expected to have a gradual border over the total periphery (in contrast to a solar lentigo/seborrhoeic keratosis) and usually to have biological symmetry without clues to melanoma (see *Sections 6.3* and *9.2*).

Benign keratinocytic

Solar lentigo: expected to be flat and to have a uniformly abrupt border which is frequently scalloped in part (*Figure 8.19*).

Seborrhoeic keratosis: expected to be raised and to have a uniformly abrupt border. Additional clues to seborrhoeic keratosis may be present.

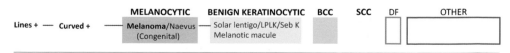

Figure 8.18: Aide-memoire for a pattern, or primary pattern of lines curved.

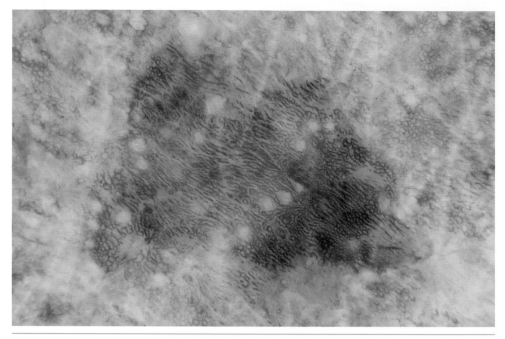

Figure 8.19: *Dermatoscopic image of a pigmented lesion with a pattern of lines curved; solar lentigo.*

Melanotic macule: may present as a pigmented lesion with a pattern, or primary pattern of lines curved, on mucosal surfaces (*Figure 8.20*). A mucosal lesion with one pattern, lines curved (and/or structureless), on the lip or genitalia, which is small and well circumscribed and confined to vermillion skin or mucosa is predictably a (non-melanocytic) melanotic macule. On the lip these lesions have a high prevalence in geographic locations of high UV index such as Australia and New Zealand. They commonly exhibit some grey colour but their specific morphology, confinement to vermillion lip and history of stability should save them from any surgical intervention (*Figure 9.72*). While penile melanotic macules should also be recognised by their symmetry, small size and demarcation, melanotic macules on the labia minora are likely to be large and poorly circumscribed and this may mandate biopsy (*Figures 8.20* and *9.73*).

8.3.2 A pattern or primary pattern of circles

A lesion with one pattern, circles, or a lesion with more than one pattern but with a primary pattern of circles will be limited to the following categories (*Figures 8.21–8.26A*)[6]:

- **melanocytic**
- **benign keratinocytic**
- **SCC**
- **DF.**

These differential options are further sorted according to specific clues as detailed below and also in Sections 9.1, 9.2, 9.4, 9.5 and 9.6.

Melanocytic

Melanoma: a pattern of *pigmented* circles-only which correlate with follicles on the head or neck is a significant clue to melanoma, regardless of colour (*Figures 8.22A* and *8.25A*)[13]. The differential diagnosis is solar lentigo if

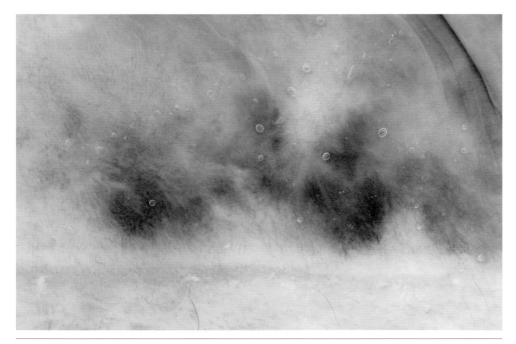

Figure 8.20: *Dermatoscopic image of a large asymmetrical pigmented lesion on the labia minora with a primary pattern of lines curved. A biopsy was necessary to establish the diagnosis; melanotic macule.*

they are brown (*Figure 8.23A*), and pigmented AK (*Figure 8.23B*), pSCC *in situ* or LPLK if they are grey. Unless the unequivocal morphology of a solar lentigo/seborrhoeic keratosis is present biopsy may be necessary to resolve the diagnosis.

While pigmented brown circles defining follicles are occasionally seen in melanomas on the trunk and extremities, they are not regarded as a clue to melanoma at these locations because they commonly occur in benign lesions (*Figure 8.26B*).

For *asymmetrical* patterns which include a primary pattern of pigmented circles defining follicles on the head or neck, the diagnosis of melanoma must be very strongly suspected[8]. Such a pattern elsewhere on the body should be assessed according to previously defined clues to melanoma (see *Section 6.3*) which

means that the pigmented circles would be regarded as a clue to melanoma only if they were grey[4].

Naevus: not expected to have a pattern of circles.

Benign keratinocytic

Solar lentigo: a pattern of brown pigmented circles on facial skin, correlating with follicular openings, in a lesion with a uniformly sharply demarcated scalloped border is consistent with a diagnosis of solar lentigo.

Unlike a pattern of pigmented *circles* on facial skin, which can be a clue to melanoma in some lesions, the pattern of structureless pigment on facial skin *interrupted by follicular openings* has no diagnostic significance at all,

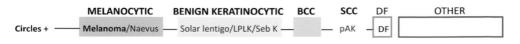

	MELANOCYTIC	BENIGN KERATINOCYTIC	BCC	SCC	DF	OTHER
Circles + ——	Melanoma/Naevus ——	Solar lentigo/LPLK/Seb K ——	——	pAK —	DF	

Figure 8.21: *Aide-memoire for a pattern or primary pattern of circles.*

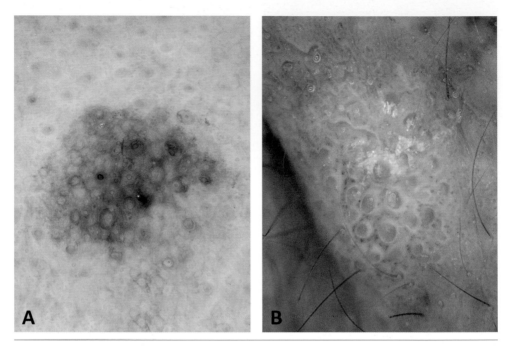

Figure 8.22: *Dermatoscopic images of two lesions each with a pattern of circles only. (A) A pigmented lesion on the face with a pattern of pigmented circles related to follicular openings; melanoma in situ. (B) A raised non-pigmented lesion on the ear with a pattern of white circles; squamous cell carcinoma.*

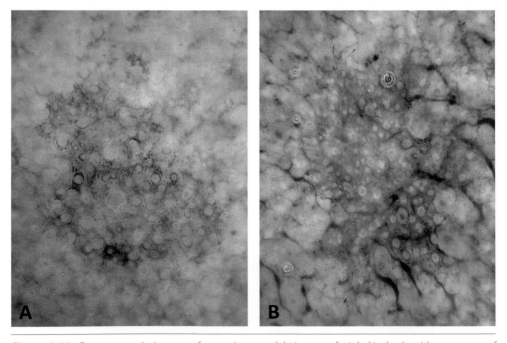

Figure 8.23: *Dermatoscopic images of two pigmented lesions on facial skin both with a pattern of pigmented circles related to follicular openings. (A) Solar lentigo and (B) pigmented actinic keratosis. In both cases chaos of border abruptness led to excision biopsy to resolve the diagnosis.*

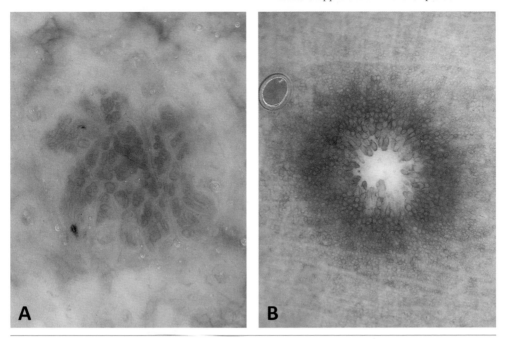

Figure 8.24: *Dermatoscopic images of two pigmented lesions each with a pattern of pigmented circles. (A) A pattern of distorted pigmented circles-only, unrelated to follicular openings, is consistent with a diagnosis of seborrhoeic keratosis; (B) a pattern of pigmented circles unrelated to follicular openings and with a gradual transition from large to small circles, combined symmetrically with a central structureless white area is consistent with a diagnosis of dermatofibroma.*

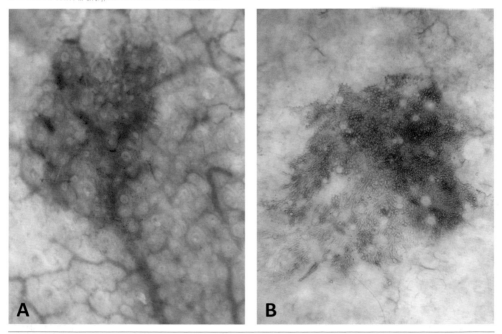

Figure 8.25: *Dermatoscopic images of two pigmented lesions located on facial skin. Predictably at this location the pigment is interrupted by follicular openings. In (A) a pattern of grey circles in a lesion with chaos of border abruptness is a compelling clue to the correct diagnosis of melanoma in situ, while in (B) the follicular openings (there are no circles) which interrupt the monotonous pigmented pattern of lines reticular/ curved are of no diagnostic significance; solar lentigo.*

apart from being a clue that the lesion is on facial skin. In fact this is the most common pattern of facial solar lentigo (*Figure 8.25B*).

Seborrhoeic keratosis: a pattern of circles pigmented by melanin can be caused by either pigment in follicular epithelium[13] or, alternatively, by basal hyperpigmentation in the presence of acanthosis which causes the individual units of the rete ridge reticular pattern to be separated from each other and appear as circles. Pigmented circles which do not correlate with follicular structures, commonly being distorted, should therefore be regarded as correlating with reticular lines altered by acanthosis, making them a compelling clue to seborrhoeic keratosis (*Figures 8.24A* and *8.26A*). They may be present in pSCC *in situ* but will be in a linear arrangement as a clue to that diagnosis.

In *Figure 8.26A* the lesion consists of one pattern circles (they are not clods because the centre is lightly pigmented compared to the periphery) with one colour brown (the degree of colour variation is not significant and there is a gradual transition, which is not consistent with the disorganised behaviour expected of malignant tissue). The circles are not related to follicles and are caused by basal hyperpigmentation of acanthotic rete ridges. Such a lesion is predictably a seborrhoeic keratosis and the sharply demarcated border is an additional clue to that diagnosis. The lesion shown in *Figure 8.26B* has a pattern of very regular fine reticular and short curved lines interrupted by a few pigmented circles which are related to follicles. Although there is some grey colour and the lesion is not perfectly symmetrical, with edges not sharply demarcated, the diagnosis of seborrhoeic keratosis was made with confidence due both to the pattern and the additional clue of a palpably rough surface texture.

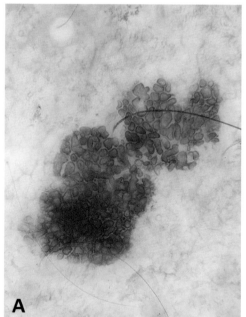 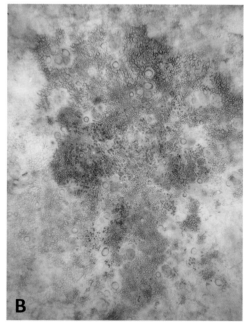

Figure 8.26: *Dermatoscopic images of two lesions on the torso which contain pigmented circles. The lesion in (A) which has one pattern, circles, not related to follicles, and one colour brown (the transition from light to dark brown is gradual), is a seborrhoeic keratosis. The lesion in (B) has circles related to follicles and the intervening pattern of very regular fine reticular and curved lines (which take priority over the pigmented circles), combined with a palpably rough texture, is consistent with a diagnosis of seborrhoeic keratosis.*

Squamous cell carcinoma

A pattern of white circles (whiter than surrounding skin) in a flat lesion on the head or neck is a clue to AK or SCC *in situ* and, if combined symmetrically or asymmetrically with a pattern of grey dots in a flat lesion on the head or neck, it is consistent with pAK or pSCC *in situ*. These dots may be randomly distributed between the white circles or they may surround them as grey circles, concentrically located around the white circles.

A pattern of white circles in a *raised* non-pigmented lesion on the head or neck had a specificity of 87% for SCC/KA in one series studied (*Figure 8.22B*)[14].

Dermatofibroma

A primary pattern of pigmented circles which is combined symmetrically as a peripheral pattern with a central structureless area, with or without the clue of central polarising-specific white lines, is consistent with a DF (*Figure 8.24B*). For practical purposes there are no other symmetrical combinations of a pattern of circles with clod, dot or structureless patterns.

8.3.3 A pattern or primary pattern of clods

A lesion with one pattern, clods, or a lesion with more than one pattern, but with a primary pattern of clods, can fall into six categories (*Figure 8.27*) but if vascular lesions (red clods), DF and pSCC *in situ* are excluded (dots-only type clods), then the differential diagnosis is limited to only three categories[6]:

- **melanocytic**
- **benign keratinocytic**
- **BCC.**

These differential options are further sorted according to specific clues as detailed below and also in Sections 9.1–9.4 (Figures 8.28 *and* 8.29).

A lesion with one pattern, clods, and one colour is assessed according to colour of the clods.

A lesion with one pattern, clods, and more than one colour is sorted according to symmetry and specific clues.

Lesions with a primary pattern of clods associated with another pattern can only be associated with structureless patterns and again the differential diagnosis will be sorted according to symmetry and specific diagnostic clues.

Melanocytic

Melanoma: if a lesion has one pattern, clods, and more than one colour, and if the dominant pigment is melanin, then asymmetry of colour combined with one or more clues to melanoma (*Figure 8.28A*) will mandate biopsy to exclude or confirm that diagnosis. Similarly, a primary pattern of clods combined asymmetrically with a structureless pattern will require biopsy on suspicion of melanoma if any clues to that diagnosis are present. If there is a secondary pattern of an eccentric structureless pattern, then that alone will constitute a clue to malignancy, either BCC (*Figure 8.29A*) or melanoma, and that differential will be sorted by specific clues.

Naevus:

A lesion with one pattern clods and one colour:

- If the clods are brown a confident prediction of naevus can be made. Most commonly this will be a congenital naevus, although Spitz naevus can also present with a pattern of brown clods.
- If the clods are skin-coloured the differential diagnosis includes congenital naevus, but also seborrhoeic keratosis. Vessels may

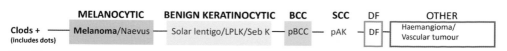

	MELANOCYTIC	BENIGN KERATINOCYTIC	BCC	SCC	DF	OTHER
Clods + (includes dots)	Melanoma/Naevus	Solar lentigo/LPLK/Seb K	pBCC	pAK	DF	Haemangioma/ Vascular tumour

Figure 8.27: *Aide-memoire for a pattern or primary pattern of clods.*

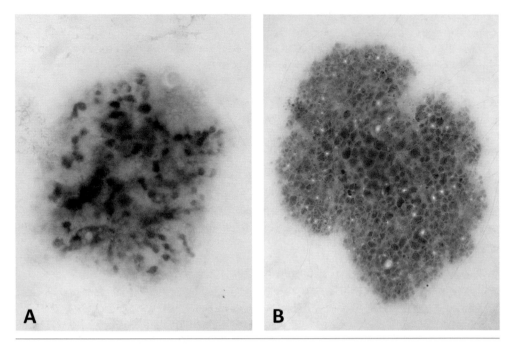

Figure 8.28: *Dermatoscopic images of two pigmented lesions each with a pattern of clods-only. (A) A pattern of clods varying in size, shape and colour, and with two colours, brown and grey, is suspicious for malignancy; melanoma in situ; and (B) a pattern of brown and white clods with symmetry – gradual transition from large to small and dark brown to light brown, is consistent with a diagnosis of (congenital) naevus.*

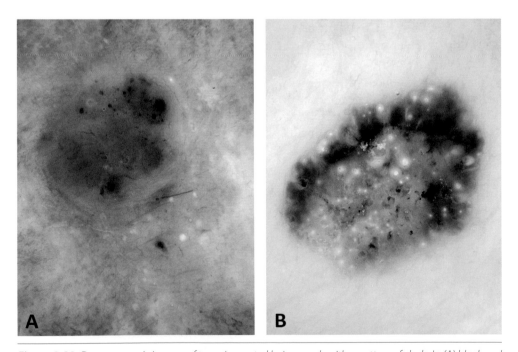

Figure 8.29: *Dermatoscopic images of two pigmented lesions each with a pattern of clods. In (A) black and blue clods/dots combined asymmetrically with a structureless pattern are consistent with a diagnosis of basal cell carcinoma; in (B) a pattern of white clods/dots supports the provisional diagnosis of seborrhoeic keratosis.*

be seen in the centre of the skin-coloured clods in both of these lesions (centred vessel pattern) and, although the historical context may be required to make the distinction, that is not critical because both are benign.

A lesion with one pattern clods and more than one colour: assessed according to whether the dominant pigment is a colour of melanin. If the dominant pigment is melanin and the lesion is symmetrical it will be predicted to be a naevus, congenital (*Figure 8.28B*) or Spitz, although if the lesion breaks the pattern of the patient's other naevi, and some clods are grey, symmetrical melanoma should be considered (*Figure 8.28A*).

A lesion with more than one pattern, with a primary pattern of clods (the other patterns being limited to structureless): if it is symmetrical it will be expected to be either a congenital (including combined), Clark or Spitz naevus. In each case a structure-less centre combined with peripheral clods is the hallmark of a growing naevus. While this is expected in adolescence and young adult-hood, the dermatoscopic clue to change, of peripheral clods, should alert the clinician to the possibility of a symmetrical melanoma at mature age (*Figure 8.14A*).

A lesion with more than one pattern, with a primary pattern of clods which is *asymmetrical* and melanin is the dominant pigment, with only *one colour present*: the diagnosis of naevus (congenital-type or Spitz) is expected.

A lesion with more than one pattern, with a primary pattern of clods which is *asymmetrical* and melanin is the dominant pigment, and *more than one colour* is present: the differential diagnosis includes melanoma, BCC (*Figure 8.29A*) and seborrhoeic keratosis (*Figure 8.29B*) and this differential will be resolved by specific clues to each of those options (see *Sections 9.1, 9.3* and *9.4*).

Benign keratinocytic
A diagnosis of solar lentigo is effectively excluded by the presence of clods.

Seborrhoeic keratosis:

A lesion with one pattern, clods, and one colour:
- If the clods are orange and the lesion has a sharply demarcated border this is consistent with a diagnosis of seborrhoeic keratosis.
- If the clods are yellow, white or skin-coloured the differential diagnosis includes seborrhoeic keratosis as well as congenital naevus.

A lesion pigmented by the colour of melanin with one pattern, clods, and more than one colour: if no clues to malignancy are present, seborrhoeic keratosis is the likely diagnosis.

A lesion with more than one pattern, with a primary pattern of clods, which is *asymmetrical*: if the clods are yellow and/or white a diagnosis of seborrhoeic keratosis will also be predicted.

BCC:

A lesion with one pattern, clods, and one colour:
- If the clods are blue a confident prediction of BCC is possible.
- If the clods are orange and the lesion does not have a sharply demarcated border this is consistent with a diagnosis of BCC, the orange clods being due to ulceration. Other clues to BCC will also be expected to be present such as absence of lines reticular/branched as well as any of: fine linear serpentine vessels set in BCC stroma; lines radial segmental converging and/ or extending from hypopigmented areas; a clod within a clod; polarising-specific white lines.

A lesion with more than one pattern, with a primary pattern of clods, which is *asymmetrical* and the clods are orange: it will be either a BCC or a seborrhoeic keratosis with those alternatives being sorted by specific clues (see *Sections 9.3* and *9.4*).

A pigmented lesion with one pattern, clods, and more than one colour, or with more than one pattern including a primary pattern of pigmented clods, which is asymmetrical: the diagnosis is resolved by clues. The presence of specific clues to BCC (as listed above) favours that diagnosis (*Figure 8.29A*).

When the pattern of clods is limited to dots only, the differential diagnosis is almost as large as for a structureless pattern (*Figures 8.30–8.33*).

A solo pattern of dots can be sorted on the basis of colour (*Figure 8.30*).

A pattern of brown dots may be seen in a Clark naevus or pSCC *in situ*. A pattern of grey dots may occur in an LPLK (*Figure 8.33A*), pigmented actinic (solar) keratosis, pSCC *in situ* (*Figure 8.33B*) or a melanoma (*Figure 8.31A*). On the face a melanoma may have only one pattern, dots, and one colour, grey – in other words it may be symmetrical (*Figure 8.31A*). A further specific clue to pSCC *in situ* is that the dots may be in a linear arrangement (*Figure 8.33B*)[11].

A pattern of dots combined with the only possible secondary pattern, structureless, is also sorted according to the colour of the dots (*Figure 8.32*). If the dots are brown then solar lentigo and congenital naevus are added to the differential diagnoses of that of a solo pattern of brown dots. If the dots are grey the options are the same as for a solo pattern of brown dots, with the addition of BCC (*Figure 8.31B*). If there are blue dots the likely diagnosis is BCC. The occurrence of black dots is a clue to melanoma if some are peripheral, with a differential diagnosis of Clark naevus.

8.3.4 A structureless pattern

A lesion with one pattern, structureless, being the least specific of all can fall into any of the six categories (*Figures 8.34–8.38*)[6]:
- **melanocytic**
- **benign keratinocytic**
- **BCC**
- **SCC**
- **DF**
- **other.**

These differential options are further sorted according to specific clues as detailed below and also throughout Chapter 9.

The possibilities are numerous but they can be sorted by colours and the arrangement of these colours, plus the clues seen due to pigmented structures, even though these are insufficient to form a pattern. In lightly pigmented structureless lesions vessels may be seen and, although they do not contribute to any pattern of pigmented structures, these vessels may provide clues to the diagnosis. For example, a structureless lesion may display a polymorphous pattern of vessels including a dot pattern as a clue to the diagnosis of melanoma (*Figure 8.38*). Small fragments of reticular lines, if also present, could add additional weight to this evidence. It is also true that any component of lesional reticular lines effectively rules out the diagnosis of BCC or SCC.

The differential diagnoses of structureless lesions according to colour are shown in *Figure 8.35*.

A structureless pattern which is one colour, black, is usually caused by an old

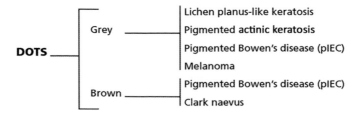

Figure 8.30: *Flowchart for the differential diagnosis of a pattern of dots. Abbreviation: pIEC (pigmented intraepidermal carcinoma). Reproduced from* Dermatoscopy, *2nd Edition, 2016*[6], *with permission.*

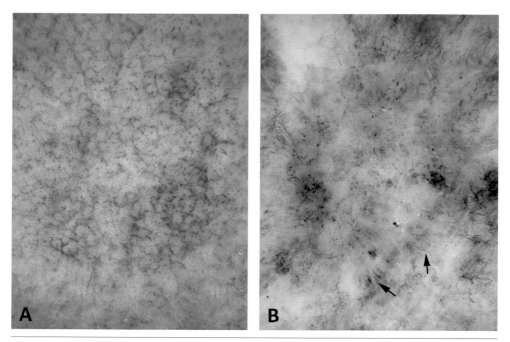

Figure 8.31: *Dermatoscopic images of two pigmented lesions each with a pattern of dots. (A) A pattern of dots-only, one colour grey, on the face, lacking the abrupt border of a solar lentigo or lichen planus-like keratosis and not having the morphology of a congenital naevus required an excisional biopsy; melanoma in situ. (B) A pattern of dots-only, one colour grey, and a clue of lines radial segmental extending from a hypopigmented area (arrows) was consistent with the diagnosis of pigmented basal cell carcinoma.*

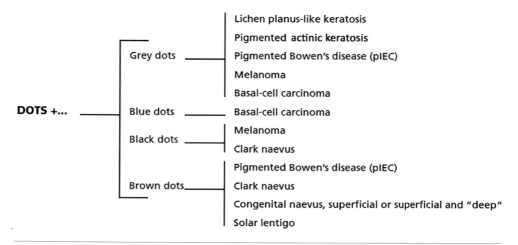

Figure 8.32: *Flowchart for the differential diagnosis of a pattern of dots combined with a structureless pattern. Abbreviation: pIEC (pigmented intraepidermal carcinoma). Reproduced from* Dermatoscopy, *2nd Edition, 2016, with permission.*

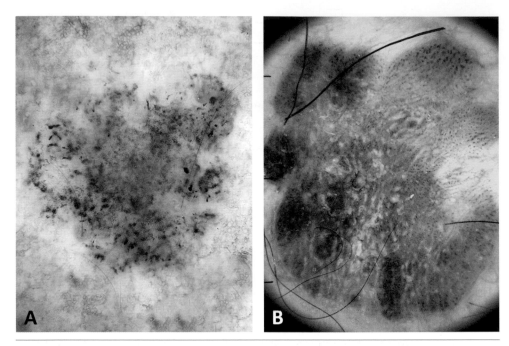

Figure 8.33: *Dermatoscopic images of two pigmented lesions each with a pattern of dots. (A) A pattern of dots-only, one colour grey, with a sharply demarcated border was consistent with a differential diagnosis of lichen planus-like keratosis. Excision biopsy was performed due to chaos of border-abruptness; lichen planus-like keratosis. (B) A primary pattern of pigmented dots (and non-pigmented dots) in linear arrangement (upper right), combined asymmetrically with an eccentric structureless pattern, was consistent with a provisional (and histological) diagnosis of pigmented squamous cell carcinoma in situ.*

haemorrhage into or onto the skin (*Figure 8.36*) or by thrombosis of a haemangioma, while one pattern structureless red is most consistent with a fresh haemorrhage into the stratum corneum. Very rarely a Clark naevus, Reed naevus or melanoma can be structureless and black. A structureless blue lesion is consistent with a blue naevus (*Figure 8.37A*) unless there is a history which raises the likelihood of melanoma metastasis. A structureless brown lesion can be an ephelis, solar lentigo or pSCC *in situ*.

A structureless pattern with more than one colour is sorted according to whether the dominant pigment is melanin or not (*Figure 8.35*). If white, yellow or orange pigment is dominant the possibilities include seborrhoeic keratosis, BCC and amelanotic melanoma. If red colour dominates then the likely diagnosis is a fresh haemorrhage in the stratum corneum. If melanin pigment is dominant and the colours are combined symmetrically then a diagnosis of naevus is expected (congenital, congenital combined,

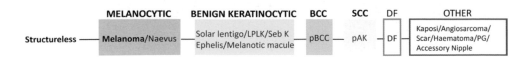

Figure 8.34: *Aide-memoire for a structureless pattern.*

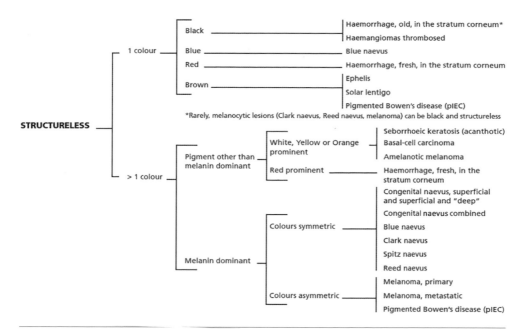

Figure 8.35: *Flowchart for the stepwise analysis of clues for pigmented lesions with one pattern, structureless. Abbreviation: pIEC (pigmented intraepidermal carcinoma). Reproduced from* Dermatoscopy, *2nd Edition, 2016, with permission.*

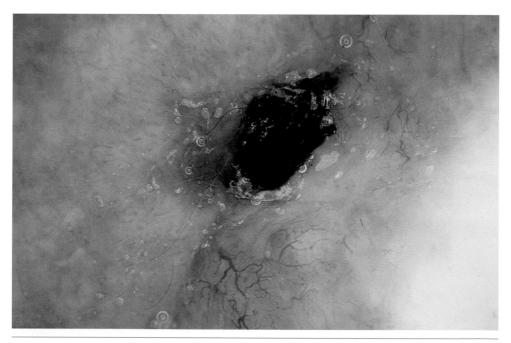

Figure 8.36: *Dermatoscopic image of a pigmented lesion with a primary structureless black pattern due to blood clot on an ulcerated BCC.*

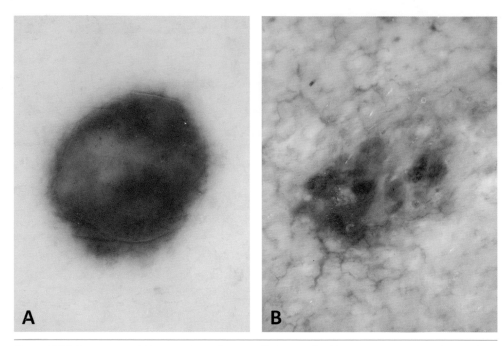

Figure 8.37: *Dermatoscopic images of two pigmented lesions each with one pattern, structureless, and one colour, blue. (A) Blue naevus (variations in colour intensity blue–grey–brown, with gradual transition, can be interpreted as one colour, blue being dominant); (B) venous lake (the pigment being haem rather than melanin), an additional clue being blanching with compression.*

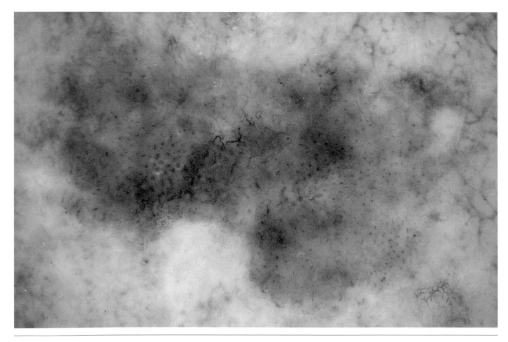

Figure 8.38: *Dermatoscopic image of a structureless pigmented lesion. There is more than one colour and colours of melanin (brown and grey) predominate, being combined asymmetrically; melanoma invasive.*

blue, Clark, Spitz, or Reed). If melanin pigment is dominant and the colours are combined asymmetrically then the differential diagnosis includes melanoma, primary or metastatic, and pSCC *in situ*.

The lightly pigmented lesion shown in *Figure 8.38* has one pattern, structureless, with the small area of grey dots constituting a clue to malignancy, although being insufficient for a pattern. In addition to the

clues of asymmetry of colour (brown, grey, pink and white), this lesion has polymorphous vessels including patterns of both linear (serpentine) and dot vessels, pointing correctly to the diagnosis of melanoma. Note the feature of peripheral structureless brown, this being reported as a clue to hypopigmented melanoma[15]. It is also of relevance that a significant proportion of melanomas, like this one, do not have any reticular lines.

References

1. Pehamberger H, Steiner A, and Wolff K. *In vivo* epiluminescence microscopy of pigmented skin lesions. I. Pattern analysis of pigmented skin lesions. *J Am Acad Dermatol*, 1987;17:571.
2. Kittler H. Dermatoscopy: introduction of a new algorithmic method based on pattern analysis for diagnosis of pigmented skin lesions. *Dermatopath Pract Concept*, 2007;13:3.
3. Kittler H, Riedl E, Rosendahl C, and Cameron A. Dermatoscopy of unpigmented lesions of the skin: a new classification of vessel morphology based on pattern analysis. *Dermatopath Pract Concept*, 2008;14:4.
4. Rosendahl C, Cameron A, McColl I, and Wilkinson D. Dermatoscopy in routine practice – "Chaos and Clues." *Aust Fam Physician*, 2012;41:482.
5. Rosendahl C, Cameron A, Tschandl P, Bulinska A, Zalaudek I, and Kittler H. Prediction without pigment: a decision algorithm for non-pigmented skin malignancy. *Dermatol Pract Concept*, 2014;4:59.
6. Kittler H, Rosendahl C, Cameron A, and Tschandl P. *Dermatoscopy*, 2nd Edition, 2016. Facultas.
7. www.scionpublishing.com/DaSC [accessed 26 August 2022].
8. https://dermoscopedia.org [accessed 26 August 2022].
9. Keir J. Dermatoscopic features of cutaneous non-facial non-acral lentiginous growth pattern melanomas. *Dermatol Pract Concept*, 2014;4(1):77.
10. Trigoni A, Lazaridou E, Apalla Z, *et al.* Dermoscopic features in the diagnosis of different types of basal cell carcinoma: a prospective analysis. *Hippokratia*, 2012;16:29.
11. Cameron A, Rosendahl C, Tschandl P, Riedl E, and Kittler H. Dermatoscopy of pigmented Bowen's disease. *J Am Acad Dermatol*, 2010;62:597.
12. Gelbard SN, Tripp JM, Marghoob AA, *et al.* Management of Spitz nevi: a survey of dermatologists in the United States. *J Am Acad Dermatol*, 2002;47:224.
13. Tschandl P, Rosendahl C, and Kittler H. Dermatoscopy of flat pigmented facial lesions. *J Eur Acad Dermatol Venereol*, 2015;29:120.
14. Rosendahl C, Cameron A, Argenziano G, Zalaudek I, Tschandl P, and Kittler H. Dermoscopy of squamous cell carcinoma and keratoacanthoma. *Arch Dermatol*, 2012;148:1386.
15. Menzies SW, Kreusch J, Byth K, *et al.* Dermoscopic evaluation of amelanotic and hypomelanotic melanoma. *Arch Dermatol*, 2008;144:1120.

CHAPTER 9

Dermatoscopic features of common and significant lesions: pigmented and non-pigmented

9.1 Melanoma: pigmented and non-pigmented

For practical purposes melanomas, both pigmented and hypo- or non-pigmented, can be subdivided into the following subtypes:
- superficial spreading melanoma (SSM)
- lentiginous melanoma (including lentigo maligna)
- nodular melanoma (NM)
- desmoplastic melanoma
- mucosal melanoma.

Superficial spreading melanoma: the most common subtype, especially in areas of relatively lower UV incidence. It typically has a prolonged radial growth phase, during which it remains *in situ*, before going into a vertical growth phase. Even if thick nodules develop it still remains defined as SSM and does not convert into NM.

Lentiginous melanoma: commonly occurs on sun-damaged skin and when on the face and still *in situ* it is known as lentigo maligna (LM), which was previously known as Hutchinson's melanotic freckle. When lentigo maligna becomes invasive it is known as lentigo maligna melanoma (LMM).

Lentiginous melanoma also occurs on the non-sun-exposed volar sites of the palms and soles (volar melanoma, commonly known as acral melanoma) and the nail matrix (nail matrix melanoma). Lentiginous melanoma, like SSM, also typically has a radial growth phase preceding a vertical (invasive) growth phase.

Nodular melanoma: differs from both SSM and lentiginous melanoma because, although it may have an epidermal component overlying the invasive component, it is believed to commence in the dermis as an invasive melanoma in vertical growth. By definition there is no superficial component beyond three rete ridges from the invasive component. Depending on Breslow thickness, NM has the same prognosis as the other subtypes but, because it is more often thicker when diagnosed, NM accounts for a higher proportion of deaths from melanoma.

Desmoplastic and mucosal (oral mucosa, vermillion lips, labia minora and glans penis) melanomas: relatively rare subtypes and mentioned here only briefly for complete-ness.

9.1.1 Pigmented melanoma

Melanoma is a proliferation of malignant melanocytes so it is not surprising that the majority of melanomas contain melanin. When present, melanin provides an abundance of diagnostic clues due to the chaotic behaviour of the melanocytes with respect to both their pigment production and their presence in various levels of the skin, apart from the expected location at the dermoepidermal junction (*Figures 9.1–9.6*).

The diagnostic clues to pigmented melanoma have been described systemat-ically in *Chapter 6* and also, with respect to those with reticular lines, in *Section 8.3.1*.

9.1.2 Hypomelanotic and amelanotic melanoma

While hypomelanotic melanoma is not uncommon (*Figure 9.7*), melanoma without any pigment at all is rare and the diagnosis of amelanotic melanoma is more likely to be delayed. In this situation recognition of the significance of a new and changing pink lesion is necessary. Compared to an amelanotic flat (junctional) naevus, a melanoma is expected to have a pinker, or even red, colour due to the increased blood flow in a malignant lesion, with irregularly defined margins compared with the expected regular well-defined margins of a naevus.

With the passage of time an amelanotic melanoma, not being constrained in its growth, will declare itself by its incongruous size. It is, however, advantageous to make the diagnosis as early as possible and this is an example of the importance of not dismissing a patient's concern without first performing dermatoscopic assessment of the lesion[1]. Dermatoscopy of such a clinically bland lesion will predictably deliver clues to the alert dermatoscopist which may include any of ulceration (rare), white lines, vessel clues and white structureless areas following regression.

The diagnostic clues to non-pigmented lesions and dermatoscopic images of examples, including of amelanotic melanoma, are presented in *Chapter 7*.

9.1.3 Metastatic melanoma

While isolated cutaneous metastases of melanoma can be diagnostically challenging (*Figure 9.8*), the clinical context of a history of melanoma, or the presence of multiple lesions, should alert the clinician to that possi-bility. Because both NM and cutaneous metas-tases may have a normal overlying epidermis, distinction may even be a challenge dermato-pathologically.

9.1.4 Melanomas on palmar and plantar skin

Volar (commonly known as acral) melanomas located on volar skin (palms and soles) have a morphology modified by the dermatoglyphic ridges and furrows (*Figures 9.9–9.11*); the pigment tends to form parallel lines prefer-entially over the broad ridges correlating with a proliferation of malignant melano-cytes in relation to the eccrine ducts. As these melanomas proliferate further, such organisa-tion is likely to be replaced by chaotic growth with clues to melanoma evolving as in other locations (*Figure 9.11*).

9.1.5 Nail apparatus melanomas

Nail matrix melanomas are hidden from view in their early stages beneath the proximal nail fold and nail plate, but they may transfer melanin into the growing nail plate and become evident due to the resulting longitu-dinal pigment stripe known as melanonychia striata or longitudinal melanonychia (*Figures 9.12–9.14*). The stripe always extends to the full length of the nail plate, affecting a band of nail from the proximal nail fold to the free edge. Unlike nail matrix naevi, the parallel lines in nail matrix melanoma are expected to vary in width, interval and colour (lines parallel chaotic).

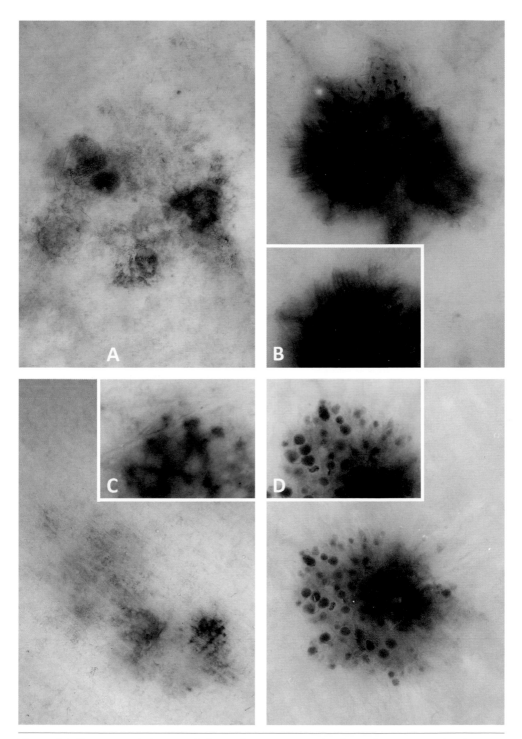

Figure 9.1: *Dermatoscopic images displaying features commonly observed in pigmented melanomas (insert images enlarged): (A) asymmetry of colours, (B) radial lines, (C) lines radial (pseudopod type) and (D) peripheral clods.*

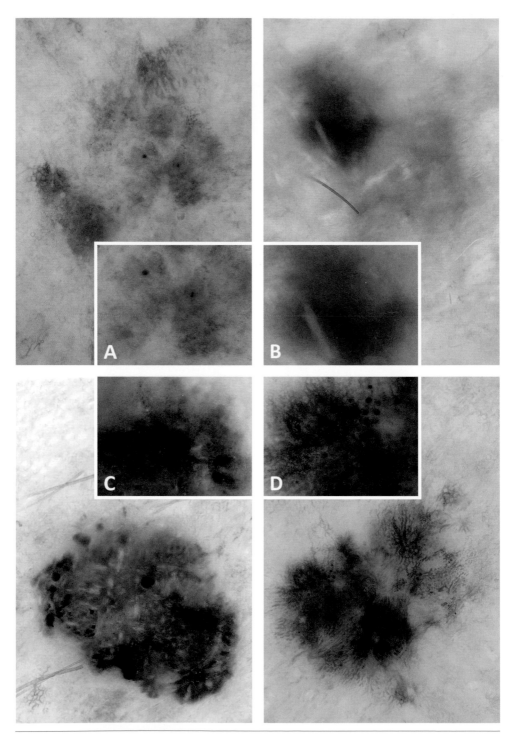

Figure 9.2: *Dermatoscopic images displaying features commonly observed in pigmented melanomas (insert images enlarged): (A) grey structures, (B) blue structures, (C) peripheral black clods and (D) peripheral black dots/clods.*

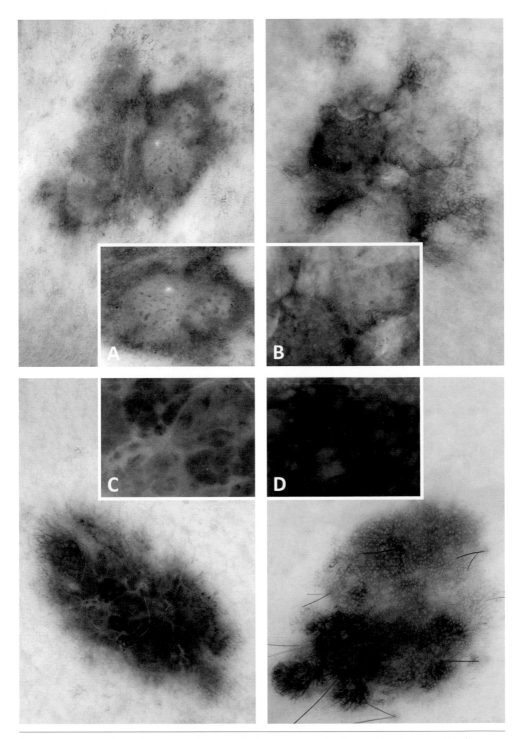

Figure 9.3: *Dermatoscopic images displaying features commonly observed in pigmented melanomas (insert images enlarged): (A) eccentric structureless areas, (B) angulated lines, (C) pigmented clods separated by skin-coloured lines ('inverse network') and (D) thick reticular lines.*

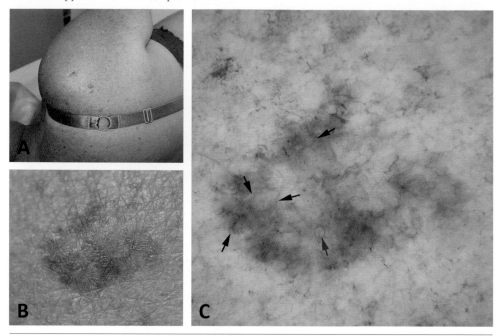

Figure 9.4: *Clinical (A), close-up (B) and dermatoscopic (C) images of a non-facial lentigo maligna (melanoma in situ) demonstrating dermatoscopic chaos plus grey structures and angulated lines (black arrows). A single grey circle (red arrow) would correlate with pigmented melanocytes extending into a follicle.*

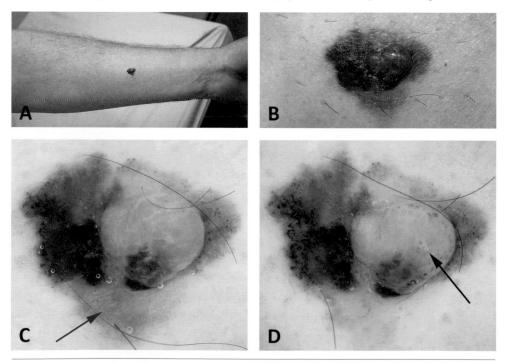

Figure 9.5: *Clinical (A), close-up (B) and dermatoscopic (C and D) images of a melanoma arising from a congenital naevus. This superficial spreading melanoma has a macular component with horizontal growth (red arrow) and an elevated portion with vertical growth (black arrow). While polymorphous linear vessels are seen in the elevated portion (D), increased footplate pressure in (C) blanches these vessels but reveals dot vessels in the macular portion.*

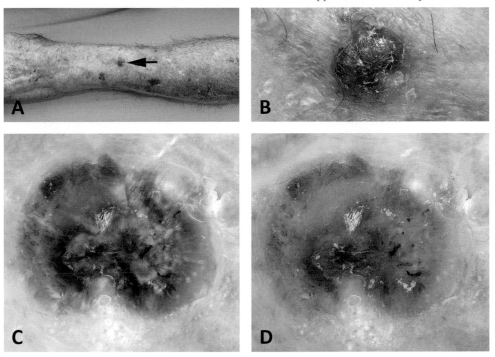

Figure 9.6: *Clinical (A), close-up (B) and dermatoscopic (C and D) images of a superficial spreading melanoma with an invasive portion. The deeply invasive portion appears as structureless blue in both polarised (C) and non-polarised (D) images, because the melanocytes in the vertical growth phase are producing melanin, whereas those that are in the horizontal growth phase are not pigmented, this portion appearing red.*

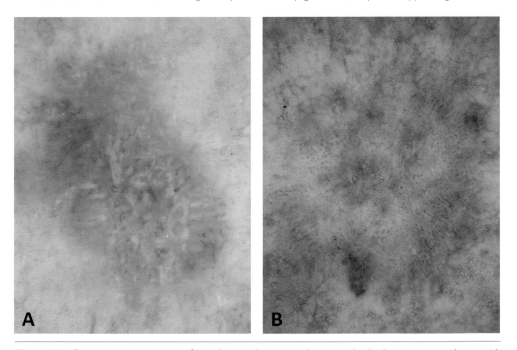

Figure 9.7: *Dermatoscopic images of two hypomelanotic melanomas, both demonstrating chaos with respect to the eccentric location of their focally pigmented components and with a polymorphous vessel pattern, including both linear and dot vessels. Polarising-specific white lines are also seen in (A).*

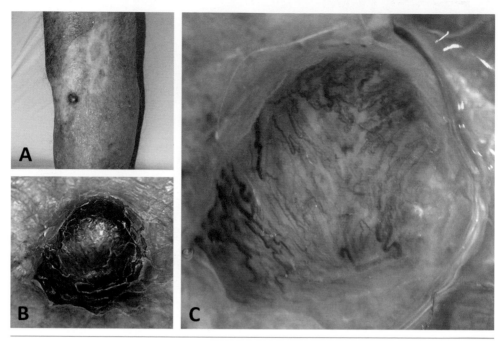

Figure 9.8: *Clinical (A), close-up (B) and dermatoscopic (C) images of a lesion of metastatic melanoma. Clinically (A and B) there is a well-defined red nodule which dermatoscopically displays linear serpentine and looped vessels over a red and white structureless background.*

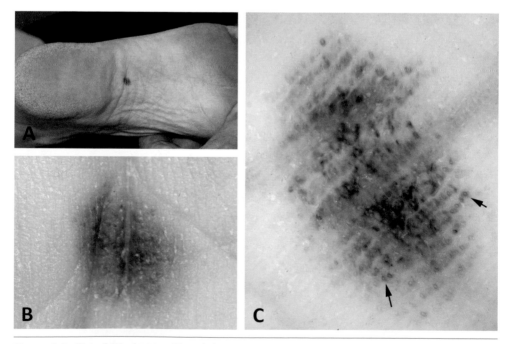

Figure 9.9: *Clinical (A), close-up (B) and dermatoscopic (C) images of a volar melanoma which has a symmetrical pattern of lines parallel on the broad dermatoglyphic ridges. This is best appreciated at the edges of the lesion. Arrows point to pigmented circles caused by the presence of pigmented melanocytes in eccrine duct openings, these eccrine openings defining the centre of the ridges.*

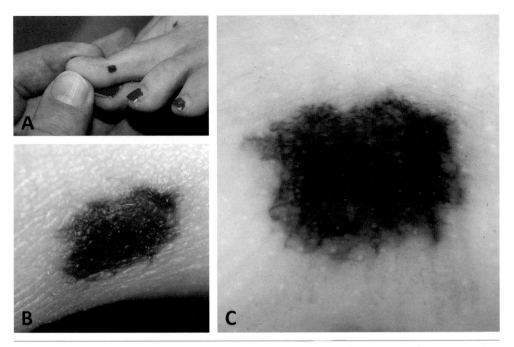

Figure 9.10: *Clinical (A), close-up (B) and dermatoscopic (C) images of a pigmented lesion situated on Wallace's line where volar (glabrous) skin meets non-glabrous skin. The volar pattern (inferiorly) is actually a parallel furrow pattern, but the lesion has irregularly dispersed portions on the non-glabrous component with thick reticular lines giving both chaos and a clue; melanoma in situ.*

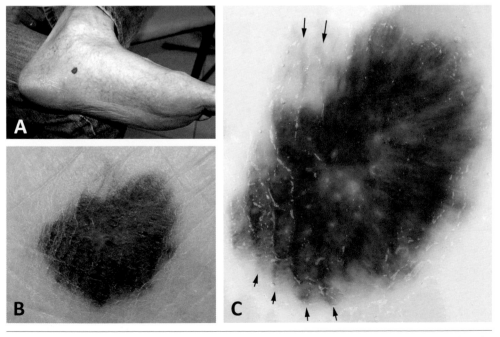

Figure 9.11: *Clinical (A), close-up (B) and dermatoscopic (C) images of a pigmented lesion situated on the foot. Dermatoscopically there is a parallel furrow pattern, best assessed at the margins (arrows), but over the upper and right sides of the image (C) a second pattern of lines radial segmental is evident; melanoma (invasive) associated with a volar naevus. Images courtesy Dr Agata Bulinska.*

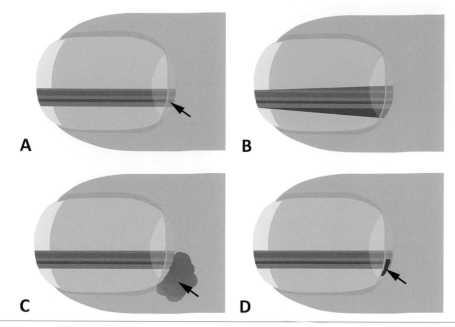

Figure 9.12: *Diagrammatic representations of nail apparatus displaying longitudinal melanonychia with lines parallel chaotic (varying in width, interval and colour) and: (A) pseudo-Hutchinson's sign – pigment visible through the translucent cuticle (arrow); (B) triangular morphology with a wider base signifying rapid growth; (C) Hutchinson's sign – pigmentation of the proximal and/or lateral nail folds (arrow); (D) micro-Hutchinson's sign – pigmentation of the cuticle (arrow).*

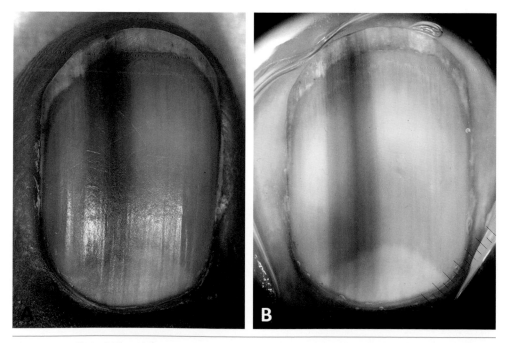

Figure 9.13: *Clinical (A) and dermatoscopic (B) images of the nail plate morphology associated with nail matrix melanoma. There is longitudinal melanonychia with lines parallel chaotic (varying in width, interval and colour) and the base is wider than the distal margin signifying growth of the lesion.*

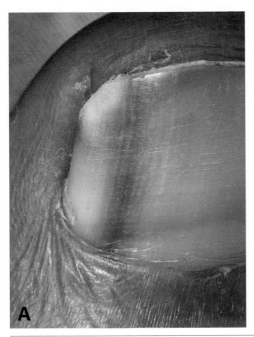
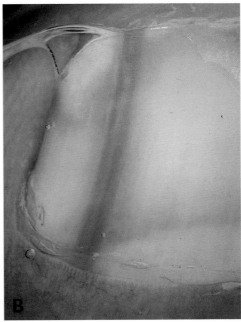

Figure 9.14: Clinical (A) and dermatoscopic (B) images of the nail plate morphology associated with nail matrix melanoma. There is longitudinal melanonychia with lines parallel chaotic (varying in width, interval and colour) but in this case the base is not evidently wider than the distal margin, consistent with a slow growth rate.

Non-pigmented nail matrix melanomas may not be recognised until they produce nail dystrophy, the clues being that the change will only involve a single nail and it will be longitudinal, affecting a band of nail from the proximal nail fold to the free edge.

Nail matrix biopsy

Biopsy to confirm nail matrix melanoma must be performed by a person trained and experienced in that technique. The location of the nail matrix is deep to the proximal nail fold and nail plate proximally and with its distal extremity defined by the lunula. Direct visualisation of the nail matrix to permit targeted examination of the nail matrix can be achieved by fenestration[2] or, more effectively, by elevation of the nail fold and nail plate analogous to lifting the bonnet of a car[3]. It is possible that nail matrix melanoma can be confirmed with histological slides stained with haematoxylin and eosin, but it cannot be excluded without immunoperoxidase stains[4].

9.2 Melanocytic naevi: pigmented and non-pigmented

Melanocytic naevi are expected to be symmetrical and, in contrast to solar lentigines and seborrhoeic keratoses, to have a gradual border over the total periphery. An exception to this may be seen with some congenital naevi which may have a seborrhoeic keratosis-like morphology, including an abrupt border over the total periphery. Melanocytic naevi may be pigmented (melanotic) or non-pigmented (amelanotic).

9.2.1 Basic classification of naevi

Basic classification of naevi:
- Acquired
  - Clark/dysplastic naevus (junctional if confined to the epidermis, otherwise compound)
  - Spitz naevus
  - Reed naevus.
- Congenital
  - superficial naevus
  - superficial and deep naevus
  - dermal
    - Miescher naevus (face)
    - Unna naevus (torso and limbs).
  - blue naevus.

We classify Clark (including so-called dysplastic), Spitz and Reed naevi as acquired naevi with others being classified as congenital. These include superficial congenital, superficial and deep congenital, dermal (Unna and Miescher) and blue naevi. The diagnosis of congenital naevi is determined by clinical, dermatoscopic and histological morphology rather than by a history of being visibly present at birth[5].

A variety of terms are used by dermatopathologists for various melanocytic naevi.

Naevi described as 'lentiginous' or 'junctional': these are acquired naevi.

'Halo naevus' and 'Meyerson's naevus': these both relate to an immune response, rather than a particular type of naevus, such processes occurring with both acquired and congenital naevi.

'Recurrent naevus': this refers to a melanocytic naevus which arises following trauma or incomplete biopsy of a pre-existing congenital or acquired naevus. Such a lesion may have a distinctive clinical, dermatoscopic and histological morphology which may overlap with the morphology of a melanoma. Clues to the diagnosis of a recurrent naevus include

a history of trauma or surgical manipulation combined with confinement of the naevus to a scar.

9.2.2 Pigmented acquired and congenital naevi

Pigmented Clark (acquired) naevi: these usually have a reticular or structureless pattern with brown colour, frequently darker centrally with any transition from dark brown (centrally) to light brown (peripherally) being gradual[6]. Clark naevi, if junctional, will be flat and if compound (the dermal component will be limited to the papillary dermis) they may be slightly raised. Examples of Clark naevi are shown in *Figures 9.15–9.19A* and *9.20*.

Pigmented congenital naevi: both compound and dermal may have a variety of symmetrical patterns, which may or may not include reticular/branched lines, clods, dots and structureless patterns, and their morphology frequently reveals their non-neoplastic, hamartomatous origin (*Figures 9.19B* and *9.21–9.29*). Terminal hair is a compelling clue to the hamartomatous nature of congenital naevi (*Figure 9.21*) and frequently other naevi with similar morphology, but lacking the terminal hair, will be seen on surrounding skin[5]. Congenital naevi, either superficial (dermal component confined to papillary dermis) or superficial and deep (dermal component extending into reticular dermis), are invariably raised or even papular and their soft consistency has led to the description of the dermatoscopic 'wobble sign'. Like Clark naevi, pigmented congenital naevi are expected to have a gradual border over the total periphery, but their dermatoscopic patterns are more variable and variants with a seborrhoeic keratosis-like morphology may have a uniformly abrupt border (*Figures 9.19B, 9.22C, 9.25C, 9.27* and *9.29*). Frequently the centre is raised and papular and this often has a pattern of clods, either skin-coloured or pigmented, with a linear pattern on any peripheral junctional component.

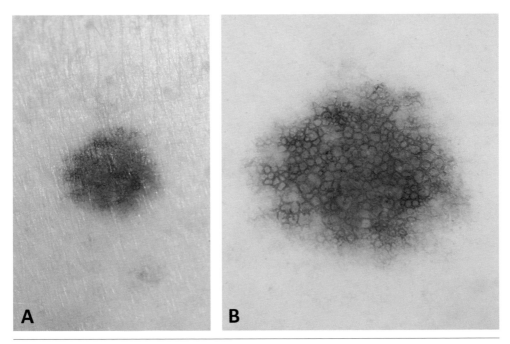

Figure 9.15: *Clinical (A) and dermatoscopic (B) images of a Clark naevus. Clinically the lesion is symmetrical and well circumscribed and dermatoscopically there is one pattern, lines reticular, and one colour, brown, with a gradual border over the entire periphery.*

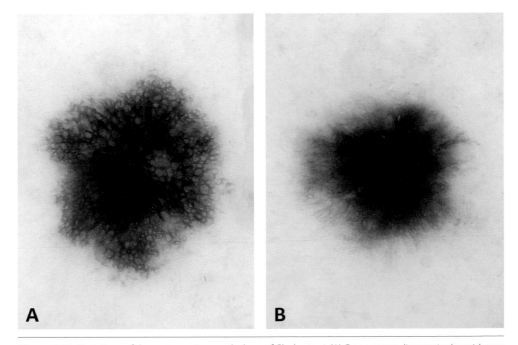

Figure 9.16: *Variations of dermatoscopic morphology of Clark naevi. (A) One pattern: lines reticular with two colours, black and brown, symmetrically combined concentrically with a darker centre, some of the central lines being thick. (B) Two patterns: central black structureless and peripheral brown lines, reticular and radial. Both lesions have a uniform gradual border over the entire periphery.*

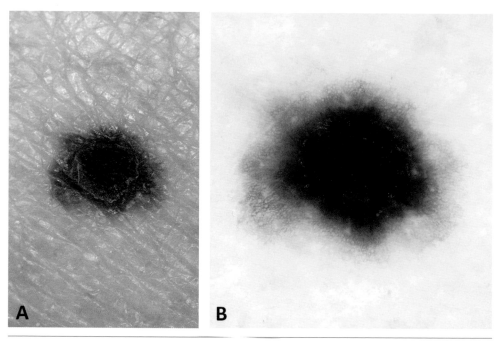

Figure 9.17: *Clinical (A) and dermatoscopic (B) images of a Clark naevus with central structureless black area due to hyperkeratosis of pigmented keratinocytes combined symmetrically/concentrically with peripheral reticular lines, the border being gradual over the total periphery.*

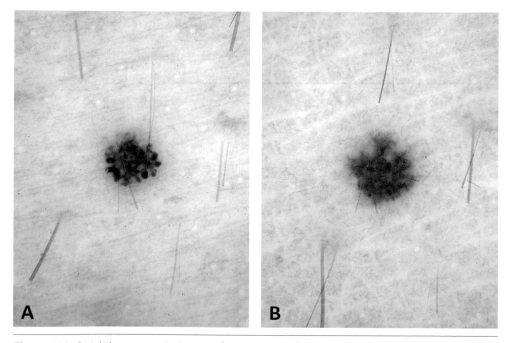

Figure 9.18: *Serial dermatoscopic images of a growing Clark naevus in a 25-year-old with central lines reticular and peripheral clods at baseline (A) and after 6 months (B) with one pattern, structureless. Both images display one colour, brown.*

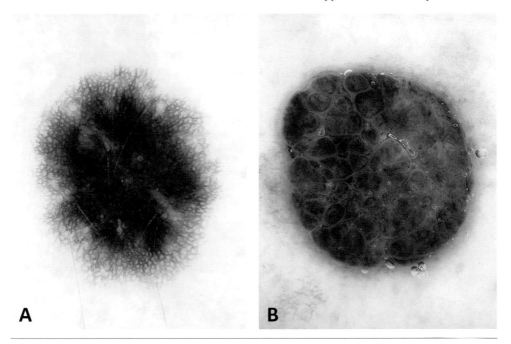

Figure 9.19: *Dermatoscopic images of a Clark naevus (A) with one pattern, lines reticular, and one colour, brown (light and dark brown with gradual transition are regarded as one colour), and a congenital naevus (B) with one pattern, clods, and one colour, brown. Both lesions have regularity of border abruptness with a gradual border in (A) and an abrupt border in (B).*

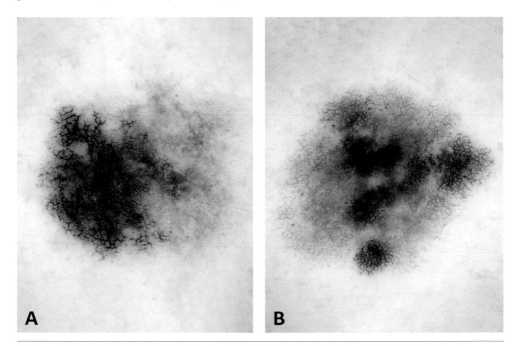

Figure 9.20: *Dermatoscopic images of Clark naevi both with chaos of border abruptness, some parts of the border being abrupt and some parts gradual. (A) Exhibits two patterns, lines reticular and structureless, asymmetrically combined and with the clue of eccentric structureless area; it was excised to exclude melanoma. (B) Displays one pattern, lines reticular, with two colours (light and dark brown with abrupt transition in some parts) and, due to asymmetry and the clue of thick reticular lines, it was also excised.*

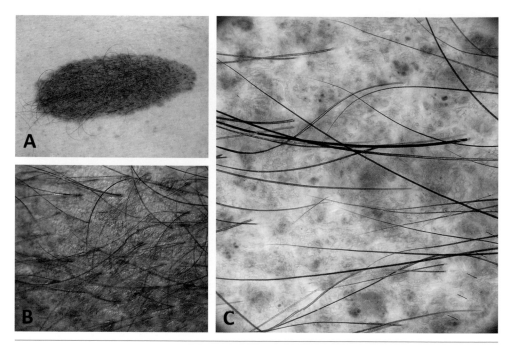

Figure 9.21: *Clinical (A), close-up (B) and dermatoscopic (C) images of a congenital naevus. The lesion is well circumscribed, with a uniform border, a structureless dermatoscopic pattern and lesional terminal hair as compelling evidence of its hamartomatous origin.*

9.2.3 Dysplastic naevus syndrome

Most patients who have been labelled as having so-called dysplastic naevus syndrome actually have multiple congenital naevi (*Figure 9.28*)[7]. The naevi on these patients are often large and morphologically variable as well as being numerous and, simply because of their high naevus count, these patients are at higher risk of melanoma (a naevus count of >100, any naevus type, confers a seven-fold relative risk of melanoma)[8]. Although most melanomas in this cohort will arise *de novo,* a small proportion may arise from the melanocytes within a naevus. When this happens, there is no transition between the naevus and the melanoma and a very frequent clue is *chaos of border abruptness*, with parts of the melanoma having an abrupt border while the naevus retains its gradual border[6]. Rapid screening for chaos of border abruptness in patients with multiple naevi has

proved fruitful for the authors in assessing such challenging patients. This does not negate the need for an assessment for chaos and clues and for digital monitoring, but it appears to be just as effective and this is worthy of further study.

With respect to a common misconception that dysplastic naevi are a precursor to melanoma, it has been shown in one study that non-dysplastic naevus remnants were more frequently associated with melanoma than dysplastic remnants (56.7% vs. 43.3%)[9]. In another study the most frequent subtype of melanoma-associated naevus remnants was the bland dermal naevus[10]. If you add the facts that the definition of 'dysplastic naevus' has changed several times, including the recent introduction of an arbitrary diameter criterion, and that concordance among pathologists in grading dysplasia is poor[11], any relevance of a diagnosis of dysplastic naevus is negated.

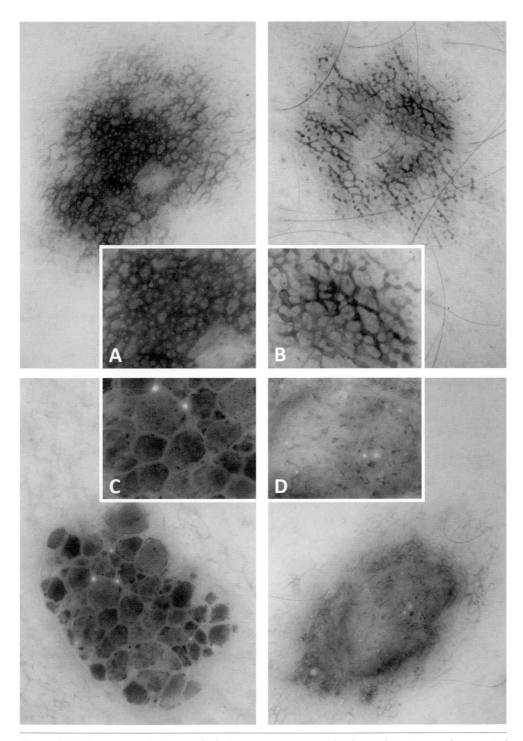

Figure 9.22: *Dermatoscopic images displaying patterns commonly observed in pigmented congenital naevi (insert images enlarged): (A) lines reticular, (B) lines branched, (C) clods, and (D) structureless.*

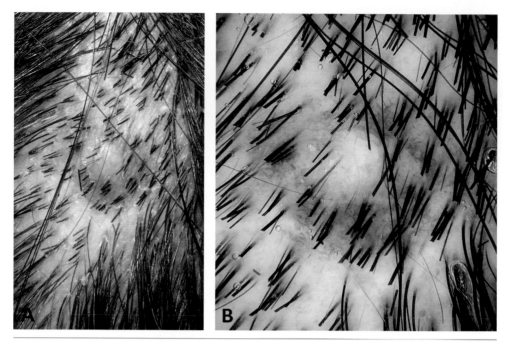

Figure 9.23: *Congenital naevi are always compound and will therefore often appear clinically raised as with this naevus on the scalp (A). Dermatoscopically (B) it is symmetrical with a hypopigmented central area, a peripheral pattern of lines, reticular/branched, and a uniformly gradual border. This morphology, commonly seen on the scalp, has been compared to a 'fried egg'.*

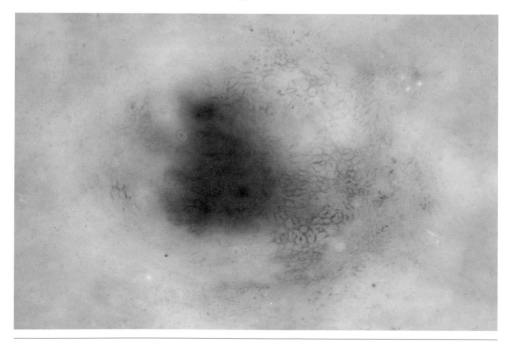

Figure 9.24: *Dermatoscopic image of a combined naevus with a central structureless blue pattern representing a blue naevus eccentrically located in combination with a peripheral pattern of brown lines, reticular, being the pattern of an associated congenital naevus. The eccentric location of the structureless blue component led to excision biopsy.*

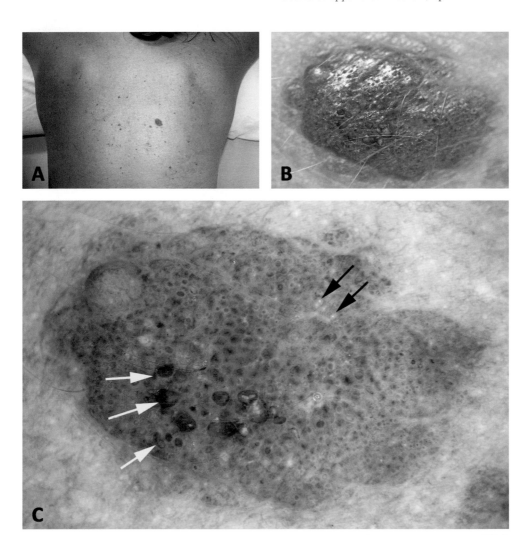

Figure 9.25: *Clinical (A), close-up (B) and dermatoscopic (C) images of a congenital naevus displaying dermatoscopic orange clods (yellow arrows) and white dots (black arrows). These structures correlate with exposed and enclosed keratin aggregations, respectively, being identical to the correlation of such structures when present in seborrhoeic keratoses. The border is uniformly abrupt, another similarity to seborrhoeic keratosis.*

9.2.4 Seborrhoeic keratosis-like features in congenital naevi

As mentioned previously, congenital naevi commonly share morphological features with seborrhoeic keratoses. One of these features, white clods due to keratin horn cysts, is further evidence of their congenital hamartomatous nature (*Figure 9.25*). In such situations other features, particularly the lack of additional clues to seborrhoeic keratosis and the presence of a gradual border, should prevent confusion. There are cases, however, where inquiry about the age of onset is necessary to distinguish congenital naevus from seborrhoeic keratosis. Although congenital naevi may not appear until teenage years the onset of a lesion in childhood effectively excludes a diagnosis of seborrhoeic keratosis.

When vessels are seen in congenital naevi they may be centred in clods (commonly seen in papillomatous components) or seen as dot or curved vessels (commonly seen in dermal naevi). In reality the so-called pattern

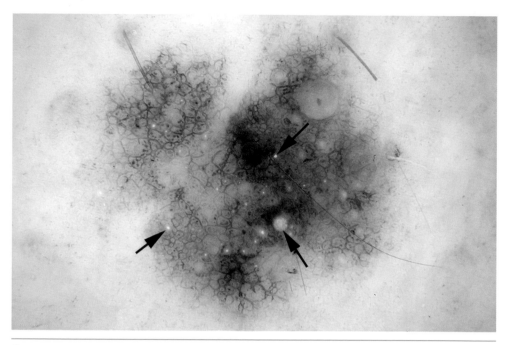

Figure 9.26: *Dermatoscopic image of a congenital naevus with a pattern of lines, reticular, and one colour, brown (light and dark brown with gradual transition are regarded as one colour), with white clods/dots (arrows). The gradual border over the majority of the periphery favours naevus over seborrhoeic keratosis, although the focally sharp border upper left (chaos of border abruptness) led to excision biopsy to exclude melanoma.*

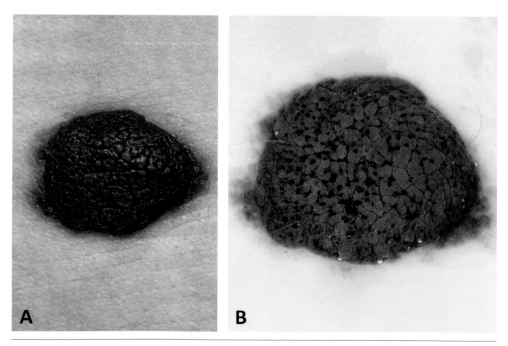

Figure 9.27: *Clinical (A) and dermatoscopic (B) images of a congenital naevus with a pattern of black and brown clods; in some places the brown clods are aggregated into thick curved lines giving a morphological appearance termed 'brain-like' by some. Black clods in the sulci between the brown clods correlate with heavily pigmented aggregates of exposed keratin.*

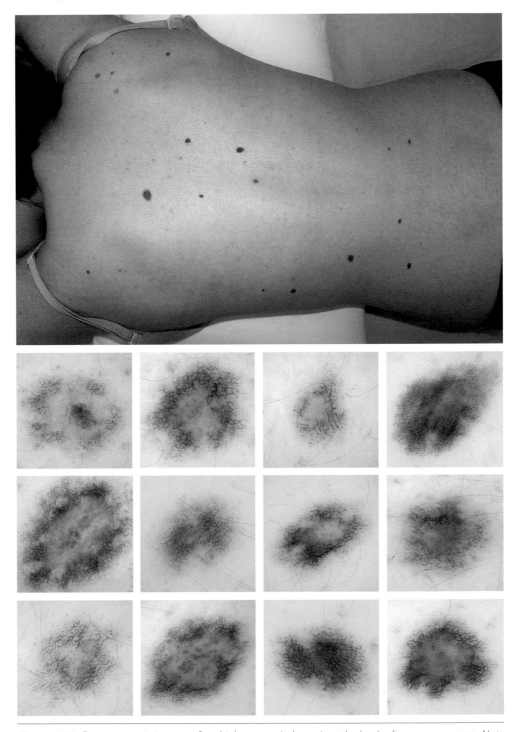

Figure 9.28: *Dermatoscopic images of multiple congenital naevi on the back of a young woman. Note that they all display concentric symmetrical combinations of pattern of lines, reticular, combined with a structureless pattern, all with a uniformly regular border. If you cannot decide whether the border is gradual or abrupt it does not matter if it is uniform. With naevi it will usually be gradual.*

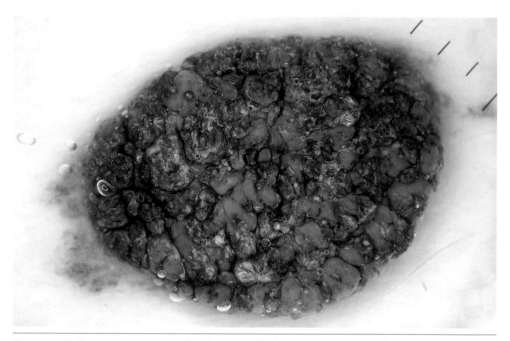

Figure 9.29: Dermatoscopic image of a pigmented skin lesion with a pattern of brown clods and evident orange clods suggesting exposed keratin aggregations as well as an abrupt border over most of the periphery. A symmetrically located macular structureless portion at each end is a clue that this is a congenital naevus rather than a seborrhoeic keratosis. A history of onset in childhood was additional evidence.

of curved vessels, especially in dermal naevi, includes serpentine vessels, but the curved vessels appear repeatedly within the pattern. The dermatoscopist is encouraged to take the opportunity to frequently examine multiple clinically obvious naevi to become familiar with the great variety of dermatoscopic appearances of vessels as well as of pigment patterns.

9.2.5 Non-pigmented naevi

Both Clark and congenital naevi may have amelanotic variants and in this situation vessels take on more significance if there is any doubt about the diagnosis[6].

Non-pigmented junctional (Clark) naevi: these are not common. When present they are expected to be well circumscribed and with a pattern of dot vessels, this being the pattern of vessels on normal skin when such vessels are seen (*Figure 9.30*). The reason they are more often seen in non-pigmented naevi than in perilesional skin may relate to the

higher metabolic demand of a proliferation of naevomelanocytes, even though benign.

Non-pigmented dermal naevi: these are the rule rather than the exception because naevomelanocytes present in the dermis have normally lost their melanin-producing capability through a process known as maturation (*Figures 9.31–9.33*). Such dermal naevi may be identifiable by the presence of terminal hair, a clue to their congenital hamartomatous origin. The archetypal vessel seen in dermal naevi is the curved vessel and, although this vessel structure is often found as a pattern, the curved structure commonly has serpentine variations. If a dermal naevus has a papillomatous surface morphology, a centred vessel pattern may be seen with various types of linear vessel seen in the centre of skin-coloured clods[6].

Dermal naevi may be pigmented (one example being shown in *Figure 9.34*). *Figure 9.35* shows a structureless melanoma arising from a pigmented clod pattern congenital naevus.

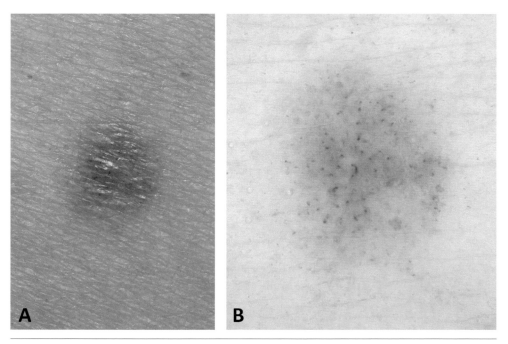

Figure 9.30: *Clinical (A) and dermatoscopic (B) images of a hypomelanotic junctional (Clark) naevus. The lesion is structureless with a monomorphous pattern of dot vessels caused by dilated but otherwise normal dermal papillary vessels not being obscured by melanin. One or two apparent linear vessels centrally do not interfere with a monomorphous pattern of dots.*

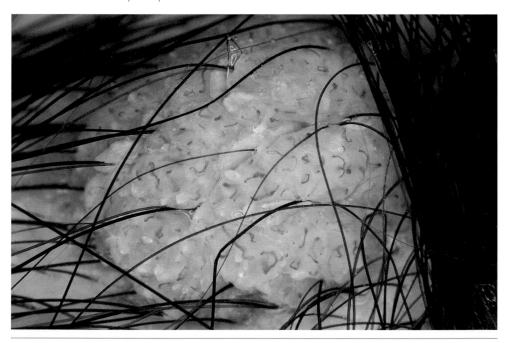

Figure 9.31: *Dermatoscopic image of a non-pigmented dermal (congenital) naevus on the scalp displaying a monomorphous pattern of curved vessels. These vessels correlate with dilated vessels in thick hypertrophic dermal papillae which have an exophytic morphology known as papillomatosis. Note the yellow clods due to exposed aggregations of keratin in between the exophytic dermal papillae.*

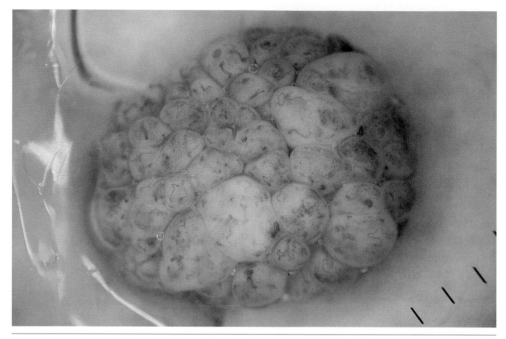

Figure 9.32: *Dermatoscopic image of a non-pigmented dermal (congenital) naevus with a centred vessel pattern, vessels of varying types being centred in skin-coloured clods. The histological correlate of this pattern is papillomatosis.*

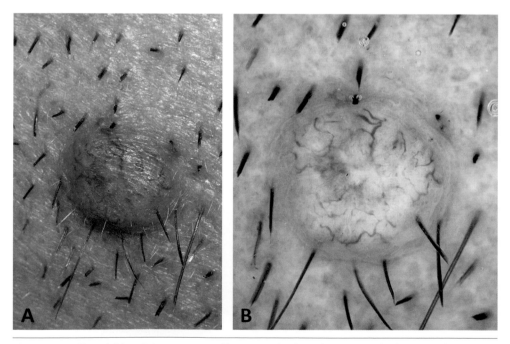

Figure 9.33: *Clinical (A) and dermatoscopic (B) images of a dermal naevus on the face (Miescher naevus). The lesion is only focally pigmented, and the 'curved' vessel pattern is, strictly speaking, serpentine, which is a common morphology for such naevi.*

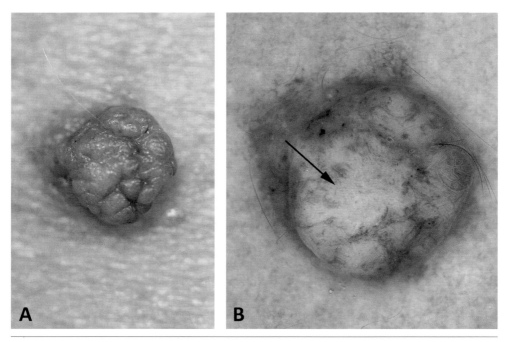

Figure 9.34: *Clinical (A) and dermatoscopic (B) images of a dermal naevus on the torso (Unna naevus). The vessel pattern is largely obscured by brown melanin, but a typical curved vessel is evident (arrow).*

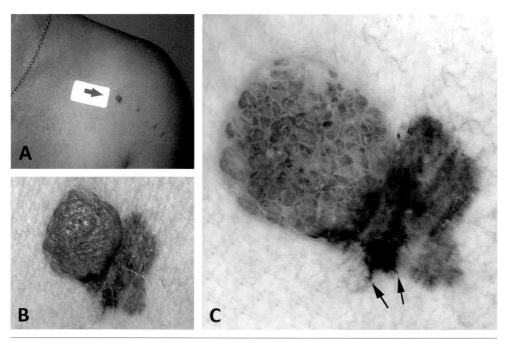

Figure 9.35: *Clinical (A), close-up (B) and dermatoscopic (C) images of a melanoma* in situ *associated with a pigmented dermal naevus (Unna naevus). The pre-existing naevus is raised and has a clod pattern while the associated melanoma is structureless, macular and chaotic with radial lines segmental (arrows).*

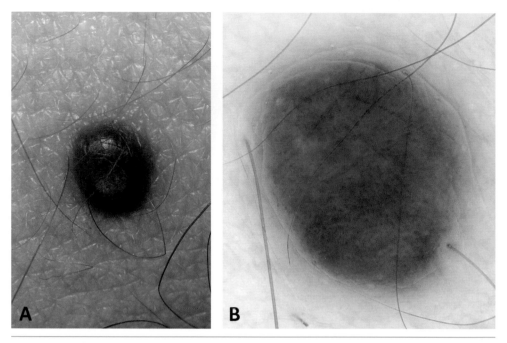

Figure 9.36: *Clinical (A) and dermatoscopic (B) images of a blue naevus. Dermatoscopically there is one pattern, structureless, and one colour, blue. Note that the transition between blue and some grey that is present is gradual, so they are regarded as one colour in this context.*

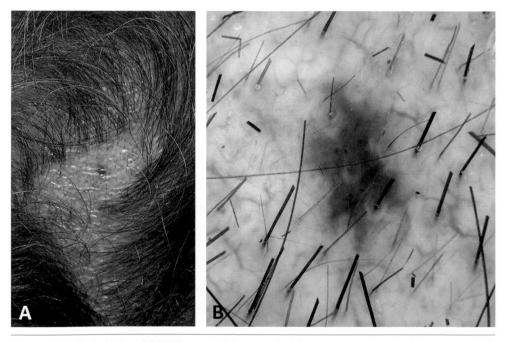

Figure 9.37: *Clinical (A) and dermatoscopic (B) images of a blue naevus on the scalp. Dermatoscopically there is one pattern, structureless, and one colour, blue.*

9.2.6 Blue naevus

This is a type of congenital naevus derived from residual 'rests' of embryonic dermal melanocytes; diagnosis is not usually a challenge with one pattern, structureless, and one colour (blue, grey or a combination of the two colours with gradual transition between them) (*Figures 9.36–9.37*). Subtle curved lines may be seen and vessels, if seen, are usually serpentine.

Amelanotic blue naevus: this is an uncommon variant presenting as a well-defined flat white lesion with fine serpentine vessels (*Figure 9.38*). The morphological criteria for the diagnosis of blue naevus are histological and do not relate to colour.

9.2.7 Halo naevus phenomenon

Naevi may undergo changes secondary to immune response including the halo naevus phenomenon (*Figure 9.39*) with immune regression (*Figure 9.40*), and also secondary to trauma as with the recurrent naevus phenomenon (*Figure 9.41*).

9.2.8 Growing naevi

These have a characteristic morphology with a central structureless, clod or reticular pattern and a symmetrical peripheral distribution of clods (*Figure 9.42A*). If there is asymmetry of pattern or colour, or if peripheral clods are seen at an age when growing naevi are not expected, peripheral clods should be interpreted as a clue to melanoma (*Figure 9.42B*).

9.2.9 Reed and Spitz naevi

Reed (pigmented spindle cell naevus of Reed) and Spitz naevi are particular types of acquired naevi which are generally recognised as new and changing lesions[5]. While the specific morphology of a Reed naevus generally facilitates a confident diagnosis

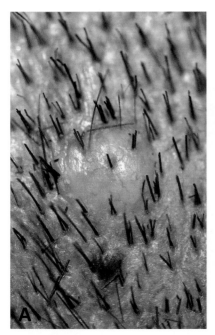
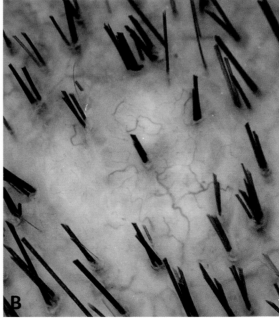

Figure 9.38: *Clinical (A) and dermatoscopic (B) images of an amelanotic blue naevus on the scalp. Dermatoscopically there is one pattern, structureless, and one colour, white, with a monomorphous pattern of serpentine vessels. The lesion was excised on suspicion of BCC. There is a small haemangioma just inferior to the naevus (A).*

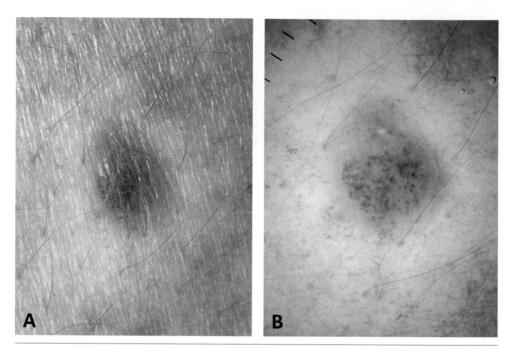

Figure 9.39: *Clinical (A) and dermatoscopic (B) images of a dermal naevus on the torso (Unna naevus) undergoing symmetrical immune regression. The lesion presents with a central pink and lightly pigmented pattern surrounded by a white structureless pattern and carries the appellation 'halo naevus'. Note the single white dot superiorly as a clue to congenital morphology.*

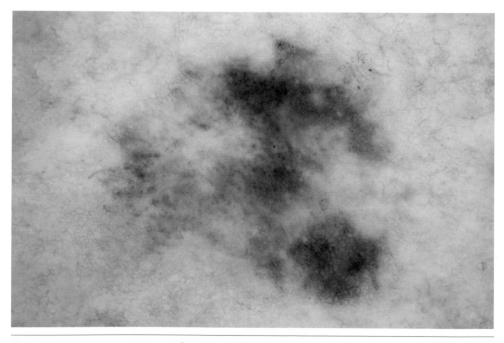

Figure 9.40: *Dermatoscopic image of a naevus undergoing asymmetrical immune regression. There are two patterns, lines reticular and structureless, and four colours, brown, grey, black and white, all asymmetrically combined. The lesion was excised on suspicion of melanoma.*

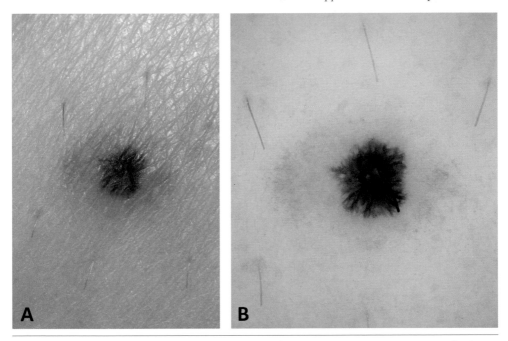

Figure 9.41: *Clinical (A) and dermatoscopic (B) images of a recurrent naevus. Dermatoscopically there is a central pattern of lines radial surrounded concentrically and symmetrically by a structureless pattern. Light and dark brown, being sharply demarcated are regarded as two colours. The peripheral structureless pattern was inconsistent with the alternative diagnoses of Reed or Spitz naevus and this, as well as the perfect symmetry, was inconsistent with a diagnosis of melanoma.*

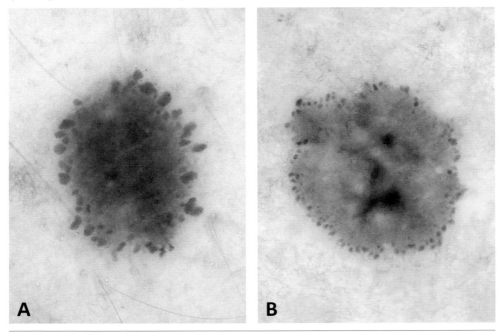

Figure 9.42: *Dermatoscopic images of two pigmented skin lesions with a structureless centre combined symmetrically with peripheral, circumferential clods/dots: (A) a growing naevus on a 24-year-old; (B) a melanoma in situ on a 55-year-old. Note that the melanoma, of concern because its pattern was unique on the patient, was a small lesion with the clue of grey colour (an exception in the 'Chaos and Clues' algorithm), even though the grey arguably did not break biological symmetry.*

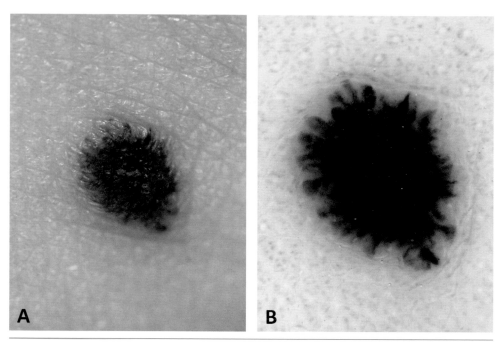

Figure 9.43: *Close-up (A) and dermatoscopic (B) images of a Reed naevus on an 8-year-old. Dermatoscopically there are two patterns, central clods (alternatively structureless) combined concentrically/symmetrically with a pattern of circumferential lines radial, and one colour, brown (alternatively black).*

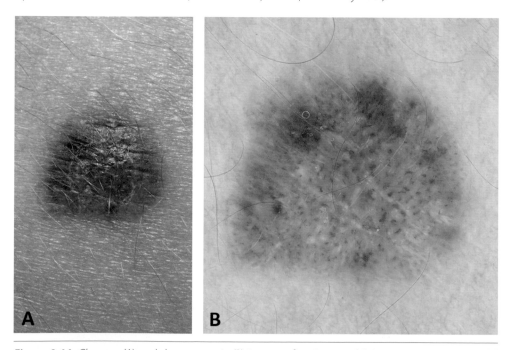

Figure 9.44: *Close-up (A) and dermatoscopic (B) images of a pigmented Spitz naevus on a 3-year-old. Dermatoscopically there is one pattern, structureless, and two colours, central pink and peripheral brown, arguably combined symmetrically. A monomorphous pattern of dot vessels is seen in the non-pigmented centre. It was excised according to the recommendation to excise lesions with the morphology of a Spitz naevus, regardless of age.*

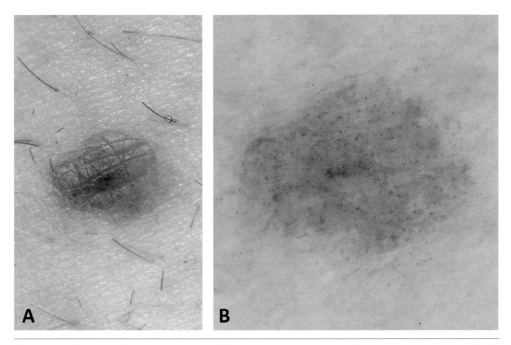

Figure 9.45: *Close-up (A) and dermatoscopic (B) images of a hypomelanotic Spitz naevus. Dermatoscopically there is one pattern, structureless, and two colours, central pink and peripheral brown, arguably combined symmetrically. A monomorphous pattern of dot vessels is seen in the non-pigmented centre.*

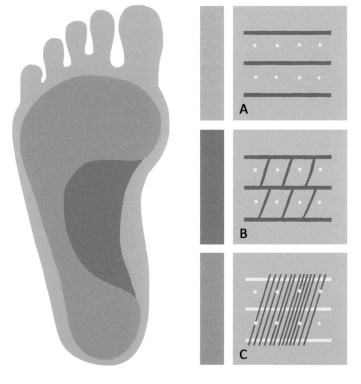

Figure 9.46: Graphic representation of various benign pigmented patterns encountered on volar skin with a colour-coded representation of the plantar foot showing the expected distribution of each pattern: (A) parallel furrow, (B) crossing (also known as lattice), (C) fine crossing (also known as fibrillar). Adapted from J Am Acad Dermatol, 2005;53:23011 and Atlas of Dermoscopy, 2nd Edition, edited by Marghoob, Malvehy and Braun, 2012, Informa.

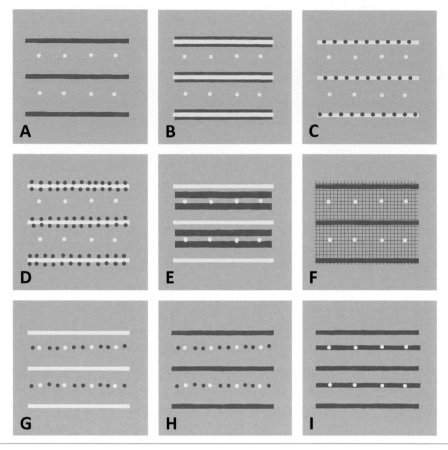

Figure 9.47: *Graphic representation of various benign pigmented patterns encountered on volar skin: (A) classic (single line in the furrows), (B) double line in the furrows, (C) single dotted line in the furrows, (D) double dotted line in the furrows, (E) tram-like lines on the ridges, (F) crista reticulated on the ridges with lines in the furrows, (G) crista dotted lines on the ridges, (H) crista dotted on the ridges and lines in the furrows (another variant – 'peas-in-a-pod' pattern), (I) fine parallel lines on ridges and in furrows. Adapted from* Atlas of Dermoscopy, *2nd Edition, edited by Marghoob, Malvehy and Braun, 2012, Informa.*

in childhood, lesions with this morphology should be excised if encountered after puberty to exclude spitzoid melanoma. Reed naevi are by definition always pigmented and they are expected to be flat or only slightly elevated. The morphology of a Reed naevus is expected to evolve[5], initially consisting solely of dark brown clods and subsequently developing a pattern of circumferential radial lines, lines radial (pseudopod type) or clods (*Figure 9.43*). Finally, they have just one pattern, reticular lines, or a structureless hyperpigmented centre and reticular lines peripherally, at which stage they are indistinguishable from a Clark naevus.

Spitz naevi, in contrast to Reed naevi, are expected to be nodular and may be pigmented or non-pigmented (*Figure 9.44*)[5]. Spitz naevi, being elevated, firm and continuously growing (EFG) should arguably be excised at any age to exclude melanoma[12].

The characteristic dermatoscopic features of pigmented Spitz naevi include a grey centre with a clod or structureless pattern and brown clods peripherally. Central white lines which may be polarising-specific are frequently present[5].

Non-pigmented Spitz naevi: these (*Figure 9.45*) may present with skin-coloured clods or

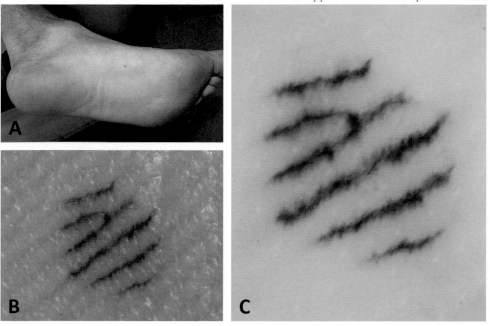

Figure 9.48: *Clinical (A), close-up (B) and dermatoscopic (C) images of a classical volar naevus with a dermatoscopic pattern of lines, parallel, in the narrow dermatoglyphic furrows. Eccrine duct openings can be seen as faint white dots marking the centre of the broad dermatoglyphic ridges.*

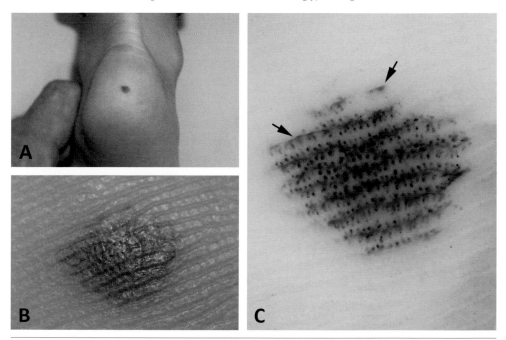

Figure 9.49: *Clinical (A), close-up (B) and dermatoscopic (C) images of a pigmented skin lesion on the volar heel of a child. The dermatoscopic pattern is of (narrow) lines parallel, lines taking priority over the dots which are adjacent to them, the centre of the dermatoglyphic ridges being hypopigmented. The lesion is symmetrical and well circumscribed as expected with a volar naevus. It is not represented by any of the varieties demonstrated graphically in Figure 9.47. Note that although there is pigment on the ridges as well as the furrows, the pigmented lines are in the furrows, this only being clearly evident at the extreme periphery at the upper part of the image (arrows).*

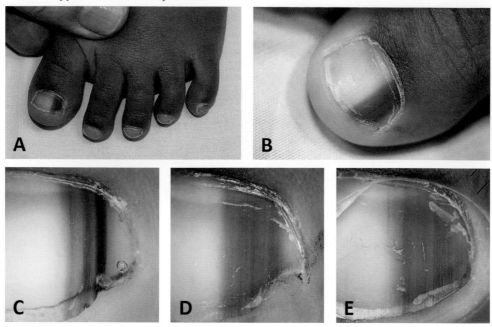

Figure 9.50: Clinical (A), close-up (B) and dermatoscopic (C, D and E) images of longitudinal melanonychia which appeared at 6 months of age (C) and was monitored at 6 months (D) and 12 months (E). Initially the lines parallel were chaotic, varying in width, interval and colour, but as predicted in infancy the pigment band became less chaotic as it widened. Provisional diagnosis: nail matrix congenital naevus; no intervention.

a skin-coloured/pink structureless area and central polarising-specific white lines[5].

9.2.10 Naevi on volar skin

These are commonly called acral naevi and have various dermatoscopic morphologies, often with pigmentation appearing as lines, parallel, in the dermatoglyphic furrows, but variations on the pattern are seen on weight-bearing plantar surfaces[13] (*Figures 9.46–9.49*).

9.2.11 Nail matrix naevi

As with pigmented nail matrix melanoma, pigmented nail matrix naevi are generally not visible if confined to the nail matrix, but the diagnostic clue is the presence of pigment stripes in the nail plate derived from the stratum corneum of the proliferating nail matrix. Typically the longitudinal melanonychia of nail matrix (congenital) naevi is a pattern of regular brown lines, but it is not unusual in very young children to see irregular lines initially, with subsequent increasing organisation (*Figure 9.50*). Although nail matrix melanoma has been reported in pre-pubertal children it is extremely rare. New nail matrix naevi are not expected in adults and the occurrence of any continually progressive widening of longitudinal melanonychia after puberty should raise suspicion of melanoma.

9.3 Basal cell carcinoma: pigmented and non-pigmented

Because the majority of BCCs are amelanotic it is useful to first consider the non-pigment clues to all BCCs, and then to discuss the specific pigment clues which may be present.

9.3.1 Non-pigment clues to basal cell carcinoma

The diagnosis of a non-pigmented BCC starts with the recognition of a non-pigmented lesion without the morphology of any of the known common benign lesions (see *Section 5.1.5*)[6].

According to 'Prediction without Pigment'[14] the first clue to be excluded or confirmed is ulceration, and if that is present a biopsy is considered on suspicion primarily of BCC.

If ulceration is not present then the next step is to assess for the presence of white lines or, in the case of a raised lesion, the keratin clues of surface keratin, white circles or white structureless areas: if any of those clues are discovered, biopsy is also considered primarily on suspicion of BCC in the case of white lines, or of SCC if keratin clues are present.

Polarising-specific white lines can support the diagnosis of both BCC and melanoma but they are much more frequently encountered in BCC. Dermatoscopic images of non-pigmented BCCs are shown in *Figures 9.51–9.62A*.

If there is no ulceration and there are no white clues then the assessment proceeds to vessel analysis and if none of the four described benign vessel patterns (clods-only, centred, serpiginous or reticular) are present, biopsy is considered on suspicion of generic malignancy. It is, however, possible in many cases to predict a specific diagnosis of BCC based on the vessel analysis.

A vessel pattern of branched serpentine vessels in a lesion which does not have the morphology of a known benign lesion is most consistent with the diagnosis of BCC[5]: the caveat about known benign lesions is necessary because any raised dermal-based cyst or tumour, benign or malignant, which displaces the dermal plexus, can result in a branched serpentine vessel pattern being evident dermatoscopically[5].

The other clue to the diagnosis of BCC which may be seen is the presence of characteristic translucent BCC jelly-like stroma: this not only throws the typical branched serpentine vessels into sharp relief but also enables very fine vessels to be seen in detail[6].

Although white clods are frequently seen in BCC they are also commonly seen in SCC and seborrhoeic keratosis so their context is important. If a white clod or clods are present in a very subtle lesion without clues to SCC or seborrhoeic keratosis, then it is a clue to BCC.

In addition to the non-pigment clues mentioned above, non-pigmented BCC of *nodular* morphology typically exhibits large-diameter clearly defined serpentine branched vessels[5]: non-pigmented *superficial* BCC may be more challenging to diagnose, but the dermatoscopic findings are similar to those for nodular BCC with the exception that vessels are typically narrower.

More *aggressive* BCC subtypes, particularly morphoeic and infiltrating BCCs, may be very subtle clinically and margins may be poorly defined: dermatoscopic margin verification at the time of surgery is particularly helpful in this situation[15].

Basosquamous BCC may have keratinising features similar to SCC, including white circles, surface keratin and white structureless areas. This is not a problem in practice because the lesion will be excised either way and the pathologist will reveal the diagnosis.

Extensively ulcerated BCC is more likely to have polymorphous vessels and signs of keratinisation[6].

9.3.2 Pigment clues to basal cell carcinoma

As for non-pigmented BCC, the diagnosis of a pigmented BCC also starts with the recognition of a lesion without the morphology of any of the known common benign lesions: in such a case the dermatoscopic assessment initially determines whether there is chaos and one or more of the defined generic clues to malignancy. If that is established, the search continues for specific diagnostic clues.

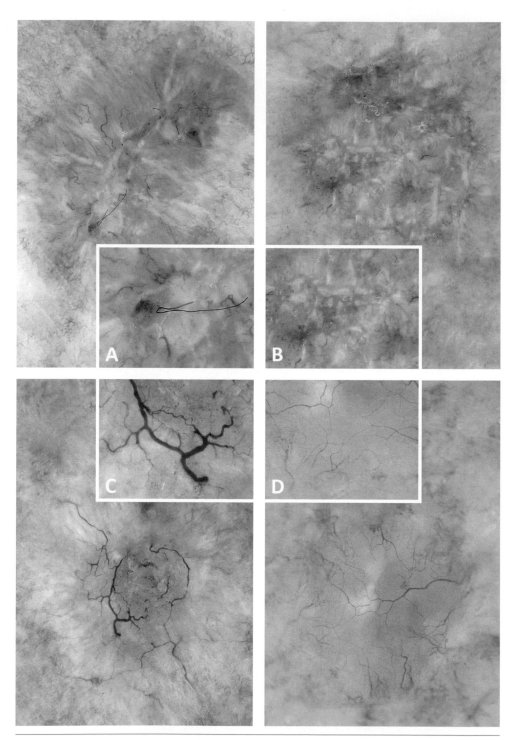

Figure 9.51: *Dermatoscopic images displaying features commonly observed in basal cell carcinomas (insert images enlarged): (A) ulceration (note 'adherent fibre' sign), (B) polarising-specific white lines, (C) linear serpentine branched vessels, and (D) semitranslucent stroma enhancing very fine serpentine vessels.*

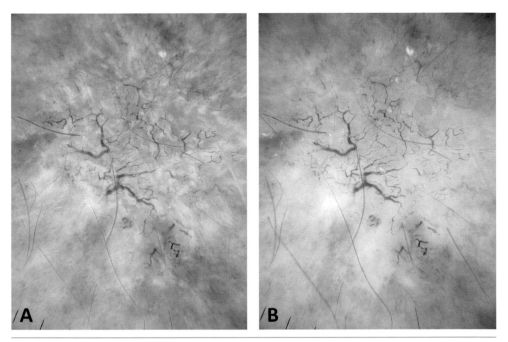

Figure 9.52: *Dermatoscopic images of a basal cell carcinoma displaying polarising-specific white areas (A) and the non-polarised correlate of this (not always present), a white structureless area (B).*

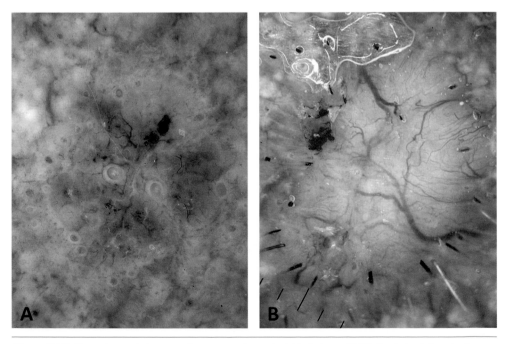

Figure 9.53: *Dermatoscopic images of two non-pigmented skin lesions. (A) White circles take priority over vessels suggesting a diagnosis of squamous cell carcinoma, while in (B) a white structureless area similarly takes priority also pointing to squamous cell carcinoma. Both cases are in fact basal cell carcinomas, being exceptions to the expected prediction.*

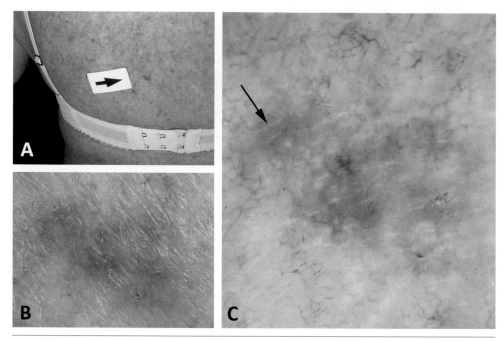

Figure 9.54: Clinical (A), close-up (B) and dermatoscopic (C) images of a superficial basal cell carcinoma displaying micro-ulceration (yellow clod – arrow), white lines and fine serpentine vessels.

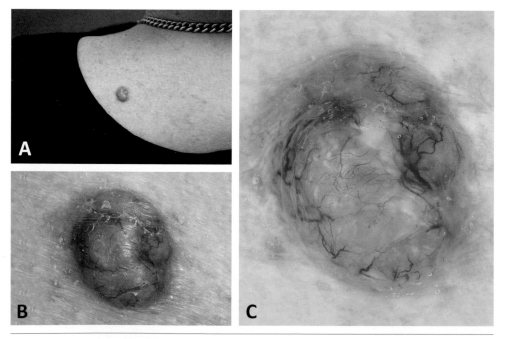

Figure 9.55: Clinical (A), close-up (B) and dermatoscopic (C) images of a nodular basal cell carcinoma displaying polarising-specific white structures and branched serpentine vessels, some being thick and some very fine, thrown into sharp relief by a translucent stroma. As is typical with this subtype the lesion is well circumscribed.

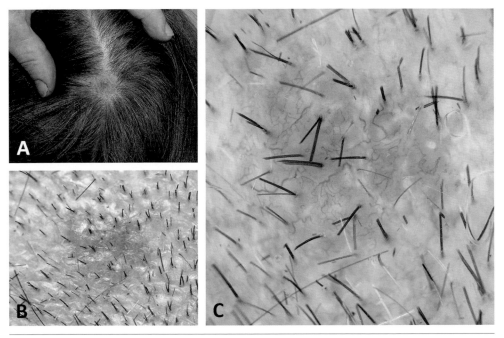

Figure 9.56: *A subtle poorly demarcated basal cell carcinoma on the scalp displaying fine serpentine vessels set in translucent stroma. Basal cell carcinomas can be found under thick hair and are not uncommon in the part-line or on the crown.*

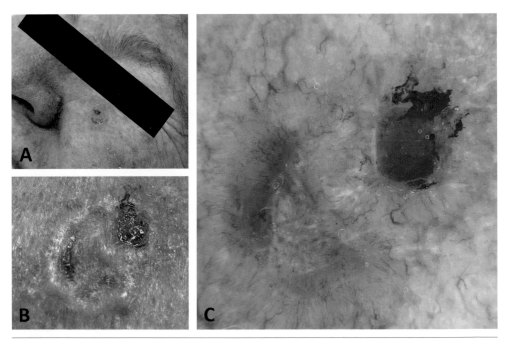

Figure 9.57: *Clinical (A), close-up (B) and dermatoscopic (C) images of a basal cell carcinoma on the cheek revealing a raised rolled border (B), evident ulceration (all images) and additional dermatoscopic clues of white lines and fine serpentine vessels.*

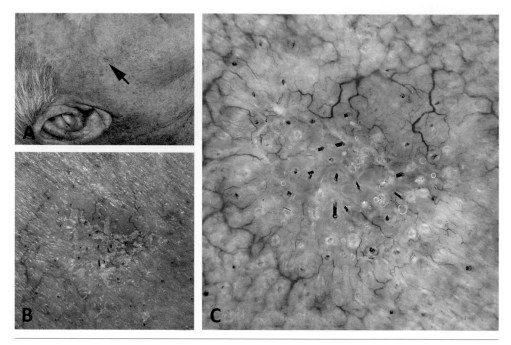

Figure 9.58: *Clinical (A), close-up (B) and dermatoscopic (C) images of a sclerosing basal cell carcinoma with evident puckering of the centre (B) due to retraction and tethering of fibrous tissue. The dermatoscopic image (C) shows a reduction of vascularity in this central portion with the more typical branched serpentine vessels, embedded in stroma, peripherally. As is typical with this aggressive subtype the lesion is poorly circumscribed.*

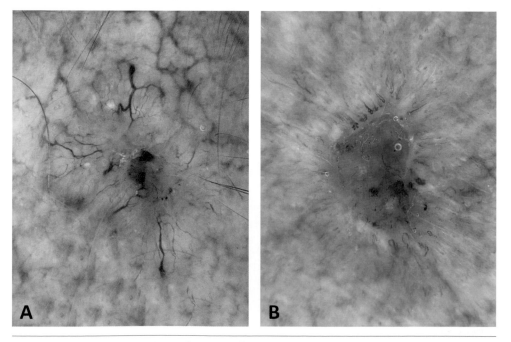

Figure 9.59: *Dermatoscopic images of two centrally ulcerated basal cell carcinomas with serpentine (A) and looped (B) vessels in a radial arrangement centred on the ulceration.*

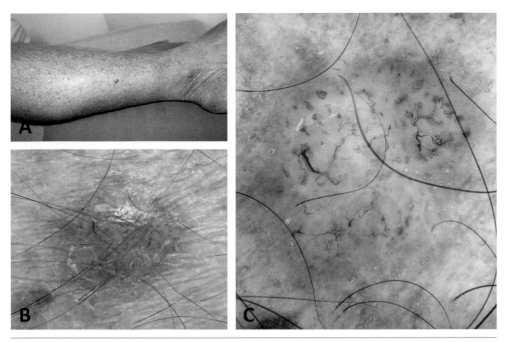

Figure 9.60: *Clinical (A), close-up (B) and dermatoscopic (C) images of a basal cell carcinoma on the distal leg displaying a polymorphous pattern of serpentine and coiled vessels, such non-typical patterns occurring more frequently at this anatomical site.*

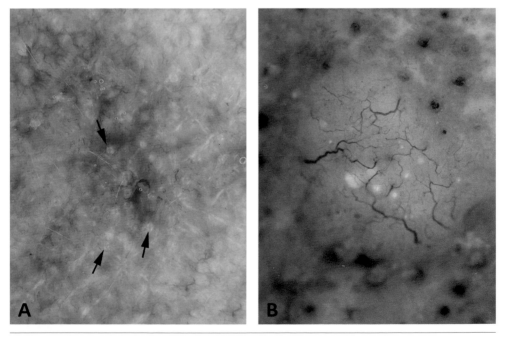

Figure 9.61: *Dermatoscopic images of two basal cell carcinomas displaying 4-dot clods (arrows in A) and white clods (B). While such structures can also be clues to actinic keratosis and squamous cell carcinoma, the presence of fine serpentine vessels favours a diagnosis of basal cell carcinoma, this being particularly true for (B) where the vessels are silhouetted by translucent stroma.*

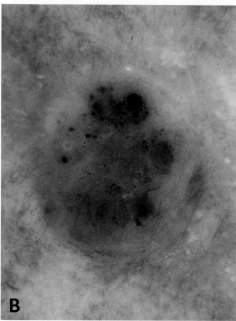

Figure 9.62: Dermatoscopic images of a non-pigmented (A) and pigmented (B) basal cell carcinoma, both displaying fine serpentine vessels set in and enhanced by translucent stroma.

The non-pigment clue of ulceration is a reasonably specific clue to BCC in pigmented as well as non-pigmented lesions because BCC, being much more prevalent than melanoma and ulcerating earlier than melanoma, is the most likely malignancy if ulceration is present.

White lines, a clue in the 'Prediction without Pigment' algorithm is also a defined clue in the 'Chaos and Clues method'[16] and with respect to pigmented malignancy it is most commonly seen in BCC.

The additional non-pigmented clues to BCC of translucent stroma highlighting very fine serpentine vessels may or may not be obscured by melanin pigment (*Figure 9.62*).

In addition to the non-pigment clues to BCC described above, there are a number of pigmented structures that can assist the specific diagnosis of BCC, including a lack of any pigmented lines apart from lines radial and the presence of one or more of (*Figures 9.62–9.66*):

- lines radial converging
- lines radial extending from a hypopigmented area
- a clod with a central dot
- blue/grey clods/dots.

9.3.3 Fibroepithelioma of Pinkus

Fibroepithelioma of Pinkus (FEP) is a type of BCC with a distinctive clinical and dermatoscopic appearance. Clinically it is a raised, soft, well demarcated non-pigmented or lightly pigmented lesion with dermatoscopic polarising-specific white lines and a vessel pattern characterised by polymorphous vessels, including fine serpentine and other linear vessel types (*Figures 9.67* and *9.68*).

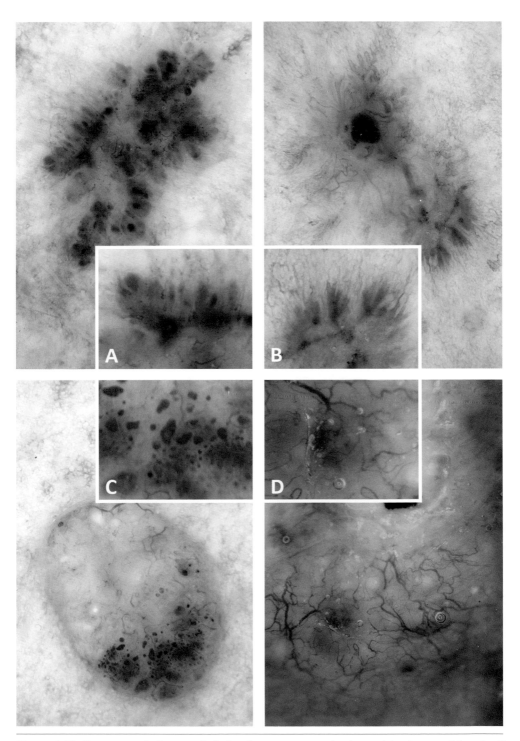

Figure 9.63: *Dermatoscopic images displaying features commonly observed in pigmented basal cell carcinomas (insert images enlarged): (A) thick lines, radial, converging to a common line (so-called 'leaf-like' structures); (B) thin lines, radial, converging to common dots (so-called 'spoke-wheel' structures); (C) grey clods and dots; (D) blue clods (so-called 'ovoid nests').*

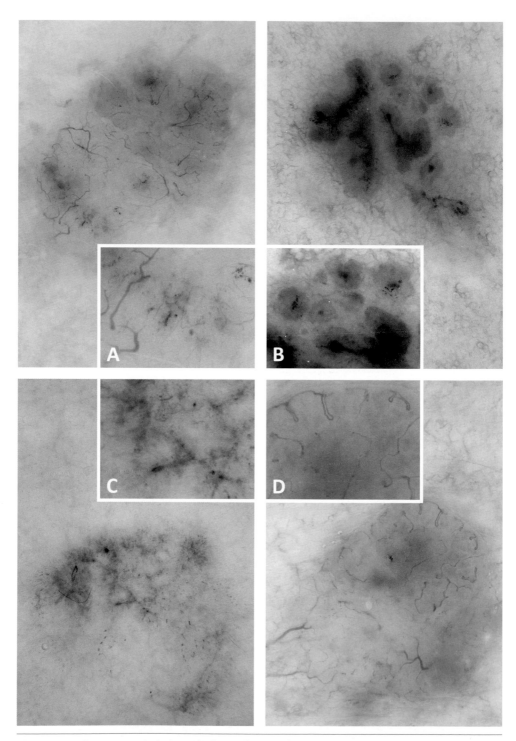

Figure 9.64: *Dermatoscopic images displaying features that may be observed in pigmented basal cell carcinomas (insert images enlarged): (A) brown dots, (B) dots/clods within clods, (C) angulated lines, and (D) structureless grey/brown.*

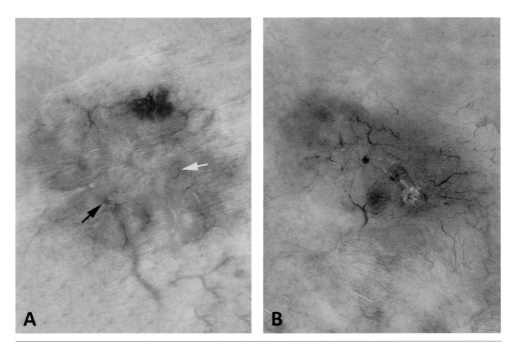

Figure 9.65: *Dermatoscopic images of two pigmented lesions each without any non-radial lines and: (A) chaos plus grey dots (black arrow) and white lines (polarising-specific) as well as the clues to basal cell carcinoma of ulceration (note adherent fibre – yellow arrow) and fine branched serpentine vessels; superficial basal cell carcinoma; (B) chaos plus blue clods as well as large-bore branched serpentine vessels in a nodular basal cell carcinoma.*

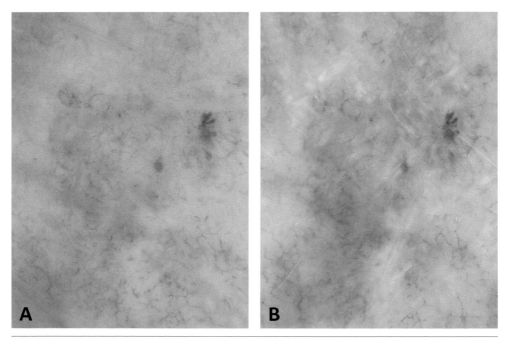

Figure 9.66: *Non-polarised (A) and polarised (B) dermatoscopic images of a pigmented superficial basal cell carcinoma showing chaos plus lines, radial, segmental (converging and projecting from a hypopigmented area) as well as polarising-specific white lines (B) and fine serpentine vessels.*

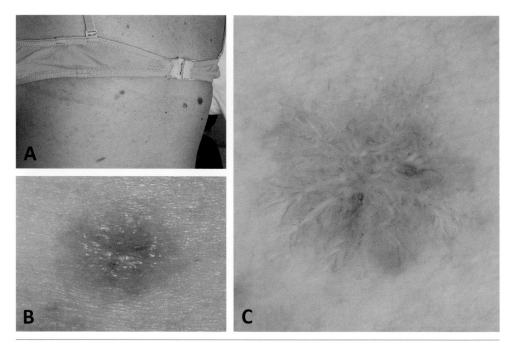

Figure 9.67: *Clinical (A), close-up (B) and dermatoscopic (C) images of a non-pigmented skin lesion with white lines and polymorphous fine linear vessels. Histological diagnosis: fibroepithelioma of Pinkus.*

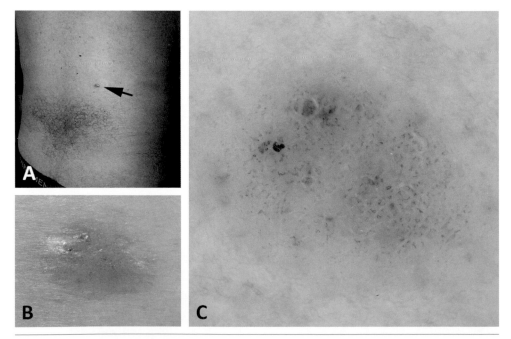

Figure 9.68: *Clinical (A), close-up (B) and dermatoscopic (C) images of a non-pigmented skin lesion with polymorphous short linear (curved, serpentine and coiled) vessels. Histological diagnosis: fibroepithelioma of Pinkus. Note that this is not a centred pattern because that pattern requires that all vessels be centred in skin-coloured clods, whereas the left half of this lesion has no such demarcated clods.*

9.4 Benign keratinocytic lesions

9.4.1 Solar lentigo, ink spot lentigo, melanotic macule and idiopathic guttate hypomelanosis

Solar lentigo, the word 'lentigo' being derived from 'lentil-like', is invariably pigmented.

Solar lentigines are brown in colour and their pattern varies according to location[5]:

- On the trunk they typically have a pattern of reticular or curved lines or a structureless pattern.
- On the dorsal hands they have a structureless pattern.
- On the face the pattern may be structureless, lines curved, lines reticular or a pattern of pigmented circles defining follicles.

The defining feature of solar lentigines is the sharply demarcated border which may be scalloped. Solar lentigines are characterised histologically by hyperpigmentation of normal basal keratinocytes and with melanocyte numbers in the normal range for sun-damaged skin. Solar lentigines arise in response to solar exposure and are regarded as a marker for UV skin damage (*Figures 9.69–9.71*).

One variant of solar lentigo is the ink spot lentigo (*Figure 9.71*) and another is melanotic macule of the lip (*Figure 9.72*).

Melanotic macules of the lip, genitalia[5] and nail matrix (*Figures 9.72-9.74*) are histologically equivalent to solar lentigo, but only melanotic macule of the lip is related to UV exposure.

Lesions of idiopathic guttate hypomelanosis are seen most commonly on the shins of fair-skinned patients of mature age who have evidence of sun damage on the adjacent skin (*Figure 9.75*). They are macules of white skin, similar in size to ephelides (freckles), and they have a sharply demarcated border causing them to be regarded as a white freckle. Histologically the lesions have a lack of melanin and may have a reduction in melanocyte numbers. The cause is believed to be a response to skin trauma, predominantly due to UV exposure.

9.4.2 Seborrhoeic keratosis: pigmented and non-pigmented

Seborrhoeic keratosis is an extremely common lesion and clinical/dermatoscopic diagnosis is seldom a challenge[5].

The majority of seborrhoeic keratoses are pigmented by melanin which has been transferred to their constituent keratinocytes from melanocytes at the dermoepidermal junction or, in the case of the melanoacanthoma variant, from benign dendritic melanocytes within the lesion.

Clinically these lesions typically occur on sun-exposed areas including primarily the face, torso (*Figure 9.76*) and lower limbs, but they are also frequently found on non-sun-exposed locations such as on the anterior chest of women at the line of pressure under the bra. They are almost never found on the buttocks, the line of demarcation from the sun-exposed back being typically abrupt. One clinical clue to seborrhoeic keratosis is that they tend occur as multiple lesions in clusters. Another very useful clue is a palpably rough surface. In contrast, melanomas and BCCs are expected to have a smooth surface and melanoma is expected to be flat unless invasive to a depth of at least 1mm, at which stage there should be evident dermatoscopic clues so that confusion with seborrhoeic keratosis is unlikely.

The not uncommon presence of transition to seborrhoeic keratosis in solar lentigines is compelling evidence that many, if not most of the ones that occur on sun-damaged skin, evolve from that precursor (*Figure 9.77*). Solar lentigines are invariably flat so any palpable thickening is a clue to seborrhoeic keratosis,

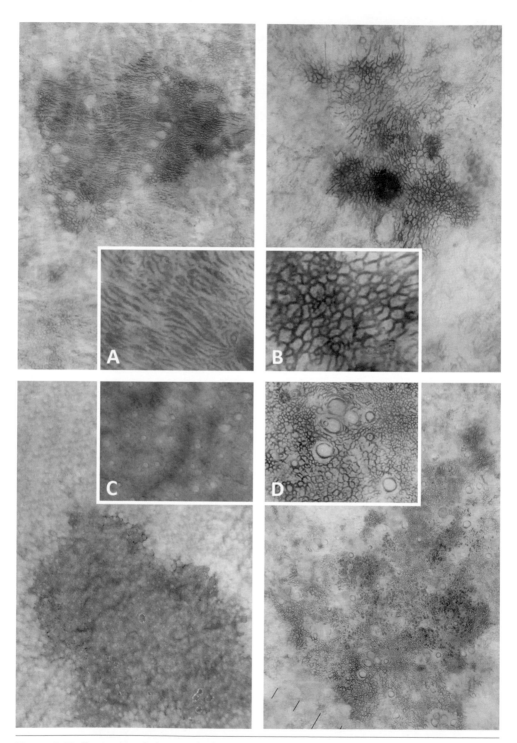

Figure 9.69: *Dermatoscopic images displaying patterns commonly observed in solar lentigines (insert images enlarged): (A) lines curved, (B) lines reticular, (C) (body site – face) structureless (interrupted by follicular openings with a very few pigmented circles; note the very sharply demarcated scalloped border), and (D) lines reticular and circles.*

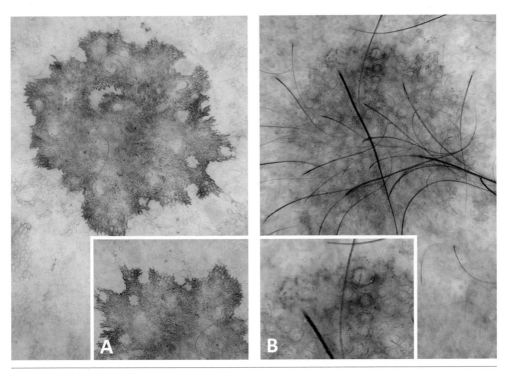

Figure 9.70: *Dermatoscopic images of two solar lentigines (inset images enlarged) demonstrating: (A) a pattern of lines reticular with some short curved lines centrally and with a very sharply demarcated scalloped border. Some of the lines at the border appear 'broken off', as distinct from lines radial. (B) A pattern of lines reticular with some follicular circles. Chaos of border abruptness as well as some chaotic grey led to excision biopsy on suspicion of melanoma.*

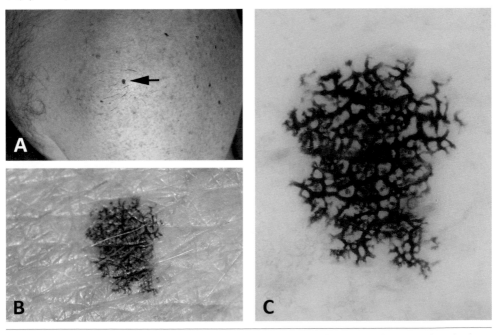

Figure 9.71: *Clinical (A), close-up (B) and dermatoscopic (C) images of an ink spot lentigo with a dermatoscopic pattern of lines branched, colour dark brown and a sharply demarcated border over the entire periphery.*

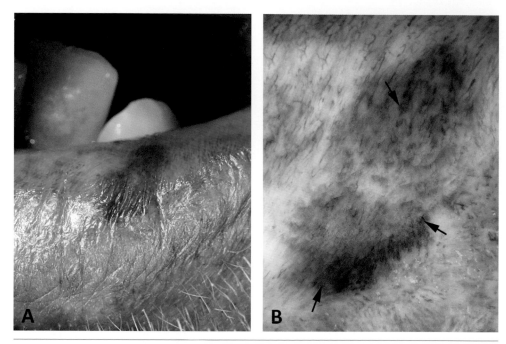

Figure 9.72: *Close-up (A) and dermatoscopic (B) images of a melanotic macule on the lip. The lesion is entirely confined to the vermillion lip with a structureless dermatoscopic pattern and two colours, brown and grey (arrows), with only focal asymmetry of colour. Apart from that focus of darker grey, the lesion exhibits biological symmetry and is well circumscribed with the typical morphology of a melanotic macule.*

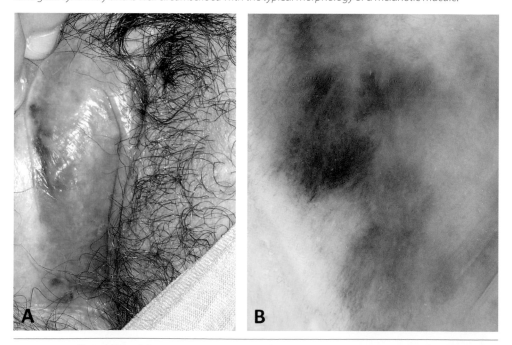

Figure 9.73: *Clinical (A) and dermatoscopic (B) images of a melanotic macule of the labia minora. This lesion exhibits chaos of structure (lines curved and structureless, asymmetrically combined) with asymmetric grey and brown colour as well chaos of border abruptness. Biopsy to exclude melanoma confirmed the diagnosis of labial melanotic macule.*

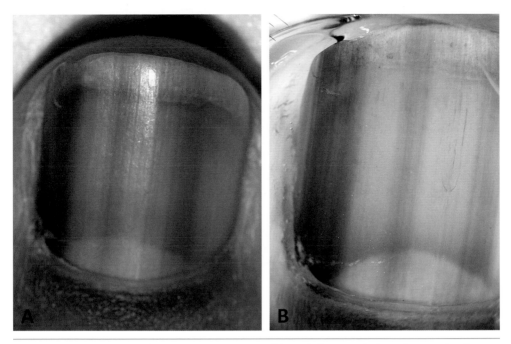

Figure 9.74: *Clinical (A) and dermatoscopic (B) images of the nail plate morphology of a case of nail matrix melanotic macule of the thumb. Longitudinal melanonychia covers most of the nail plate. The involvement of multiple nails on both fingers and toes was compelling evidence to the diagnosis of nail matrix melanotic macule.*

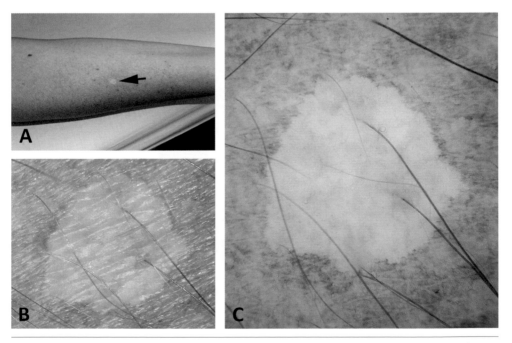

Figure 9.75: *Clinical (A), close-up (B) and dermatoscopic (C) images of idiopathic guttate hypomelanosis with dermatoscopic structureless white and a very sharply demarcated border.*

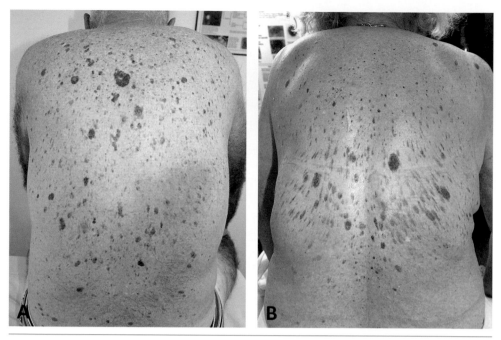

Figure 9.76: *Clinical images of the backs of two individuals both with multiple seborrhoeic keratoses. The distribution appears more random in (A) while in (B) there is a pattern roughly parallel to the dermatome pattern which has been likened variously to a Christmas tree or to the appearance of drizzled wax.*

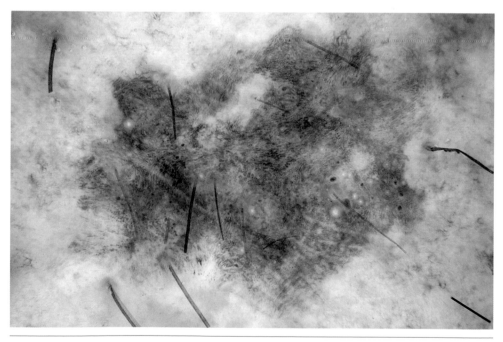

Figure 9.77: *Dermatoscopic image of a solar lentigo with a very characteristic pattern of short curved lines in which an arising seborrhoeic keratosis is identified by white clods.*

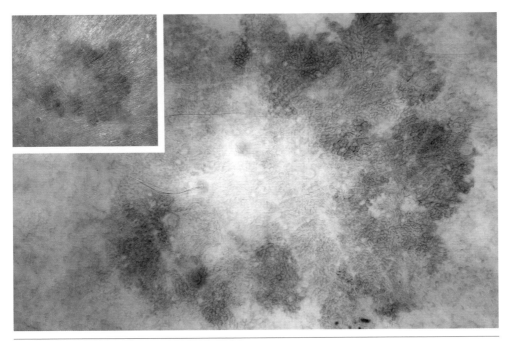

Figure 9.78: *Clinical (insert) and dermatoscopic images of a reticulated seborrhoeic keratosis which is distinguished from a solar lentigo only by its palpably rough texture due to acanthosis. Dermatoscopically a central structureless white area is surrounded by a pattern of very characteristic fine regular reticular lines. The border is sharply demarcated and scalloped.*

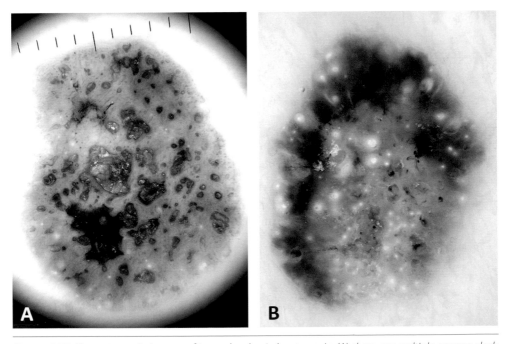

Figure 9.79: *Dermatoscopic images of two seborrhoeic keratoses. In (A) there are multiple orange clods and a few white dots (inferiorly) and the border is uniformly sharply demarcated. In (B) there are numerous white clods and dots and there is chaos of border abruptness, but in spite of this the lesion can confidently be diagnosed as an unequivocal seborrhoeic keratosis.*

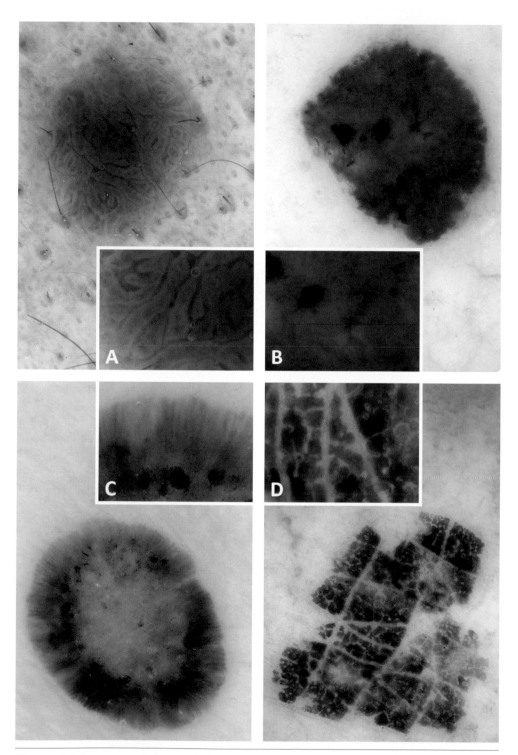

Figure 9.80: *Dermatoscopic images displaying patterns that may be observed in seborrhoeic keratoses (insert images enlarged): (A) thick curved lines (compared to a brain-like pattern in metaphoric terminology); (B) structureless pattern; (C) radial lines; (D) clods (the interruption to that pattern by natural skin markings of the lower limb is not part of the pattern and is ignored).*

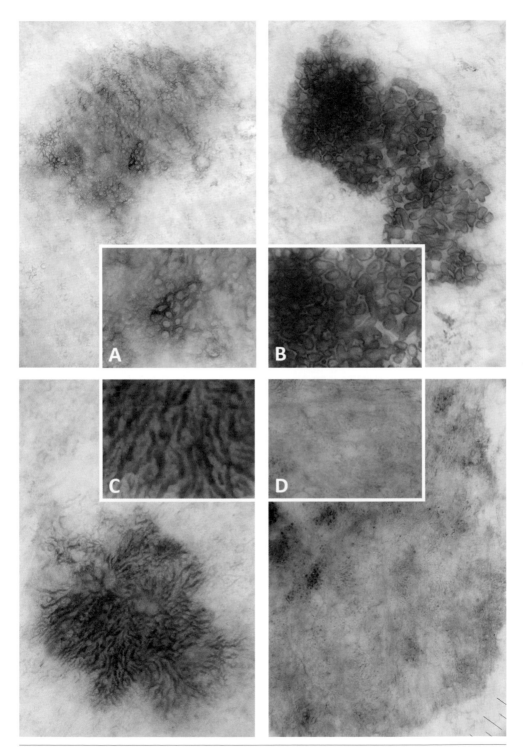

Figure 9.81: *Dermatoscopic images displaying patterns that may be observed in seborrhoeic keratoses (insert images enlarged): (A) reticular lines; (B) circles (reticular lines modified by acanthosis of pigmented rete ridges); (C) thin curved lines; (D) structureless pattern in which none of the basic structures predominate.*

as is the presence of any thick curved lines, clods whether white, yellow, orange, brown or black, or pigmented circles not related to hair follicles.

Dermatoscopic clues to seborrhoeic keratosis, distinguishing them from solar lentigines, include (*Figures 9.78–9.83*):

- thick curved lines
- multiple orange or yellow clods.

If the differential diagnosis is melanoma, then a sharply demarcated border over the total periphery should be present for the diagnosis of seborrhoeic keratosis to even be considered.

Clonal seborrhoeic keratoses cannot normally be distinguished clinically or dermatoscopically from other subtypes. They are characterised histologically by intraepithelial nests of basaloid keratinocytes (*Figure 9.84*).

The loosely woven orthokeratotic keratin overlying seborrhoeic keratosis may absorb and retain exogenous substances such as copper and fake tan and this phenomenon has been described as the St Tropez sign[17] (*Figure 9.85*).

The vessels seen in seborrhoeic keratosis typically include looped, coiled and even dot vessels, this polymorphous pattern being overshadowed in the presence of otherwise compelling evidence in the form of keratin clues to the diagnosis (*Figure 9.86*).

Non-pigmented seborrhoeic keratosis is a common variant and when the surface is palpably rough on a lesion with sharply demarcated margins the diagnosis will not be a problem. They may also be identified by clues described above for pigmented variants, such as a sharply demarcated border and yellow or white clods. Polymorphous vessels, including coiled and looped vessels, are often seen and the dermatoscopist is encouraged to examine clinically evident non-pigmented

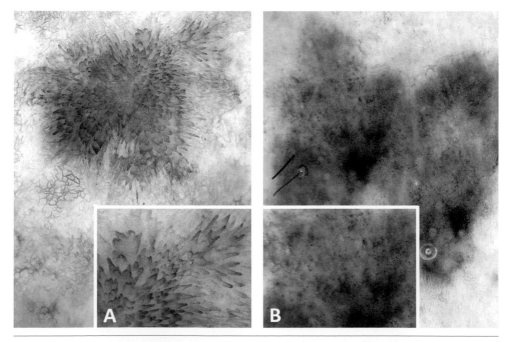

Figure 9.82: *Dermatoscopic images displaying patterns that may be observed in seborrhoeic keratoses (insert images enlarged): (A) radial lines, and (B) dots.*

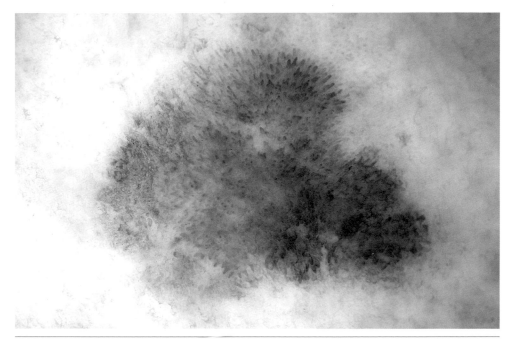

Figure 9.83: *Dermatoscopic image of a seborrhoeic keratosis with three patterns combined asymmetrically: lines radial (superior), lines reticular (left) and structureless (centre and right), as well as chaos of border abruptness. The lesion was excised to exclude melanoma.*

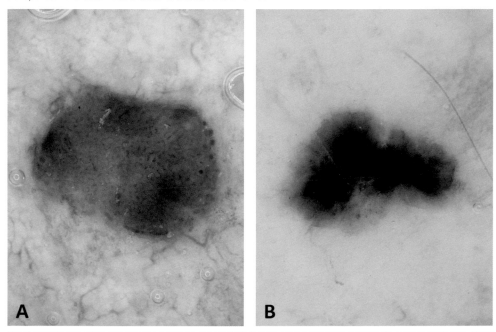

Figure 9.84: *Dermatoscopic images of two seborrhoeic keratoses classified histologically as clonal. (A) A pigmented lesion with a pattern of blue clods overlying structureless brown pigment (the pattern is clods). The clods are blue because they are composed of horn cysts of pigmented keratin which, although epidermal, are in rete ridges which are angled beneath dermis, thus inducing the Tyndall effect. (B) A pigmented lesion with the sharply demarcated border of a seborrhoeic keratosis and a combination of a pattern of dots and structureless areas.*

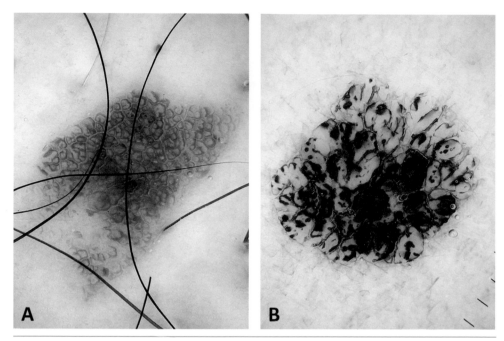

Figure 9.85: *Dermatoscopic images of two seborrhoeic keratoses, each exhibiting the St Tropez sign. (A) Uptake by keratin of green pigment from a copper stud in a pair of jeans, and (B) uptake of fake tan.*

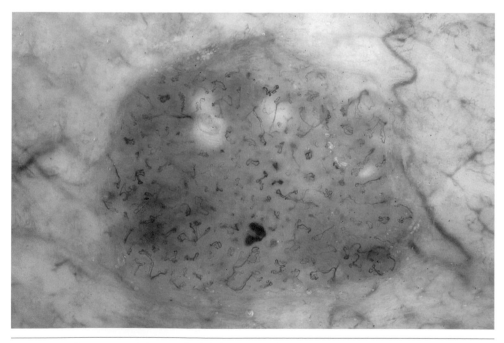

Figure 9.86: *Dermatoscopic image of a lightly pigmented acanthotic seborrhoeic keratosis. The pattern is structureless with focal brown and grey pigment and with one yellow (left side) and two white clods. There is a polymorphous pattern of linear curved, coiled and serpentine vessels.*

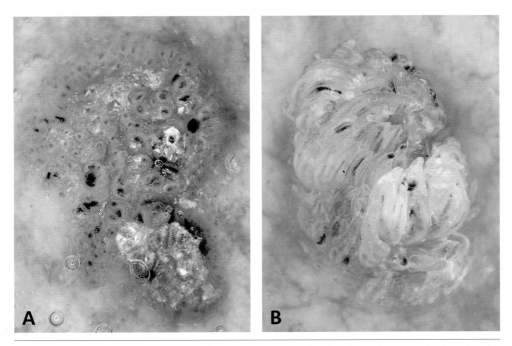

Figure 9.87: *Dermatoscopic images of two non-pigmented seborrhoeic keratoses both exhibiting papillomatosis. A centred vessel pattern is evident in (A), but the hypertrophic dermal papillae are so elongated in (B) that the centred pattern is distorted.*

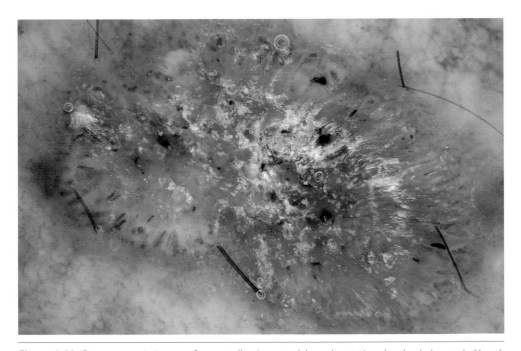

Figure 9.88: *Dermatoscopic image of a centrally pigmented, hyperkeratotic seborrhoeic keratosis. Vessels are only displayed peripherally and are seen on a background of structureless white. The lesion was excised to exclude SCC.*

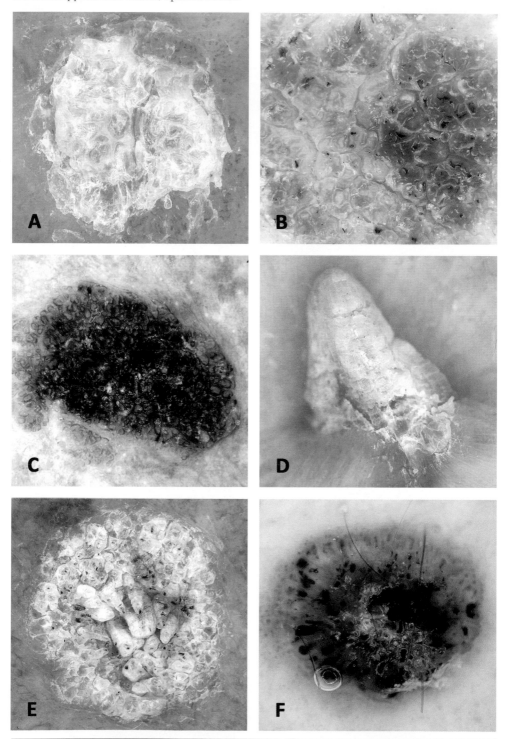

Figure 9.89: *Dermatoscopic images of six hyperkeratotic seborrhoeic keratoses illustrating the variations in surface keratin colour and morphology: (A) thick white structureless scale, (B) yellow and orange clods and structureless scale, (C) brown clods and structureless scale, (D) a laminated white keratin horn, (E) scale projecting from underlying papillomatosis, and (F) blood spots in a keratin plaque. Features also seen in squamous cell carcinoma may mandate biopsy.*

seborrhoeic keratoses frequently to become familiar with their morphology. A centred vessel pattern when present is a compelling clue to benignity, this pattern sometimes being present in hypertrophic dermal papillae, giving the lesion a papillomatous contour (*Figure 9.87*)[6].

Flat non-pigmented seborrhoeic keratoses may be confused with BCC and SCC *in situ* and, if clues to these are present, biopsy may be necessary. The polarising-specific white lines, stroma and serpentine vessels characteristic of superficial BCC are not expected in seborrhoeic keratosis, nor are the prominent monomorphous clustered coiled vessels of SCC *in situ*.

Seborrhoeic keratoses, both pigmented and non-pigmented, may be hyperkeratotic. Pigmented invasive (raised) SCC is very rare, but hyperkeratotic non-pigmented seborrhoeic keratosis may mimic SCC[18] (*Figures 9.88* and *9.89*).

9.4.3 Lichen planus-like keratosis

LPLK usually represents solar lentigines or seborrhoeic keratoses that have undergone immune regression[5]: these precursor lesions may still be evident when regression is incomplete, otherwise the lesion may be recognised by its uniformity and sharply demarcated border, reminiscent of the precursor lesion (*Figure 9.90*). Several of the precursor lesions are expected to be in the vicinity.

A typical LPLK has one pattern, dots, and one colour, grey (*Figure 9.91*): earlier in their evolution they may present as an erythematous inflamed solar lentigo which is frequently symptomatic as itchy and visible to the patient (*Figures 9.92–9.94*).

Non-pigmented LPLK is the lesion most commonly mistaken for BCC (in the authors' experience): this lesion typically presents on the torso or limbs as a small pink lesion with polarising-specific white lines and short fine

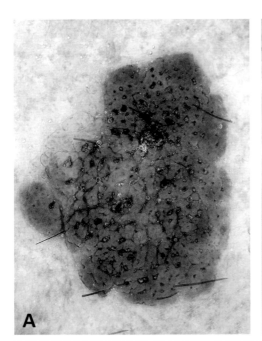
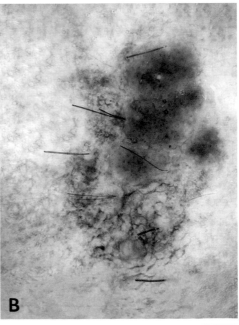

A **B**

Figure 9.90: *A pigmented skin lesion at presentation (A) and an image taken after 2 years of monitoring (B). Although there are numerous clues to seborrhoeic keratosis in the initial image, the chaos evident in the follow-up image led to excision biopsy; lichen planus-like keratosis.*

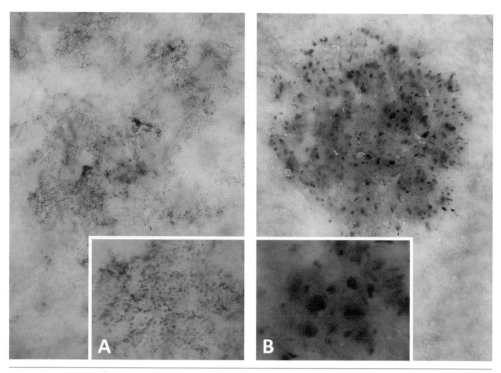

Figure 9.91: *Dermatoscopic images (insert images enlarged) of two lichen planus-like keratoses, each demonstrating the commonly seen morphology of grey dots (A and B) and grey dots and clods (B).*

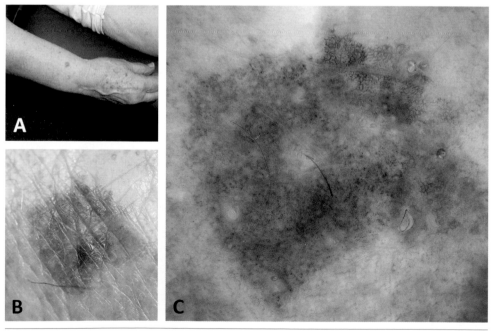

Figure 9.92: *Clinical (A), close-up (B) and dermatoscopic (C) images of a lichen planus-like keratosis arising from an evident solar lentigo (right side of image).*

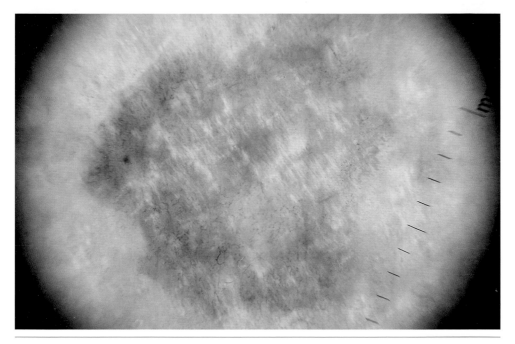

Figure 9.93: *Dermatoscopic image of a hypopigmented lichen planus-like keratosis with chaos of border abruptness, polarising-specific white lines and polymorphous linear and dot vessels which led to excision biopsy on suspicion of melanoma.*

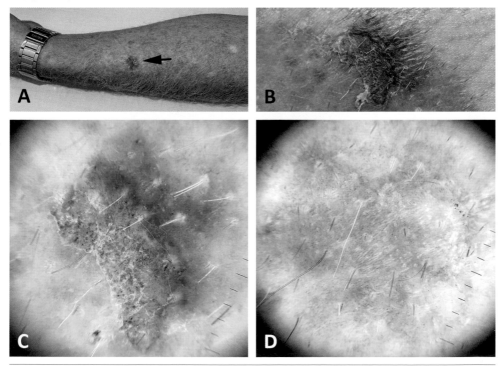

Figure 9.94: *Clinical (A), close-up (B) and dermatoscopic (C) images of a lesion which presented with evident erythema due to apparent inflammation. Evolving lichen planus-like keratosis was suspected and the lesion subsequently developed the reassuring morphology of a more typical lichen planus-like keratosis (dermatoscopic image D).*

serpentine vessels. The translucent jelly-like BCC stroma is not present (*Figures 9.93–9.95*). These lesions can also mimic SCC *in situ* (*Figure 9.96*).

9.4.4 Porokeratosis

Porokeratosis may present as a solitary lesion which has a distinct morphology, most evident clinically as a flat lesion surmounted by fine scale and with a cornoid lamella presenting as a raised border around the periphery (*Figure 9.97*).

Disseminated actinic porokeratosis is characterised by multiple lesions of porokeratosis on sun-exposed areas on both upper and lower limbs.

9.4.5 Stucco keratosis

Stucco keratosis presents typically as multiple small sharply demarcated keratotic lesions on the distal legs, more commonly of males (*Figure 9.98*). It is named for its 'stuck-on'

appearance ('stucco' being a variety of wall plastering). This should not be confused with idiopathic guttate hypomelanosis which lacks palpable surface keratin (*Figure 9.75*).

9.4.6 Viral wart

Viral wart (verruca vulgaris) is generally diagnosed clinically as a skin-coloured plaque or papule, usually present in company with other warts. If a vessel pattern is seen it will be centred in skin-coloured clods which may be present in hyperplastic dermal papillae extending as finger-like projections, a morphology known as papillomatosis (*Figure 9.99*).

9.4.7 Clear cell acanthoma

Clear cell acanthoma is an acanthoma which has a specific serpiginous vascular pattern – one of the four benign patterns of the 'Prediction without Pigment' decision algorithm (*Figure 9.100*)[6].

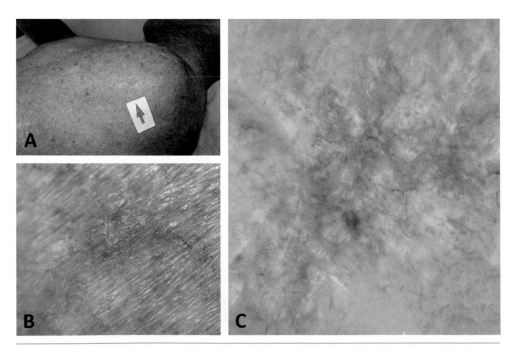

Figure 9.95: *Clinical (A), close-up (B) and dermatoscopic (C) images of a lichen planus-like keratosis presenting as a non-pigmented lesion with polarising-specific white lines and fine serpentine vessels, leading to treatment on suspicion of basal cell carcinoma.*

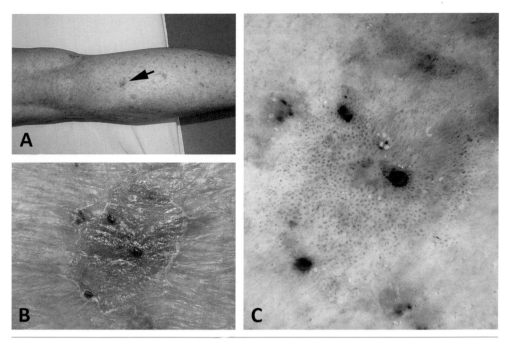

Figure 9.96: *Clinical (A), close-up (B) and dermatoscopic (C) images of a lichen planus-like keratosis presenting as a non-pigmented lesion with ulceration and a monomorphous pattern of coiled vessels, leading to treatment on suspicion of squamous cell carcinoma in situ.*

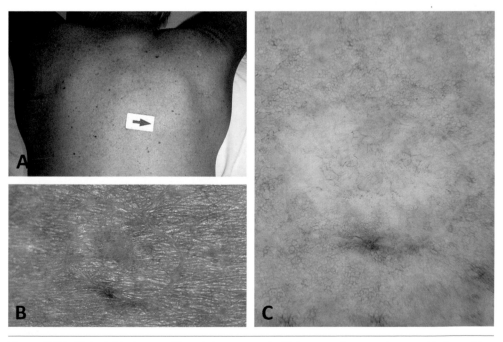

Figure 9.97: *Clinical (A), close-up (B) and dermatoscopic (C) images of a non-pigmented lesion with a sharply circumscribed elevated margin as a clue to porokeratosis (not excised).*

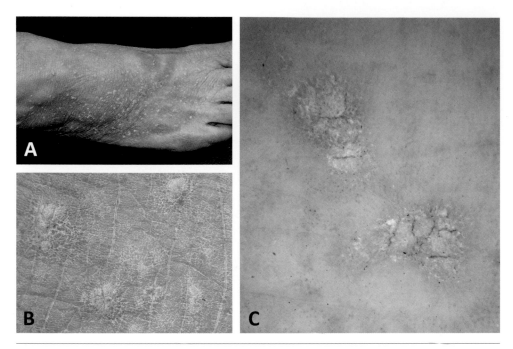

Figure 9.98: *Clinical (A), close-up (B) and dermatoscopic (C) images of stucco keratoses. The clinical appearance shown in (A) is very characteristic for this condition, and the dermatoscopy in this case is characterised by central white clods and peripheral white dots.*

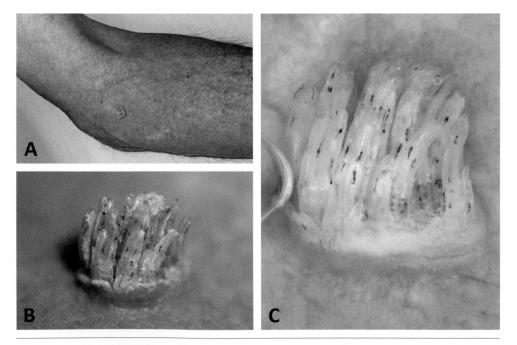

Figure 9.99: *Clinical (A), close-up (B) and dermatoscopic (C) images of a wart (verruca vulgaris) with the characteristic morphology of papillomatosis, where each finger-like projection represents a hypertrophic dermal papilla containing a single papillary vessel. If these structures are shorter this can give rise to a centred vessel pattern.*

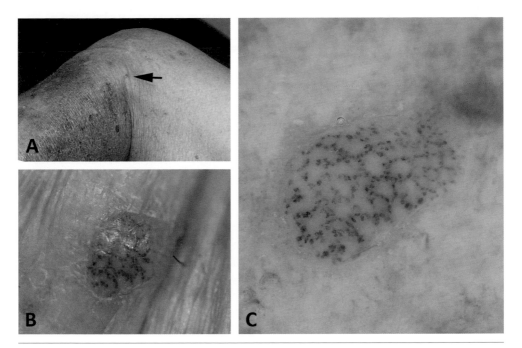

Figure 9.100: *Clinical (A), close-up (B) and dermatoscopic (C) images of a clear cell acanthoma exhibiting a characteristic serpiginous (also known as 'string of pearls') vessel pattern.*

9.5 Actinic keratosis, squamous cell carcinoma *in situ* and squamous cell carcinoma

The majority of AK and SCC *in situ* are non-pigmented and invasive SCC is only very rarely pigmented.

9.5.1 Actinic keratosis

Most AK present on sun-damaged skin as flat lesions with visible or palpable surface scale. If the lesion is visible beneath the scale it will be pink from increased blood flow and the vascular plexus will be prominent with fine linear or coiled/dot vessels. The translucent jelly-like stroma often present in BCC will not be seen. There will be an absence of looped vessels, such vessels only being seen in raised lesions as described in *Section 4.7.3*[6]. The presence of polarising-specific 4-dot clods is a supporting clue to AK, but the diagnosis should not be made from that clue alone because it can be seen on any sun-damaged skin, including on melanoma.

On the face AK will commonly present with dermatoscopic white circles on a pink background and vessels may be prominent between the circles.

Dermatoscopic images of non-pigmented actinic keratoses are presented in *Figures 9.101–9.104*.

Pigmented AK presents as for non-pigmented AK, with the addition of pigment clues in the form of structureless pigment, pigmented dots and occasionally polygons[5]. The pigment may be brown or grey and rarely black. The follicles remain non-pigmented and the stark contrast to interfollicular pigment makes them very evident, a distinguishing feature compared to both solar lentigo and lentigo maligna (see *Section 9.5.3*).

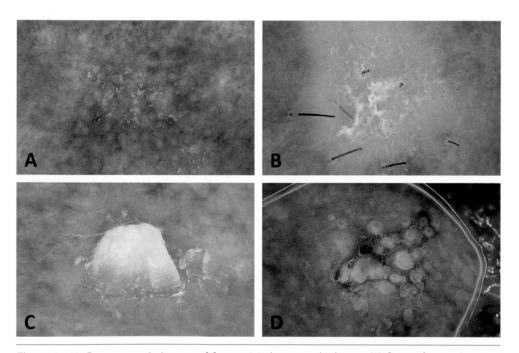

Figure 9.101: *Dermatoscopic images of four actinic keratoses displaying: (A) fine surface scale over a structureless pink area, (B) fine surface scale over a structureless white area (excised on suspicion of SCC), (C) a thick laminated keratin horn, and (D) white clods and white circles on a red eroded background in an actinic keratosis on facial skin.*

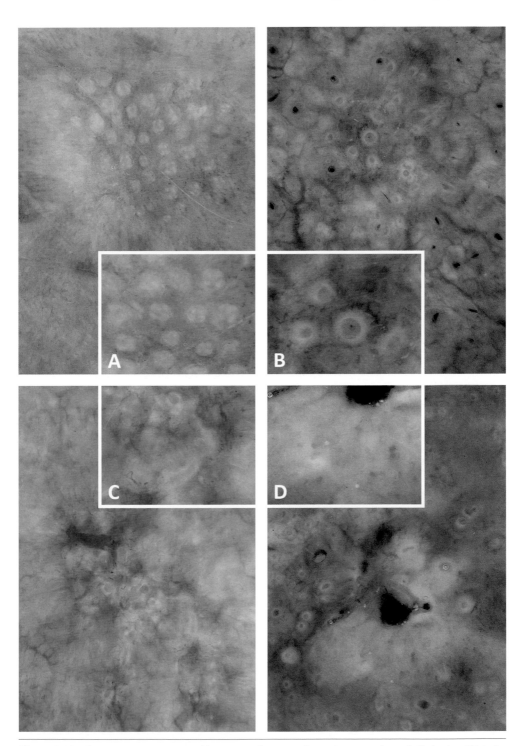

Figure 9.102: *Dermatoscopic images of four actinic keratoses (insert images enlarged) displaying: (A) 4-dot clods (also known as rosettes), (B) white circles in an actinic keratosis on facial skin, (C) white circles and polarising-specific white lines, and (D) white circles and a white structureless area in an actinic keratosis on facial skin.*

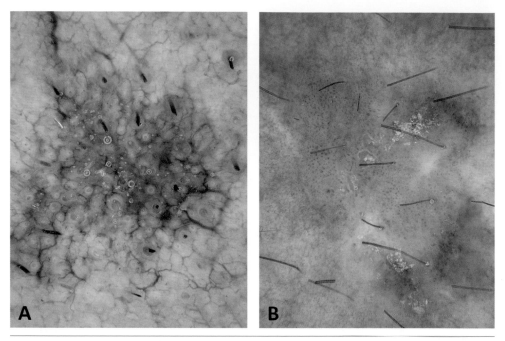

Figure 9.103: *Dermatoscopic images of two solar keratoses displaying: (A) dilated dermal plexus vessels and background redness, and (B) monomorphous coiled (or dot depending on resolution) vessels.*

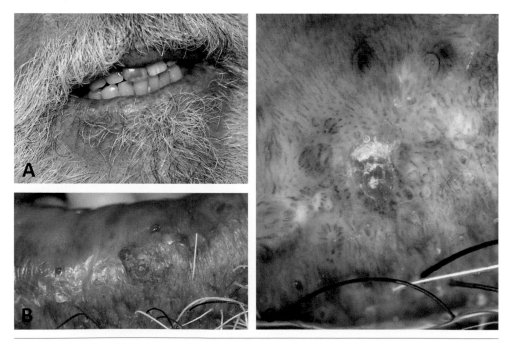

Figure 9.104: *Clinical (A), close-up (B) and dermatoscopic (C) images of a solar keratosis on vermillion lip which was biopsied due to an elevated profile, ulceration and other overlapping features, to exclude squamous cell carcinoma.*

9.5.2 Squamous cell carcinoma *in situ*

SCC *in situ* shares features with AK, which is not surprising because histologically they only differ with respect to a few layers of cells beneath the stratum granulosum, these being spared from dysplasia in AK. Clinically and dermatoscopically, however, there are differences including a tendency for SCC *in situ* to present as a large macule or plaque with well-defined margins. Usually SCC *in situ* appears on sun-damaged skin, but there is a variant associated with human papilloma virus (HPV) infection which presents in sun-protected locations, usually in proximity to the genitalia such as in the crural fold.

SCC *in situ* often has surface keratin, although this is generally less evident than with AK, and 4-dot clods are often present. With non-pigmented SCC *in situ* the erythema is more pronounced than with non-pigmented AK. A distinctive dermatoscopic feature usually observed in non-facial, non-pigmented SCC *in situ* is the presence of coiled/dot vessels which will either be in a clustered or linear arrangement. On facial SCC *in situ* white circles are frequently seen.

Images of lightly pigmented and non pigmented SCC *in situ* are presented in *Figures 9.105–9.109*.

Pigmented SCC *in situ* is not uncommon, accounting for 3–5% of all SCC *in situ* and it is a lesion frequently mistaken for melanoma[19]. Clinical and dermatoscopic features are similar to those of non-pigmented variants with respect to the features of flat morphology and sharply defined margin, the frequent presence of surface keratin, 4-dot clods, white circles on facial skin, and coiled/dot vessels in clustered or linear arrangement. Pigment may occur as structureless brown and/or grey (*Figure 9.110A*), as brown and/or grey dots (*Figure 9.110D*), or as lines angulated (polygons) (*Figure 9.110C*). The presence of dots, with red dots merging into pigmented dots in linear and/or radial arrangement, is a compelling clue to pSCC *in situ*. Images of a variety of cases of pSCC *in situ* are presented in *Figures 9.109–9.114*.

In a study of 52 consecutive cases of pSCC *in*

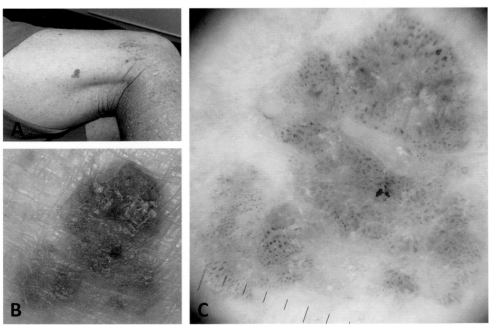

Figure 9.105: *Clinical (A), close-up (B) and dermatoscopic (C) images of a lightly pigmented SCC in situ on the thigh. Clinically it is a well demarcated pink plaque with surface scale. Dermatoscopically, where not obscured by keratin scale, there is a monomorphous pattern of coiled (or dot, depending on your perception) vessels in linear arrangement.*

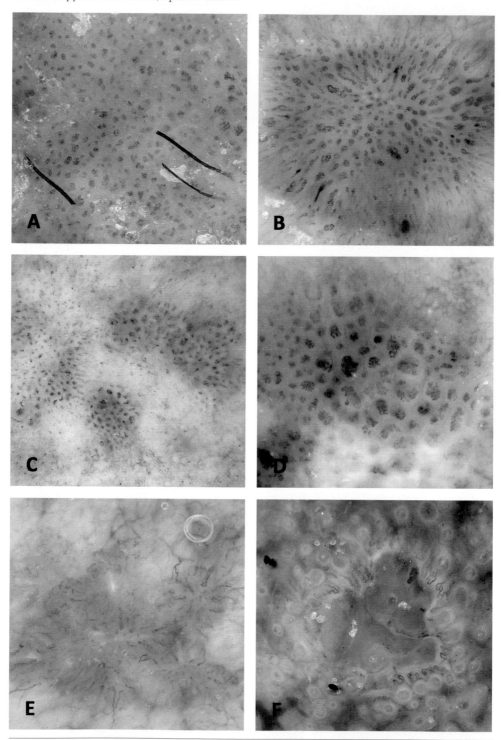

Figure 9.106: *Dermatoscopic images of portions of six examples of squamous cell carcinoma* in situ: *(A) monomorphous coiled vessels in random arrangement; (B) monomorphous coiled vessels in linear/radial arrangement; (C) monomorphous coiled vessels in clustered arrangement; (D) monomorphous coiled vessels in linear arrangement; (E) linear serpentine vessels (unusual); (F) linear looped vessels around a central focus, associated with white circles in a squamous cell carcinoma* in situ *on facial skin.*

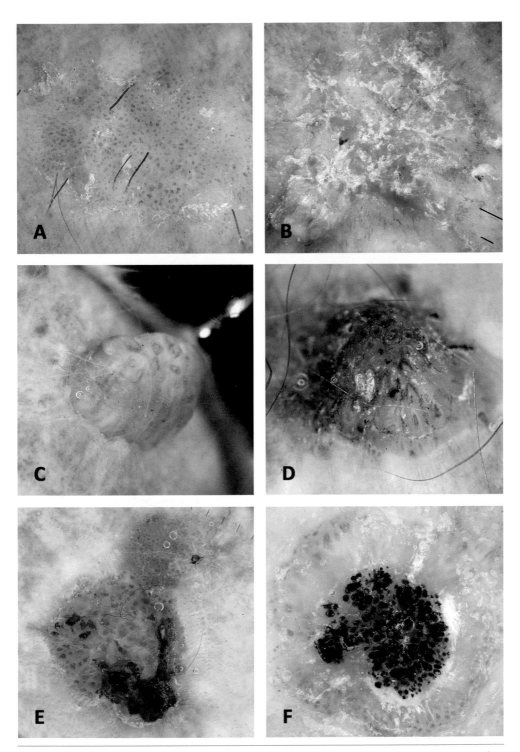

Figure 9.107: *Dermatoscopic images of six squamous cell carcinomas* in situ *with variations in surface morphology: (A) minimal white surface scale; (B) thick yellow and white surface scale; (C) keratin horn; (D) verrucous morphology with central thick yellow keratin; (E) crusting and adherent fibre secondary to ulceration and serum exudation; (F) central thick keratin plaque with blood spots.*

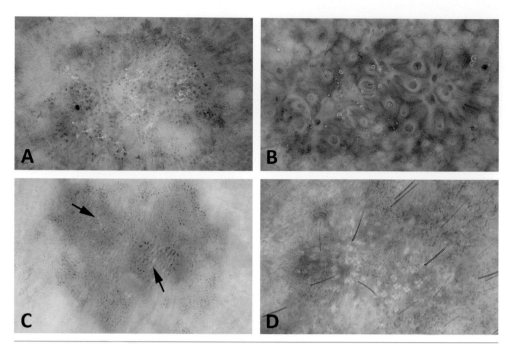

Figure 9.108: *Dermatoscopic images of four squamous cell carcinomas* in situ *displaying various white structures: (A) white structureless areas; (B) white circles in a squamous cell carcinoma* in situ *on facial skin; (C) white lines (arrows); (D) 4-dot clods.*

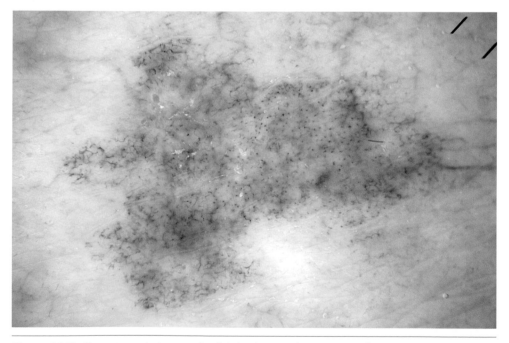

Figure 9.109: *Dermatoscopic image of a lightly pigmented squamous cell carcinoma* in situ *with a polymorphous pattern of vessels including short linear vessels and dots. As is frequently the case with pigmented squamous cell carcinoma* in situ, *the differential diagnosis is melanoma.*

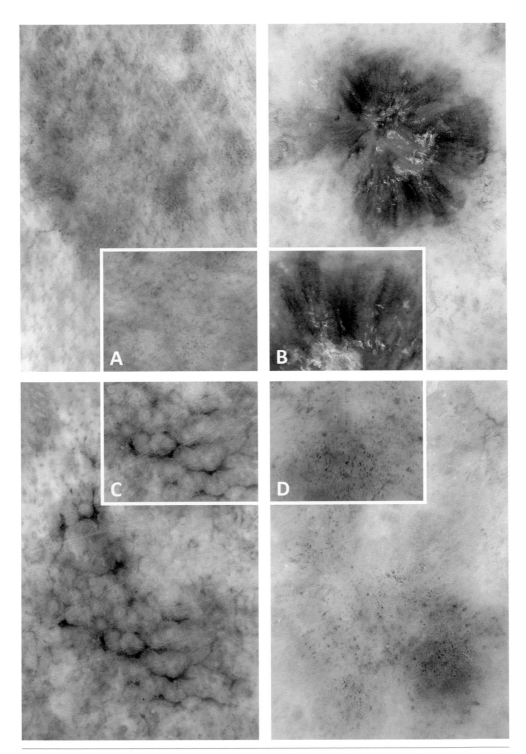

Figure 9.110: *Dermatoscopic images of four examples of pigmented squamous cell carcinoma* in situ *displaying various patterns (insert images magnified): (A) structureless (vessels as red dots are not regarded as a pattern for this purpose); (B) dots in radial arrangement; (C) lines angulated; (D) dots.*

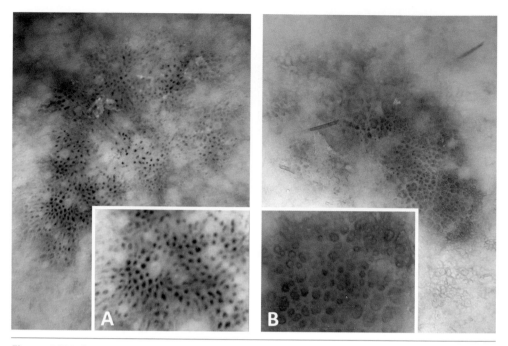

Figure 9.111: *Dermatoscopic images of two examples of pigmented squamous cell carcinoma* in situ *displaying various patterns (insert images magnified): (A) clods/dots in linear arrangement; (B) circles (not related to adnexae).*

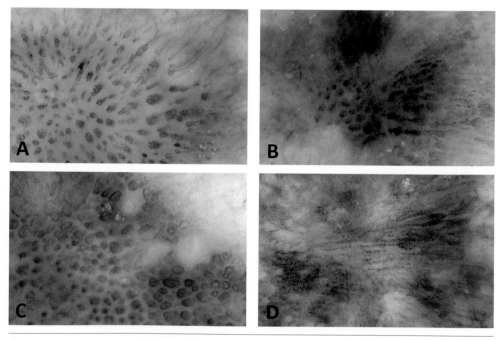

Figure 9.112: *Dermatoscopic images of four examples of squamous cell carcinoma* in situ *with structures in linear arrangement: (A) non-pigmented squamous cell carcinoma* in situ *with coiled vessels in linear arrangement, and three pigmented squamous cell carcinomas* in situ *with (B) linear clods, (C) linear circles, and (D) linear dots.*

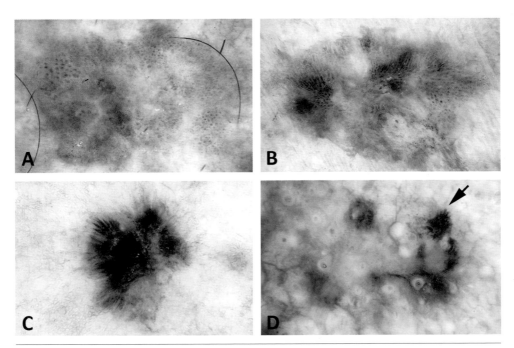

Figure 9.113: *Dermatoscopic images of four pigmented squamous cell carcinomas in situ displaying various patterns: (A) a pattern of brown dots/clods in linear arrangement combined asymmetrically with a structureless area; (B) a pattern of brown dots in linear arrangement combined asymmetrically with a structureless area; (C) a pattern of lines radial segmental combined asymmetrically with a structureless area; (D) a structureless pigmented lesion on the face with the clue of lines radial segmental (arrow) and white circles.*

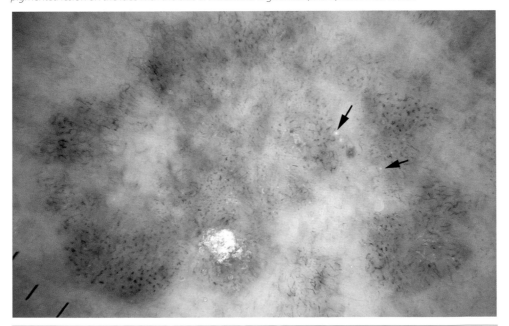

Figure 9.114: *Dermatoscopic image of a pigmented squamous cell carcinoma in situ. Pattern is structureless with a polymorphous pattern of short linear and coiled vessels predominantly in a clustered arrangement, with some vessels in linear arrangement (lower left) as a clue to squamous cell carcinoma in situ rather than melanoma. A few white dots (arrows) are the only dermatoscopic clue to a precursor seborrhoeic keratosis.*

situ, the lesions were typified by the absence of a pattern of reticular lines and by the presence of a pattern of dots and/or structureless zones. A single pattern was present in 53.8% with 48.1% being only structureless. Hypopigmented (pink, skin-coloured or white) structureless areas were present in 67.3%. Brown or grey dots in a linear arrangement were present in 21.2% and a linear arrangement of coiled vessels was found in 11.5%[19].

9.5.3 Distinguishing flat pigmented facial lesions: solar lentigo, pAK/SCC *in situ* and LM

Probably the most important consideration about flat pigmented facial lesions on sun-damaged skin at mature age is that the differential diagnosis is not expected to include acquired (Clark) naevus[20]. Congenital naevi occur on the head and neck and although usually dermal (Miescher) or compound they may sometimes be visibly

and palpably flat. Such congenital naevi are generally evident by their symmetrical morphology, uniformly gradual border and long-standing history of stability (*Figure 9.115*).

Especially at mature age, in the context of an excision biopsy of a lesion from sun-damaged skin on the head or neck, a histological report of lentigo simplex, Clark naevus or so-called dysplastic naevus should prompt a discussion with the reporting dermatopathologist and a request for review of the histology[20].

The differential diagnosis of flat pigmented lesions on the head or neck includes solar lentigo (including LPLK), pigmented AK (pAK)/SCC *in situ* and LM[21]. Histology is the gold standard to distinguish these lesions[22] but there are clues which will lead to a correct diagnosis in most situations. These will be discussed in the order of commonality, which is appropriate for the context of what is encountered during an examination for skin cancer.

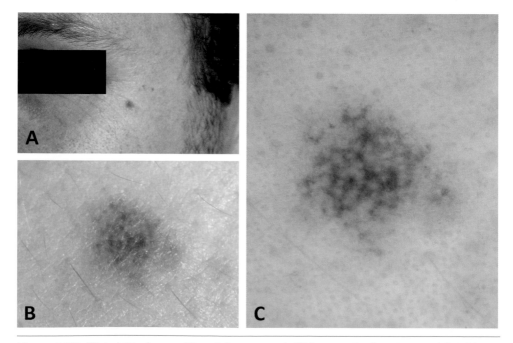

Figure 9.115: *Clinical (A), close-up (B) and dermatoscopic (C) images of a flat pigmented facial lesion. Whether you call the pattern lines, clods or structureless, it is symmetrical and fades gradually towards the periphery which is consistent with the morphology of a congenital naevus, this being confirmed by long-term stability.*

Solar lentigo and lichen planus-like keratosis

If solar lentigo can be diagnosed on clinical and dermatoscopic grounds then a biopsy is avoided.

A flat pigmented lesion on the head and neck with the following features will predictably be a solar lentigo (*Figure 9.116*)[21]:

- one colour, brown
- no palpable scale
- a sharply demarcated border over the total periphery, scalloped in some parts
- a structureless, lines reticular or lines curved, pattern
- no prominent vessels.

Another compelling clue is the presence of a *monotonous regular* pattern of short curved or reticular lines: such a regular pattern not being expected in a malignant condition (*Figure 9.116*).

There may be some parts of the border which are not abrupt and this may warrant a closer look, but if there is no grey colour and no other clues to pAK or LM then solar lentigo can be predicted.

If the pattern includes lines it is not uncommon for these to end abruptly at parts of the periphery as a 'broken-off' appearance. Solar lentigo is a precursor to seborrhoeic keratosis and an elevated component with clues to seborrhoeic keratosis can provide additional evidence. It should always be remembered, however, that melanoma can occur in collision with seborrhoeic keratosis because the latter are so common. Pigmented circles were found to favour a diagnosis of melanoma in one study, but the lesions in that study were all excised on suspicion of malignancy, so solar lentigines with pigmented circles were often not included because of other benign features as outlined above[21]. Pigmented circles may be found in solar lentigines, in which case the dermatoscopist must look carefully at the other clues to decide whether biopsy is indicated (*Figure 9.116*).

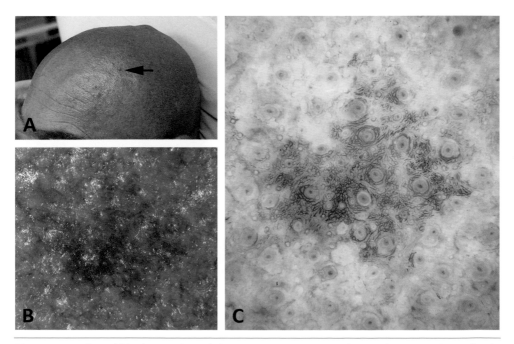

Figure 9.116: Clinical (A), close-up (B) and dermatoscopic (C) images of a solar lentigo on the scalp. The primary pattern is of reticular lines, lines taking priority over circles which are therefore relegated to the status of a clue. The very regular fine reticular lines favour a diagnosis of solar lentigo, but because there were pigmented circles and the border was not uniformly abrupt an excision biopsy was considered necessary.

Solar lentigines being subjected to an immune attack are known as LPLK and such lesions may have dermatoscopic grey dots or grey circles. In many cases these grey structures will mandate biopsy if pAK cannot be diagnosed with confidence (*Figures 9.117–9.119*). On the face symmetry cannot generally be relied upon to exclude melanoma if a confident alternative diagnosis is not possible, considering all criteria (*Figures 9.127* and *9.128*).

Pigmented AK and pigmented SCC *in situ*
Pigmented AK (and pSCC *in situ*) can share some features with solar lentigo such as a sharply demarcated border which may include some scalloping and 'broken-off' lines at some parts of the periphery.

Distinguishing features may include any or all of (*Figures 9.120–9.124*)[23]:
- palpable scale

- very evident pale follicles which may be enlarged or variable in size
- interfollicular erythema
- white circles and 4-dot clods.

It is the fact that the follicles themselves are almost invariably not pigmented that creates this valuable distinguishing feature contrasting pAK with LM and also from many solar lentigines. Although pAK may exhibit pigmented circles, the very pale follicles that these circles surround, and which they throw into sharp contrast, strongly favours a diagnosis of pAK rather than of either solar lentigo or LM[23]. It is also common to see grey structures in pAK, and these may include grey circles made up of grey dots in a circle surrounding the very evident pale follicles. Images of pAK and pSCC *in situ* are displayed in *Figures 9.120–9.124*.

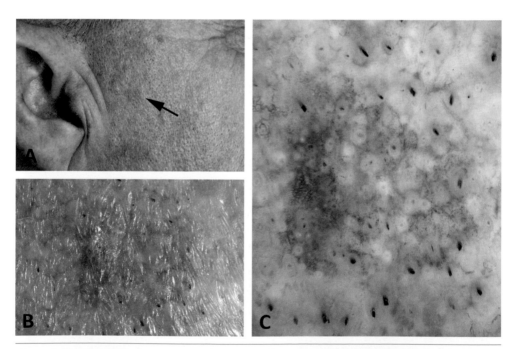

Figure 9.117: Clinical (A), close-up (B) and dermatoscopic (C) images of a flat pigmented facial lesion. On the right-hand side there are evident pale follicles with interfollicular grey dots. Very regular fine reticular brown lines on the left with a few bright white dots are evidence of a pre-existing seborrhoeic keratosis. Excision biopsy was, however, performed because the border was not uniformly abrupt; lichen planus-like keratosis.

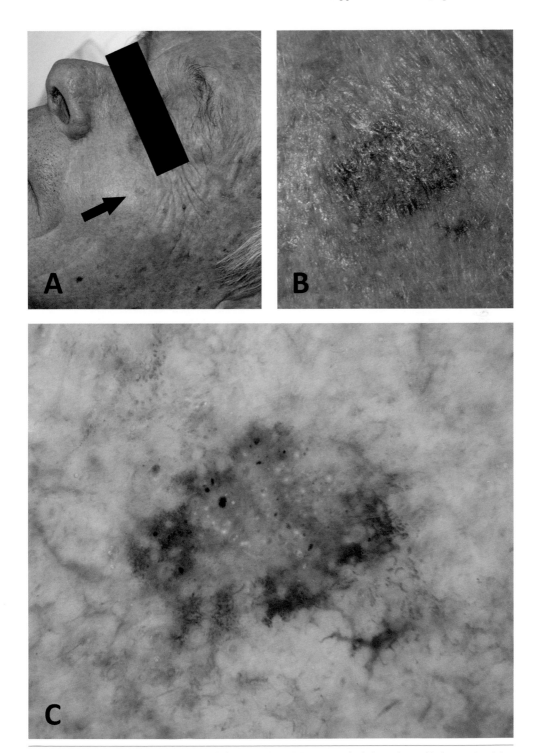

Figure 9.118: *Clinical (A), close-up (B) and dermatoscopic (C) images of a lichen planus-like keratosis arising from a seborrhoeic keratosis. Residual elements of the seborrhoeic keratosis (white dots) are evident.*

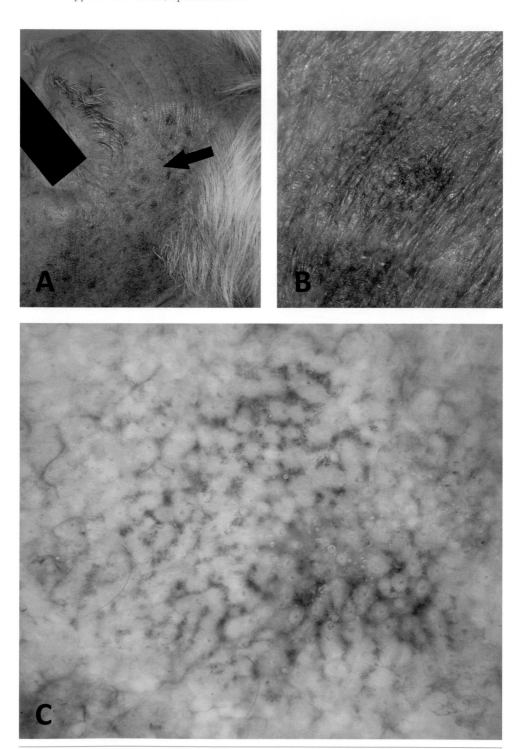

Figure 9.119: *Clinical (A), close-up (B) and dermatoscopic (C) images of a lichen planus-like keratosis in which a poorly defined border as well as evident angulated lines (polygons) led to suspicion of melanoma and subsequent biopsy.*

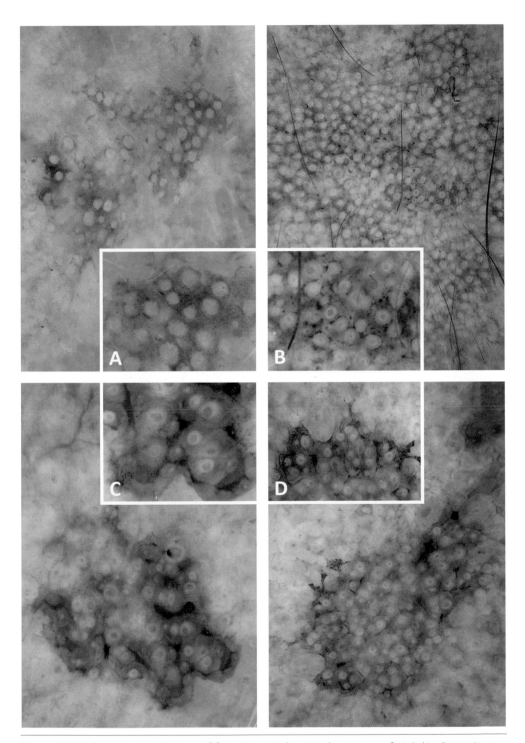

Figure 9.120: *Dermatoscopic images of four pigmented actinic keratoses on facial skin (insert images enlarged) displaying: (A) structureless pigmentation interrupted by very evident pale follicular openings; (B) a pattern of white circles overlying pigmented dots; (C) a pattern of interfollicular angulated lines combined with the clue of white circles; (D) a pattern of very prominent white circles overlying structureless pigment. Very sharp borders consistent with pigmented surface keratin scale are evident in (C) and (D).*

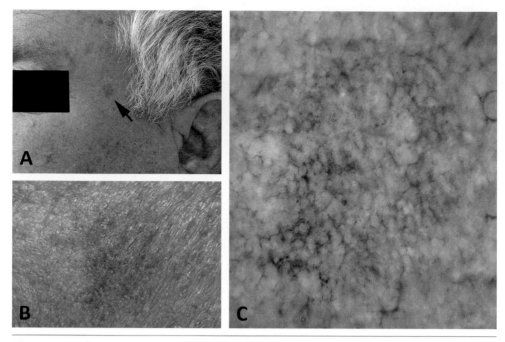

Figure 9.121: *Clinical (A), close-up (B) and dermatoscopic (C) images of a pigmented actinic keratosis in which histologically reported regression resulted in dermatoscopic clues to melanoma, including chaos of colour, chaos of border abruptness and polygons.*

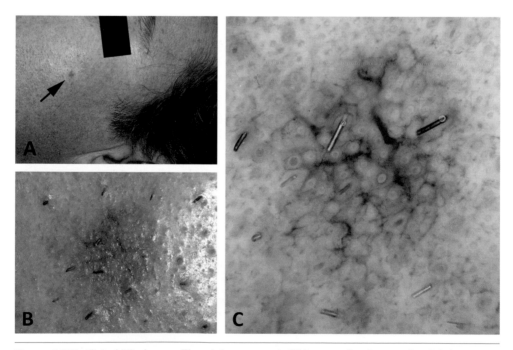

Figure 9.122: *Clinical (A), close-up (B) and dermatoscopic (C) images of a pigmented actinic keratosis in which pigmented circles and a poorly defined border resulted in excision on suspicion of melanoma. Note the dilated vessels and very pale follicles, both of which are consistent with pigmented actinic keratosis.*

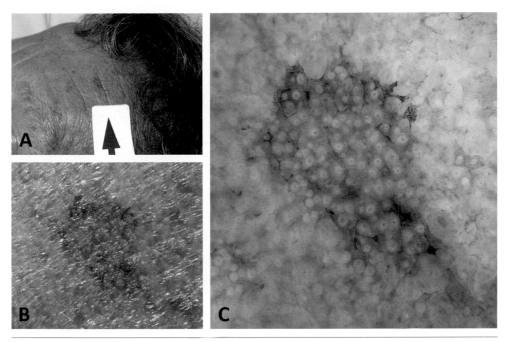

Figure 9.123: *Clinical (A), close-up (B) and dermatoscopic (C) images of a pigmented actinic keratosis on the forehead. In this case the primary pattern is of white circles and there is interfollicular pigmentation. The follicles, unlike those of the solar lentigo in Figure 9.116, are very pale and therefore visually evident, in stark contrast to the surrounding pigment, and some peripheral pigmented lines are sharply 'broken-off', both of these features not being expected in lentigo maligna.*

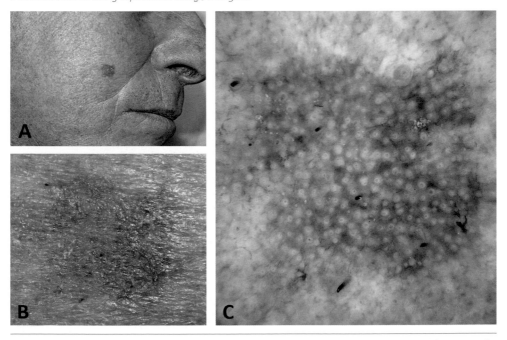

Figure 9.124: *Clinical (A), close-up (B) and dermatoscopic (C) images of a flat pigmented lesion on the cheek. Dermatoscopic features of very pale follicles in stark contrast to interfollicular pigment and erythema are consistent with a diagnosis of pigmented actinic keratosis. In this case histology revealed full-thickness epidermal dysplasia; pigmented squamous cell carcinoma* in situ.

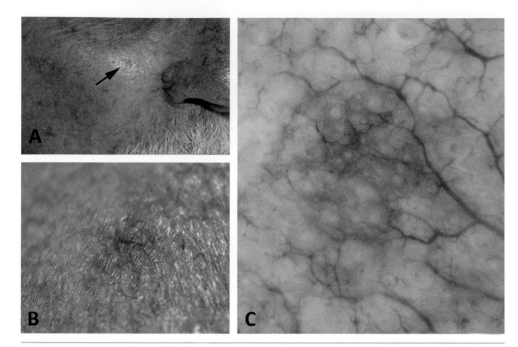

Figure 9.125: Clinical (A), close-up (B) and dermatoscopic (C) images of a very subtle flat pigmented lesion on the cheek. There is structureless pigment with poorly defined borders and although there are a few pigmented circles, the follicular openings are not as evident as those seen in the pigmented actinic keratosis and squamous cell carcinoma in situ *in Figures 9.123 and 9.124, respectively. The poorly defined border precludes a provisional diagnosis of solar lentigo; lentigo maligna (melanoma* in situ*).*

Lentigo maligna

Lentigo maligna, being a form of melanoma *in situ*, is the most important flat pigmented lesion on the head and neck for the purpose of diagnosis and management. In its early stages it is often a clinically unremarkable lesion which may be overlooked if the dermatoscope is not applied.

Dermatoscopic clues which raise suspicion for LM include the following.

- A poorly defined border which fades out in contrast to the well-defined sharp border of both solar lentigo and pAK[23].
- There may be some areas of border abruptness in a more advanced LM but this will only involve a portion of the border and is not expected in a small early lesion.
- A light brown structureless pattern, the brown pigmentation being spread across both interfollicular and follicular structures (*Figures 9.125–9.127*), this being in contrast to pAK where the follicles are very evident because of their pallor[23].

- When pigmented circles are present they are expected to surround pigmented follicles so that the follicles would not be evident except for the presence of pigmented circles (*Figures 9.125–9.127*).
- One uncommon feature strongly favouring a diagnosis of LM is the dermatoscopic observation of a double pigmented circle; a circle within a circle (*Figure 9.126B*).

As a LM develops there may be a progression from pigmented circles, through angulated lines (polygons or rhomboid structures), to obliteration of follicles in some parts and at such a stage the LM will start taking on the morphological features of melanomas on the body in general (*Figure 9.126A, B* and *D*). At this stage the differentiation from solar lentigo and pAK should no longer be an issue. Sometimes the only clue to LM will be a pattern of grey dots without a sharply demarcated border, which if present would support the alternative diagnosis of LPLK (*Figure 9.128*).

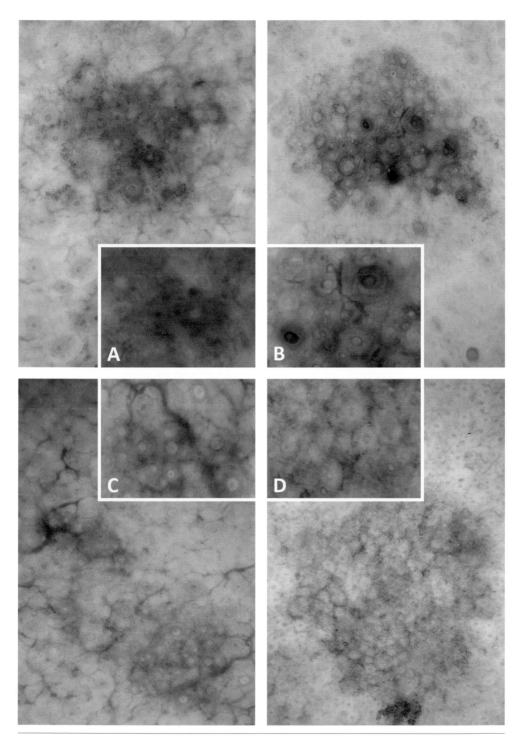

Figure 9.126: *Dermatoscopic images displaying patterns commonly observed in lentigo maligna (insert images enlarged): (A) grey structures, (B) pigmented circles related to follicles, (C) poorly defined ('fading') border, and (D) angulated lines. None of these lesions have a border consistent with a naevus or solar lentigo/seborrhoeic keratosis and the follicles are less pale and therefore not as evident as in the examples of pigmented actinic keratosis or squamous cell carcinoma* in situ *shown in* Figures 9.120–9.124.

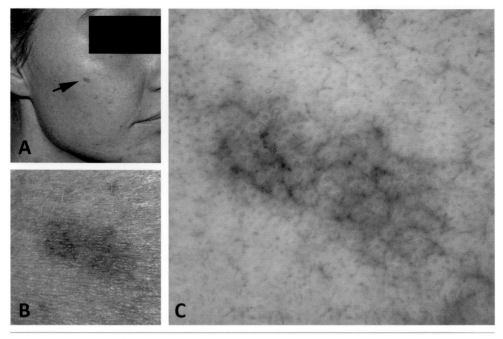

Figure 9.127: *Clinical (A), close-up (B) and dermatoscopic (C) images of facial lentigo maligna (melanoma in situ) on a young woman, demonstrating minimal dermatoscopic chaos, plus angulated lines (polygons). Note how the polygons coincide with the dermal vessel plexus.*

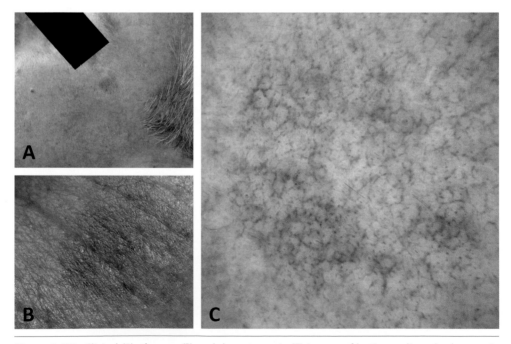

Figure 9.128: *Clinical (A), close-up (B) and dermatoscopic (C) images of lentigo maligna (melanoma in situ) demonstrating an absence of convincing chaos but with grey dots as a clue to malignancy. This case demonstrates the importance of responding to grey colour on the face. The morphology, especially with regard to the border, does not support the alternative diagnosis of lichen planus-like keratosis.*

9.5.4 Squamous cell carcinoma and keratoacanthoma

The vast majority of invasive SCC and all keratoacanthoma (KA) are non-pigmented: although a history of rapid growth of a recently occurring keratotic lesion favours KA, it is been shown that the two cannot be reliably distinguished by dermatoscopic criteria[24].

Invasive SCC and KA typically present as a flesh-coloured nodule with one or more of[24]:

• surface keratin
• a white structureless area
• white circles.

Looped vessels, with or without a white surround, are expected and serpentine branched vessels are also frequently seen. The presence of serpentine branched vessels adjacent to keratin is a reliable clue to SCC/KA[24].

Examples of SCC and KA are presented in *Figures 9.129–9.136*.

Pigmented invasive SCC is very rare: a report of one case with a review of all five preceding reported cases revealed that dermatoscopically all had an absence of any reticular lines, and all but one had structureless blue colour[25]. White circles were present in the lesion reported (*Figure 9.137*) and it also had serpentine vessels as did at least one of the other cases reviewed.

Poorly differentiated SCC will be devoid of keratin clues (surface keratin, white circles and white structureless areas) and is expected to have a polymorphous pattern of linear vessels (coiled, looped and serpentine) covering the majority of the lesion[26]. Ulceration is frequently present (*Figure 9.138*).

Squamous cell carcinoma should be suspected in cases of nail plate dystrophy involving a single nail: changes can include longitudinal dystrophy, a triangular lunula (*Figure 9.139*) and bony erosions of the underlying distal phalanx visible on X-ray.

With respect to management decisions it is important to ensure that all SCC are adequately excised because of the small but real risk of metastasis, even of well differentiated lesions. Given that KA cannot reliably be distinguished, clinically or dermatoscopically, without a biopsy which demonstrates the complete architecture, excision biopsy is the preferred diagnostic procedure when a diagnosis of either SCC or KA is suspected, at any site apart from nail matrix and mucosal surfaces. Alternatively on the distal leg, where primary closure following elliptical excision may be challenging, a vertically oriented incisional biopsy through the centre of the lesion, including a portion of normal skin on each side, is acceptable, after which histologically identified KA can be observed until resolution is confirmed. Such observation of KA on the face is not acceptable because KA can have an aggressive behaviour causing significant damage to facial structures, prior to resolution.

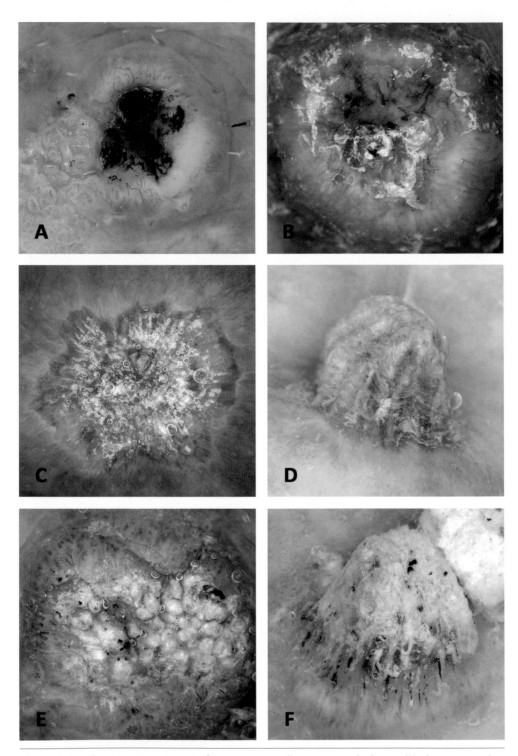

Figure 9.129: *Dermatoscopic images of six squamous cell carcinomas displaying: (A) ulceration, a white structureless area, white circles and linear serpentine vessels; (B) white structureless areas, surface keratin and polymorphous linear vessels; (C) keratin plaque; (D) a laminated cutaneous horn; (E) keratin overlying papillomatosis; (F) blood spots on a keratin horn with white structureless areas and linear vessels in the base.*

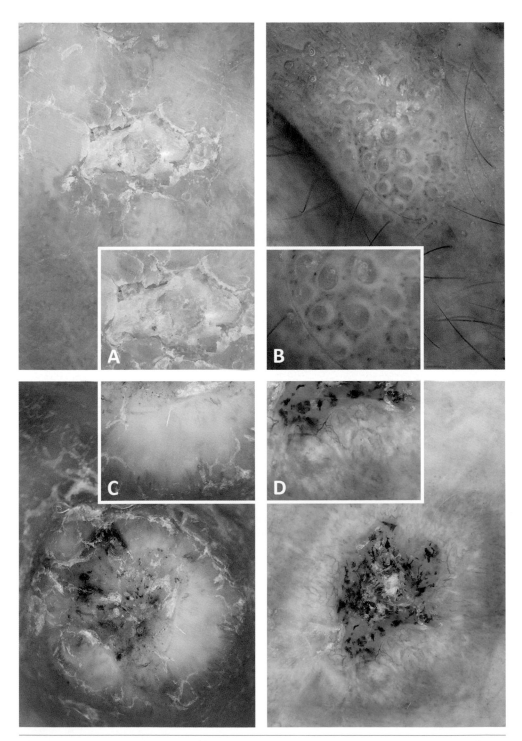

Figure 9.130: *Dermatoscopic images of four squamous cell carcinomas (insert images enlarged) displaying: (A) surface keratin; (B) white circles in a squamous cell carcinoma on the ear; (C) white structureless area and blood spots; (D) blood spots, white structureless areas and white lines.*

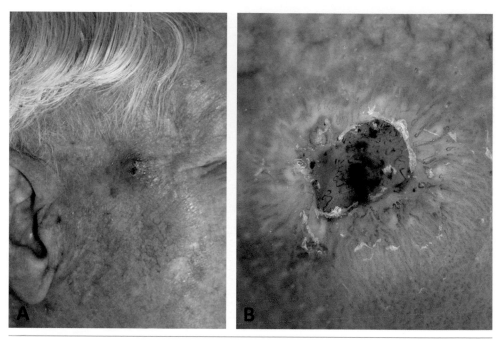

Figure 9.131: *Clinical (A) and dermatoscopic (B) images of a squamous cell carcinoma with central ulceration surrounded by a white structureless area and radially arranged looped vessels.*

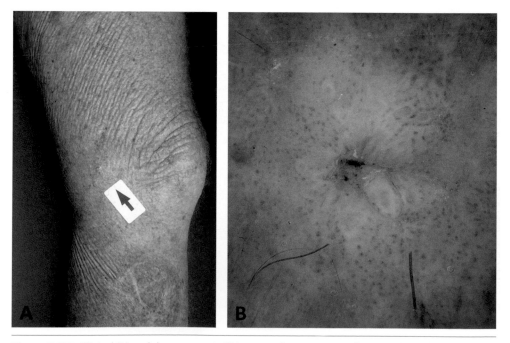

Figure 9.132: *Clinical (A) and dermatoscopic (B) images of a squamous cell carcinoma with a large white structureless area, white circles and a monomorphous pattern of coiled vessels (resolving as dot vessels depending on magnification/visual acuity).*

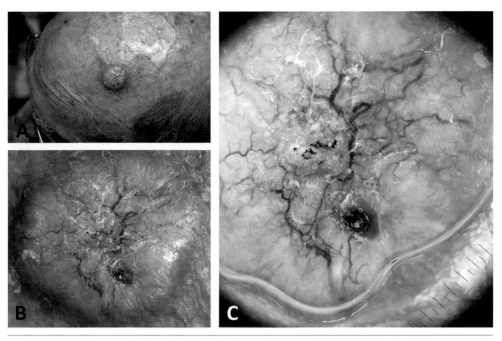

Figure 9.133: *Clinical (A), close-up (B) and dermatoscopic (C) images of a squamous cell carcinoma reported as having perineural invasion, showing ulceration, white structureless areas and branched serpentine vessels.*

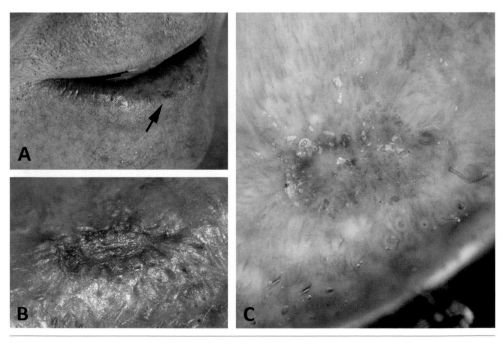

Figure 9.134: *Clinical (A), close-up (B) and dermatoscopic (C) images of a squamous cell carcinoma on the lower lip showing ulceration and white circles present at the vermillion border where hair shafts are evident. This is a high-risk location for metastasis.*

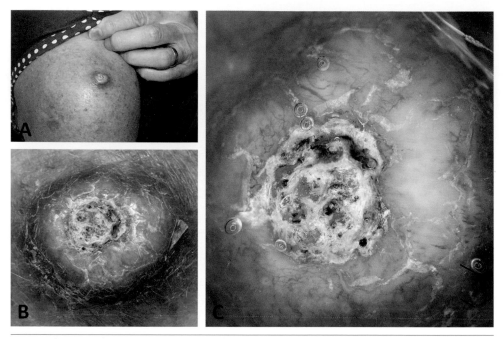

Figure 9.135: *Clinical (A), close-up (B) and dermatoscopic (C) images of a typical keratoacanthoma showing central keratin surrounded by a white structureless area with linear serpentine vessels.*

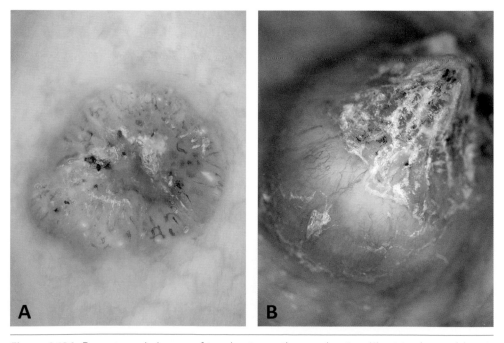

Figure 9.136: *Dermatoscopic images of two keratoacanthomas showing: (A) minimal central keratin surrounded by a skin-coloured structureless area and a radial pattern of polymorphous linear vessels; (B) a central keratin horn surrounded by a white structureless area and a radial pattern of linear serpentine vessels.*

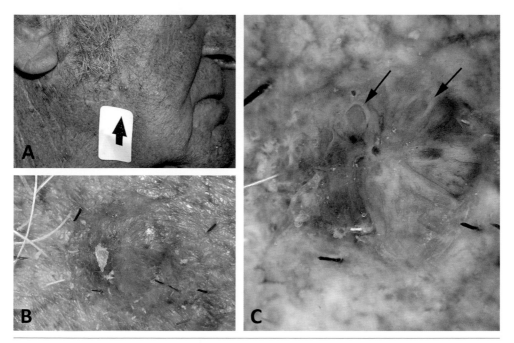

Figure 9.137: *Clinical (A), close-up (B) and dermatoscopic (C) images of an invasive pigmented squamous cell carcinoma with surface scale (B) and a dermatoscopic blue and white structureless area as well as white circles (arrows).*

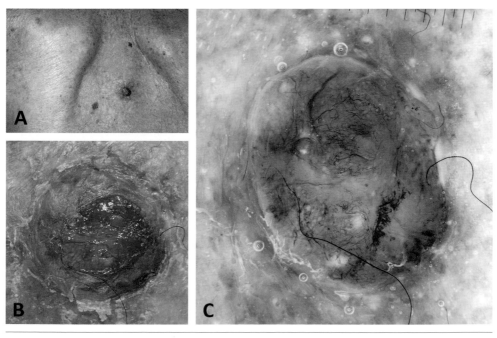

Figure 9.138: *Clinical (A), close-up (B) and dermatoscopic (C) images of a moderately to poorly differentiated squamous cell carcinoma with broad ulceration (note adherent fibre), polymorphous linear vessels and minimal keratinisation in the form of isolated white clods.*

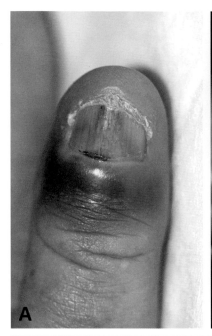
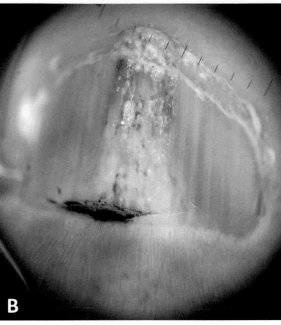

Figure 9.139: Clinical (A) and dermatoscopic (B) images of an invasive squamous cell carcinoma of the nail matrix. The patient presented because of a painful acute abscess combined with a history of progressive changes in the nail plate over the preceding 3 years. This history, in addition to monodactylic progressive hypertrophic dystrophy and the triangular lunula, led to nail matrix biopsy which released pus from the abscess and confirmed squamous cell carcinoma of the nail matrix. Biopsy was preceded by an X-ray which revealed no erosion of the underlying terminal phalanx.

9.6 Dermatofibroma and dermatofibrosarcoma protuberans

The diagnosis of DF can usually be confidently confirmed by a symmetrical combination of virtually any dermatoscopic pattern peripherally, combined with a central hypopigmented structureless area in which vessels of almost any type may be seen. Commonly, polarising-specific white lines are also seen in the central hypopigmented area. A history of stability of a clinical palpable nodule which characteristically retracts when the lesion is laterally compressed is usually compelling additional support for the diagnosis of DF (*Figures 9.140–9.144*)[5].

Dermatofibroma is frequently non-pigmented clinically but some pigment will usually be seen peripherally on dermatoscopy. The diagnosis is not difficult with a small nodular symmetrical pink skin lesion with vessels of various structures centrally, with or without polarising-specific white lines also in a central location. Dimpling on lateral compression assists diagnostic confidence as does a history of stability.

Dermatofibrosarcoma protuberans is a dermal-based skin tumour which shares some morphological features with DF[27]. It usually comes to biopsy either because of symptoms (redness and pain occur in 15% of cases) and/or because it is an elevated, firm, and growing (EFG) lesion. The lesion has a tendency to recur, necessitating wide surgical margins, but it rarely metastasises.

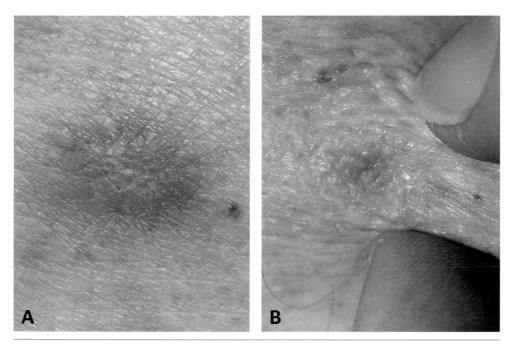

Figure 9.140: *Clinical image of a dermatofibroma (A) and an image (B) demonstrating puckering of the skin caused by lateral compression (the pinch test).*

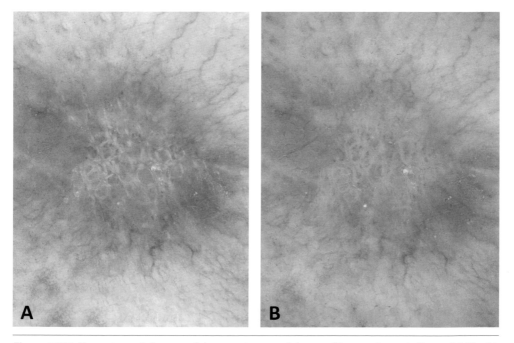

Figure 9.141: *Dermatoscopic images of the non-pigmented dermatofibroma shown in* Figure 9.140 *with (A) polarised light showing central polarising-specific white lines orientated perpendicularly to each other but not crossing, and (B) with non-polarised light showing central reticular white lines.*

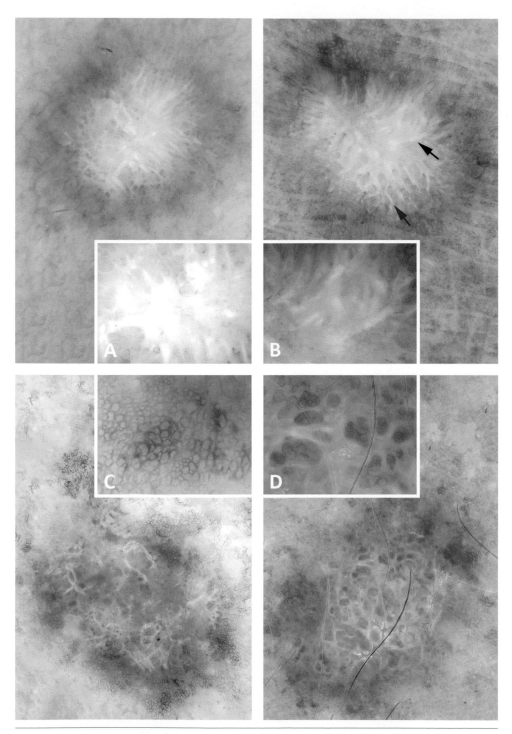

Figure 9.142: *Dermatoscopic images displaying features that may be observed in dermatofibromas (insert images enlarged): (A) central structureless white area and polarising-specific white lines; (B) polarising-specific white lines (black arrow) and other white lines (red arrow); (C) reticular lines peripherally and polarising-specific white lines centrally; (D) pigmented clods and circles, some of which are separated by polarising-specific white lines.*

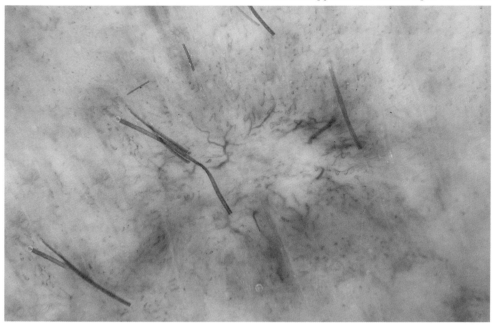

Figure 9.143: *Dermatoscopic image of a lightly pigmented dermatofibroma with central structureless white and peripheral structureless brown areas. Polymorphous vessels are clearly seen with patterns of both (linear) branched serpentine vessels and dot vessels. The symmetry of the pigment distribution and of the vessel patterns is consistent with the diagnosis of dermatofibroma rather than melanoma.*

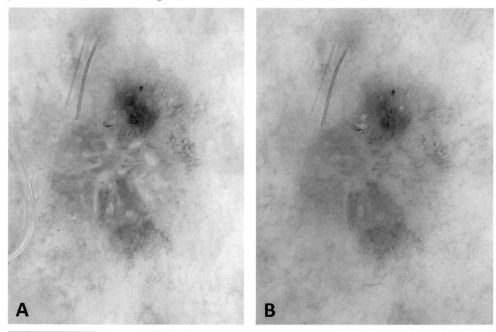

Figure 9.144: *Polarised (A) and non-polarised (B) dermatoscopic images of a dermatofibroma. The peripheral pigment, lines reticular and structureless light and dark brown areas, combined asymmetrically, surround a non-pigmented centre of polarising-specific white lines in (A), and of a skin-coloured structureless pattern in (B). This lesion exhibited asymmetry produced by a small eccentric structureless grey area superiorly, with the additional clue to malignancy of polarising-specific white lines (A), but palpation and lateral compression by squeezing suggested the diagnosis of (asymmetrical) dermatofibroma which was consistent with a history of stability over more than 20 years.*

9.7 Haemangioma and other vascular lesions

Haemangioma is one of the most common lesions encountered on the skin. In a skin cancer-oriented practice it will be seen on the skin of many patients every day. Haemangiomas are benign lesions and most of them are probably not even noticed in the search for malignancies. The archetypal clods-only pattern is one of the four benign vascular patterns in the 'Prediction without Pigment' algorithm[6]. The clods are commonly red and purple and some may be blue. A haemangioma will usually only be examined dermatoscopically if there is some specific cause for concern, such as reported change, bleeding or itch. The presence of any lesional brown colour or polarising-specific white lines are causes for concern and, although very small haemangiomas may

have some small linear vessels, the presence of any linear vessels within blood-coloured clods should lead to excision biopsy[6]. Large haemangiomas may have the clods separated by white fibrous septa projecting as white lines. Dermatoscopic images of a variety of vascular lesions are presented in *Figures 9.145–9.149*.

Another reasonably common vascular lesion is pyogenic granuloma (PG) (*Figures 9.150 and 9.151*). These typically have either a clods-only pattern or a structureless red pattern with white or skin-coloured lines crossing the red structureless pattern[5]. PG are predictably new and changing and therefore should always undergo excision biopsy as EFG lesions and should never have ablative therapy without biopsy[28,29].

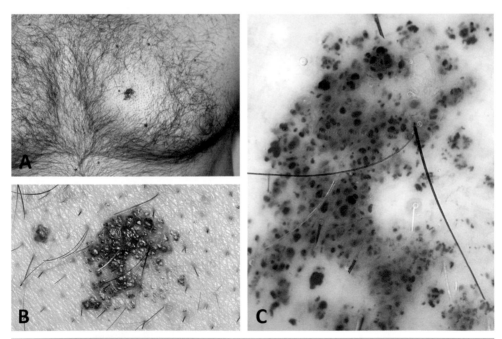

Figure 9.145: *Clinical (A), close-up (B) and dermatoscopic (C) images of a congenital haemangioma exhibiting a dermatoscopic clods-only pattern.*

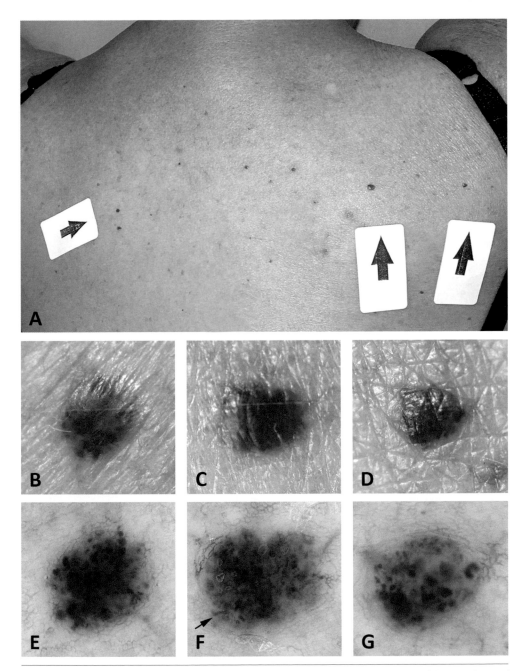

Figure 9.146: *Clinical (A), close-up (B, C and D) and dermatoscopic (E, F and G) images of three archetypal acquired haemangiomas. These three lesions all show variations of a 'clods-only' pattern. Note that some short linear vessels do not change the pattern (arrow F) and may be more numerous in very small haemangiomas, however, any linear vessel within a red clod is not consistent with this benign pattern.*

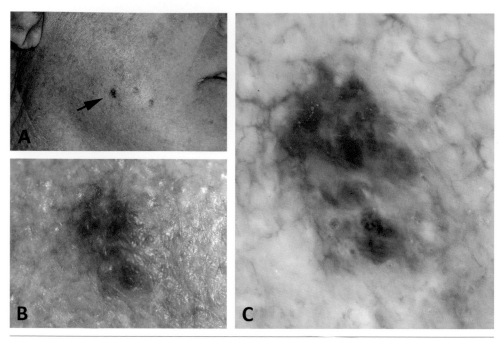

Figure 9.147: *Clinical (A), close-up (B) and dermatoscopic (C) images of a venous lake exhibiting a structureless blue pattern. Blanching of the lesion when compressed, as well as its compressibility, distinguishes it from a blue naevus.*

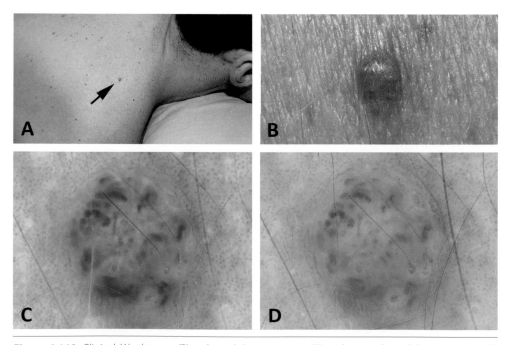

Figure 9.148: *Clinical (A), close-up (B), polarised dermatoscopic (C) and non-polarised dermatoscopic (D) images of a vascular lesion with a sparse clods-only pattern. Some of the clods have a somewhat linear morphology as is not uncommon. Histology revealed that there were acanthotic down-growths of the epidermis separating the vessels, which accounted for the fact that they were dermatoscopically sparse, the lesion being classified as an angiokeratoma.*

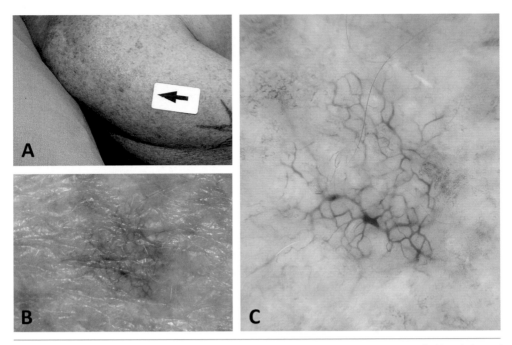

Figure 9.149: *Clinical (A), close-up (B) and dermatoscopic (C) images of a cluster of dilated dermal plexus vessels known as a telangiectasia. The vessel pattern is reticular as is commonly seen on atrophic sun-damaged skin.*

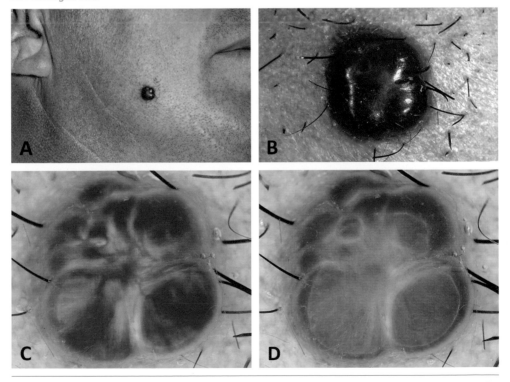

Figure 9.150: *Clinical (A), close-up (B), polarised dermatoscopic (C) and non-polarised dermatoscopic (D) images of a rapidly growing vascular lesion with large red clods separated by white lines evident with both polarised and non-polarised dermatoscopy; pyogenic granuloma.*

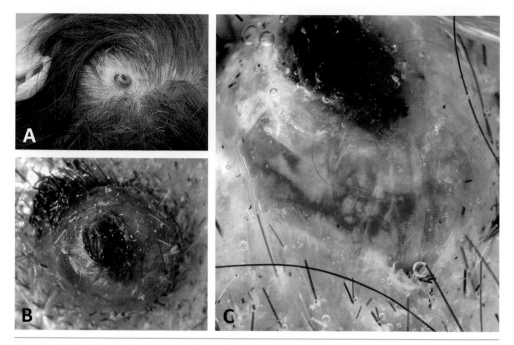

Figure 9.151: *Clinical (A), close-up (B) and dermatoscopic (C) images of a rapidly growing raised non-pigmented lesion which had bled spontaneously. Dermatoscopically there was a polarising-specific white structureless area on a red background and central ulceration; pyogenic granuloma.*

9.8 Merkel cell carcinoma

Merkel cell carcinoma (MCC) is a rare neuroendocrine cell tumour with aggressive behaviour and an unfavourable prognosis. It often responds well to radiotherapy and prompt initiation of that therapy is a priority. MCC typically has a distinctive clinical appearance of a well-defined nodular, shiny red lesion having the clinical appearance of a 'glazed cherry' (*Figure 9.152*)[29]. Dermatoscopically, serpentine vessels are seen poorly defined from surrounding stroma, in contrast to BCC in which the vessels are well defined. In one published series no polarising-specific features were observed[30].

9.9 Atypical fibroxanthoma

Atypical fibroxanthoma is a red tumour of sun-damaged skin only expected at advanced age[5]. Frequently ulcerated, it is characterised by a high degree of vascularity with numerous randomly arranged polymorphous vessels (dot and linear – looped and serpentine) with calibre varying from thin to thick (*Figure 9.153*)[31]. Polarising-specific white lines may obscure the vessels.

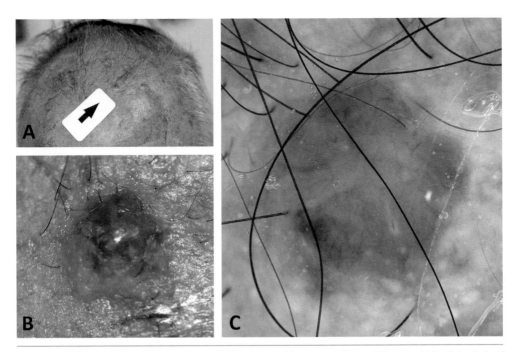

Figure 9.152: *Clinical (A), close-up (B) and dermatoscopic (C) images of a small lesion which clinically had a deep red colour with an apparent collaret (B). Dermatoscopically (C) it was structureless pink with fine serpentine branched vessels, but without the basal cell carcinoma-type stroma to cast the vessels in sharp relief; Merkel cell carcinoma. Reproduced from* Dermatologic Surg, *2009;35:1005[29] with permission from the American Society for Dermatologic Surgery.*

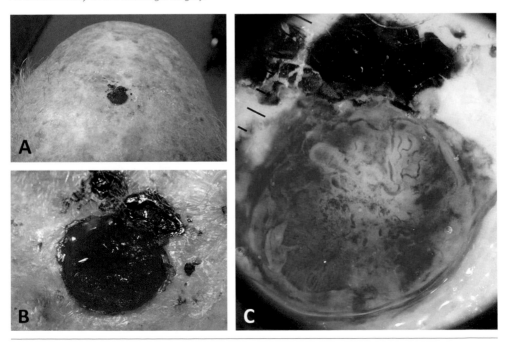

Figure 9.153: *Clinical (A), close-up (B) and dermatoscopic (C) images of a bright red and clinically ulcerated vascular tumour on a severely sun-damaged bald scalp of an elderly man. Dermatoscopically it is red with polymorphous serpentine vessels, fresh blood and adjacent clot; atypical fibroxanthoma.*

9.10 Adnexal tumours

9.10.1 Sebaceous gland hyperplasia

Sebaceous gland hyperplasia is a benign hair follicle tumour most commonly seen on the face at mature age[5]. It is characterised by dermatoscopic dull white, yellow or skin-coloured central clods surrounding a vellus hair follicle which may not be clinically or dermatoscopically evident. Serpentine blood vessels are prominent and this sometimes causes confusion with BCC, but the vessels do not cross the centre and, in the context of prominent but poorly demarcated white, yellow or skin-coloured clods and the absence of BCC-type stroma, the diagnosis should not be a problem (*Figure 9.154*)[32].

9.10.2 Trichoepithelioma

Trichoepithelioma, including desmoplastic trichoepithelioma, is a benign follicular tumour which by virtue of its translucent stroma, fine serpentine vessels and white clods mimics BCC. It may also have dermatoscopic white structureless areas. Clues to the specific diagnosis may include a central dell and numerous dermatoscopic small white clods as well as a history of long-term stability (*Figures 9.155* and *9.156*)[33].

9.10.3 Trichilemmoma

Trichilemmoma is another benign follicular tumour and it has a distinctive dermatoscopic appearance with coiled vessels centrally and coiled/looped vessels in radial arrangement peripherally, in what has been described as the 'iris' sign (*Figure 9.157*)[34].

9.10.4 Cysts – trichilemmal (pilar) cyst/wen and epidermal cyst

Trichilemmal cyst typically presents as a large, soft, fleshy raised lesion. Dermatoscopically it is likely to have a structureless skin-coloured

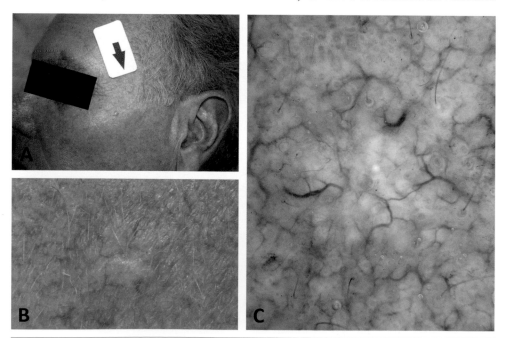

Figure 9.154: Clinical (A), close-up (B) and dermatoscopic (C) images of sebaceous gland hyperplasia presenting as a non-pigmented lesion with the very characteristic dermatoscopic morphology of skin-coloured and white clods with linear serpentine vessels which do not cross the centre of the lesion.

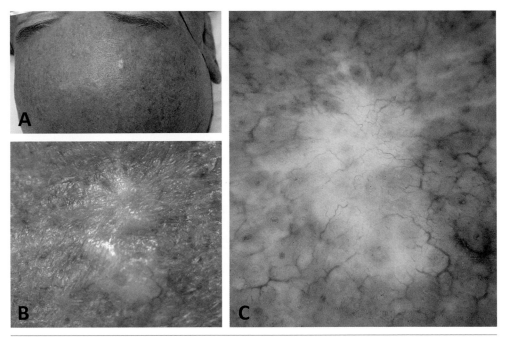

Figure 9.155: *Clinical (A), close-up (B) and dermatoscopic (C) images of a trichoepithelioma presenting as a non-pigmented lesion with a shiny surface (A, B) and with a dermatoscopic white structureless area with fine serpentine branched vessels.*

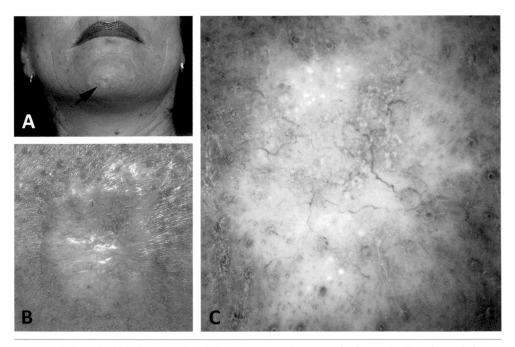

Figure 9.156: *Clinical (A), close-up (B) and dermatoscopic (C) images of a desmoplastic trichoepithelioma. Clinically (A and B) there is a well circumscribed non-pigmented lesion with loss of normal skin markings and a central dell (depression) which is characterised dermatoscopically by multiple white dots and clods with fine serpentine branched vessels.*

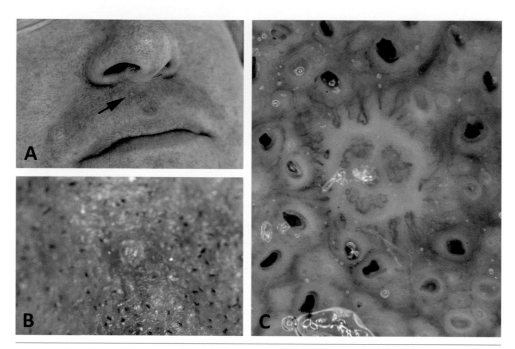

Figure 9.157: *Clinical (A), close-up (B) and dermatoscopic (C) images of a trichilemmoma, presenting as a non-pigmented lesion characterised dermatoscopically by a central white structureless area with coiled vessels surrounded by radially arranged looped vessels as well as some white circles.*

morphology with poorly defined serpentine vessels of the dermal plexus[35].

Epidermal cysts have a very characteristic appearance of a white raised lesion with a smooth contour, which may exhibit dermatoscopic branched serpentine vessels of the outwardly displaced dermal vascular plexus (*Figure 9.158*).

9.10.5 Pilomatrixoma

This presents at any age, including childhood, typically as a solitary firm (hard) lesion with a structureless white and blue zone, blue, if present, being due to haemorrhage. Vessels are serpentine (*Figure 9.159*)[36].

9.10.6 Eccrine poroma

Eccrine poroma, a benign tumour of the sweat gland duct may have a polymorphous vessel pattern including thin serpentine, coiled and branched vessels (*Figure 9.160*). It may resemble BCC but frequently occurs on non-sun-dam-aged skin, especially in a volar location on the palms and soles where BCC is not expected[37].

9.10.7 Sebaceous adenoma and carcinoma

Sebaceous adenoma and carcinoma are rare tumours of sebaceous glands which may occur in syndromes that are also character-ised by internal malignancies (Muir–Torre and Lynch syndrome).

Sebaceous adenomas appear as yellow papules most commonly encountered on the face, scalp and eyelids. Dermatoscopically, sebaceous adenoma has been depicted as a non-pigmented raised tumour with yellow clods on a pink background with looped vessels at the periphery (*Figure 9.161*)[38].

Sebaceous carcinoma most commonly appears as a firm yellow nodule on the eyelids which is often ulcerated. It has a high risk of metastasis. Dermatoscopically, it is charac-terised by polymorphous vessels on a yellow background[39].

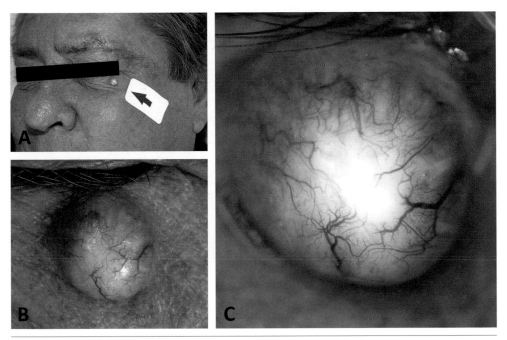

Figure 9.158: *Clinical (A), close-up (B) and dermatoscopic (C) images of an epidermal cyst presenting as a raised non-pigmented white structureless lesion with dermatoscopic branched serpentine vessels.*

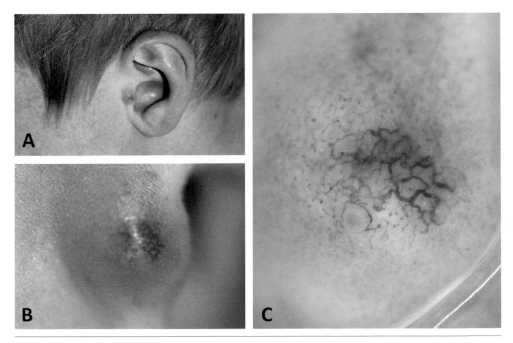

Figure 9.159: *Clinical (A), close-up (B) and dermatoscopic (C) images of a pilomatrixoma on the tragus of a child which presents as a raised non-pigmented lesion with a dermatoscopic orange clod, dilated branched serpentine vessels centrally and dot vessels peripherally.*

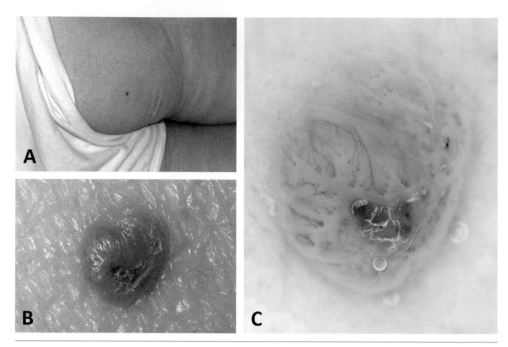

Figure 9.160: *Clinical (A), close-up (B) and dermatoscopic (C) images of an eccrine poroma, a non-pigmented lesion on non-sun-damaged skin with ulceration and dermatoscopic thin serpentine, coiled and branched vessels with a characteristic morphology including terminal loops.*

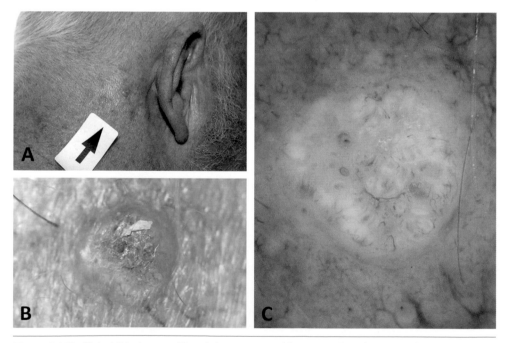

Figure 9.161: *Clinical (A), close-up (B) and dermatoscopic (C) images of a sebaceous adenoma exhibiting dermatoscopic white and yellow clods as well as white and yellow structureless areas with a few fine linear (curved and serpentine) vessels.*

Neurofibroma

This benign tumour is commonly mistaken for a dermal naevus, being raised and soft with a wrinkled appearance to the overlying epidermis. Dermatoscopically, it presents as

a raised, skin-coloured lesion with very fine serpentine branched vessels without any evidence of BCC-type stroma (*Figure 9.162*)[40].

9.12 Molluscum contagiosum

Molluscum contagiosum, a viral lesion, is normally diagnosed clinically without difficulty and is only likely to be a diagnostic issue when presenting as a solitary and large lesion. Dermatoscopically, it typically displays

radial vessels with a central white, orange or skin-coloured clod or with several of such clods (*Figure 9.163*).

9.13 Cutaneous lymphoma

Cutaneous T-cell lymphoma (mycosis fungoides) can present as a lesion with surface scale mimicking psoriasis, parap-

soriasis, eczema, photodermatitis, drug reactions, etc.

When compared to chronic dermatitis in

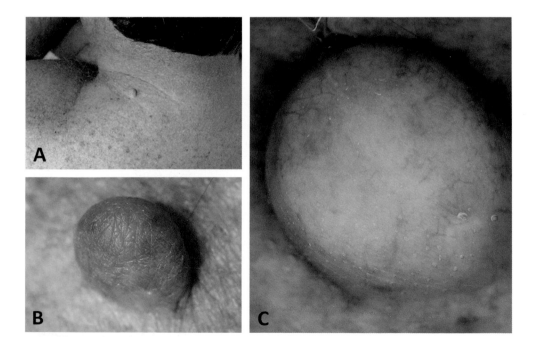

Figure 9.162: *Clinical (A), close-up (B) and dermatoscopic (C) images of a neurofibroma. These lesions have a very characteristic skin-coloured polypoid clinical appearance (B) often with evident unaltered skin markings. Dermatoscopically, the lesions are skin-coloured (whiter if blanched by footplate pressure) with vessels with the calibre and pattern of the normal dermal plexus.*

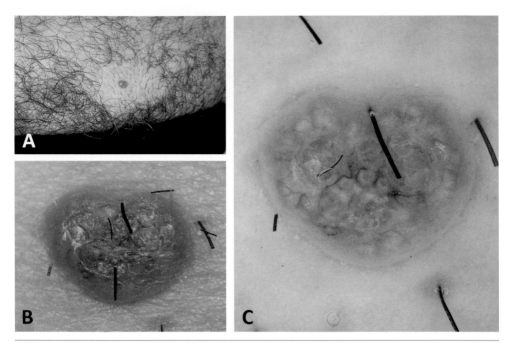

Figure 9.163: *Clinical (A), close-up (B) and dermatoscopic (C) images of an isolated lesion of molluscum contagiosum. Dermatoscopically, it exhibits central orange clods as well as white clods and circles. The vessels are linear serpentine, not being in the expected radial arrangement. Due to diagnostic uncertainty excision biopsy was performed.*

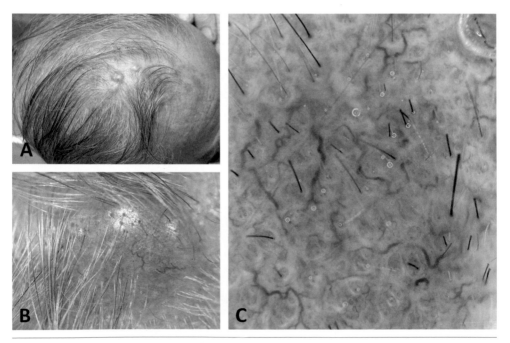

Figure 9.164: *Clinical (A), close-up (B) and dermatoscopic (C) images of one of several raised non-pigmented skin-coloured lesions on the scalp with a vascular pattern consistent with dilated vessels of the dermal plexus. The individual lesions are poorly demarcated. Biopsy revealed T-cell lymphoma.*

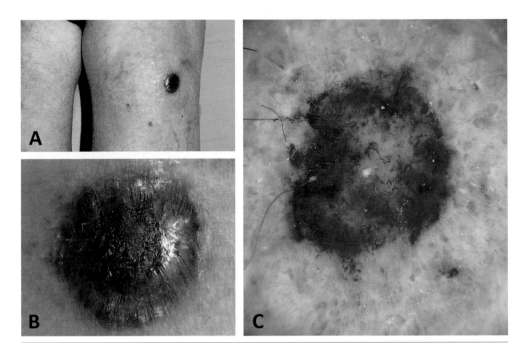

Figure 9.165: *Clinical (A), close-up (B) and dermatoscopic (C) images of a raised non-pigmented ulcerated purple lesion on the popliteal fossa of the same patient as shown in* Figure 9.164. *Dermatoscopically, the lesion is structureless red with fine polymorphous linear vessels; T-cell lymphoma.*

one study, mycosis fungoides lesions exhibited a characteristic dermatoscopic pattern consisting of fine short linear vessels and orange–yellowish patchy areas. A characteristic vascular structure resembling spermatozoa was also found to be highly specific for the diagnosis of mycosis fungoides. In contrast, chronic dermatitis was typified by a different dermatoscopic pattern, usually consisting of dotted vessels[41].

Two examples of cutaneous T-cell lymphoma are shown in *Figures 9.164* and *9.165.*

9.14 Kaposi sarcoma

Kaposi sarcoma is a herpes virus-associated condition that may occur as single or multiple purple-coloured skin lesions. There are several subtypes, one of which is HIV-associated.

Examination with polarised dermatoscopy typically reveals multicoloured areas showing various colours of the rainbow spectrum. This so-called 'rainbow pattern' was found in six out of seven patients with Kaposi sarcoma and was not observed in other vascular tumours. In addition, in the majority of Kaposi sarcoma lesions, there was an absence of dermatoscopic features specific for other vascular and non-vascular skin tumours, such as well-defined red clods or a structured vascular pattern[42].

An example of a lesion of Kaposi sarcoma is shown in *Figure 9.166.*

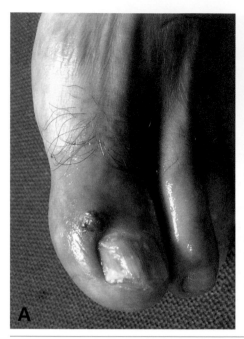
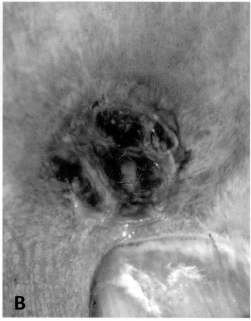

Figure 9.166: Clinical (A) and dermatoscopic (B) images of a lesion of Kaposi sarcoma with the clinical presentation of a purple nodule and with dermatoscopy exhibiting red, white and blue merging colours as well as linear serpentine vessels. Image courtesy Professor Nisa Akay.

References

1. Bourne P, Rosendahl C, Keir J, and Cameron A. BLINCK—A diagnostic algorithm for skin cancer diagnosis combining clinical features with dermatoscopy findings. *Dermatol Pract Concept*, 2012;2(2):12.

2. Braun RP, Baran R, Le Gal FA, *et al*. Diagnosis and management of nail pigmentations. *J Am Acad Dermatol*, 2007;56:835.

3. Rtshiladze M, Stretch J, Stewart D, and Saw R. Pigmented lesions of the nail bed – Clinical assessment and biopsy. *Aust Fam Physician*, 2016;45:810.

4. Weedon D, Van Deurse M, and Rosendahl C. "Occult" melanocytes in nail matrix melanoma. *Am J Dermatopathol*, 2012;34:855.

5. Kittler H, Rosendahl C, Cameron A, and Tschandl P. *Dermatoscopy*, 2nd Edition, 2016. Facultas.

6. https://dermoscopedia.org [accessed 26 August 2022].

7. Kittler H, and Tschandl P. Dysplastic nevus: why this term should be abandoned in dermatoscopy. *Dermatologic Clinics,* 2013;31:579.

8. Gandini S, Sera F, Cattaruzza MS, *et al*. Meta-analysis of risk factors for cutaneous melanoma: common and atypical nevi. *Eur J Cancer*, 2005;41:28.

9. Lin WMMD, Luo SMD, Muzikansky AMA, *et al*. Outcome of patients with *de novo* versus nevus-associated melanoma. *J Am Acad Dermatol*, 2014;72:54.

10. Pampena R, Kyrgidis A, Lallas A, Moscarella E, Argenziano G, and Longo C. A meta-analysis of nevus-associated melanoma: prevalence and practical implications. *J Am Acad Dermatol*, 2017;77:938.e4.

11. Elmore JG, Barnhill RL, Elder DE, *et al*. Pathologists' diagnosis of invasive melanoma and melanocytic proliferations: observer accuracy and reproducibility study. *BMJ*, 2017;357:j28139.

12. Gelbard SN, Tripp JM, Marghoob AA, *et al*. Management of Spitz nevi: a survey of dermatologists in the United States. *J Am Acad Dermatol*, 2002;47:224.

13. Miyazaki A, Saida T, Koga H, Oguchi S, Suzuki T, and Tsuchida T. Anatomical and histopathological correlates of the dermoscopic patterns seen in melanocytic nevi on the sole: A retrospective study. *J Am Acad Dermatol*, 2005;53:230.

14. Rosendahl C, Cameron A, Tschandl P, Bulinska A, Zalaudek I, and Kittler H. Prediction without Pigment: a decision algorithm for non-pigmented skin malignancy. *Dermatol Pract Concept*, 2014;4(1):9.

15. Caresana G, and Giardini R. Dermoscopy-guided surgery in basal cell carcinoma. *J Eur Acad Dermatol Venereol*, 2010;24:1395.

16. Rosendahl C, Cameron A, McColl I, and Wilkinson D. Dermatoscopy in routine practice – "Chaos and Clues." *Aust Fam Physician*, 2012;41:482.

17. Orpin SD, Preston PW, and Salim A. "The 'St. Tropez' sign; a new dermoscopic feature of seborrhoeic keratoses?" *Clin Exp Dermatol*, 2006;31:707.

18. Rizk M, Alian M, Tschandl P, *et al*. A prospective diagnostic study on povidone-iodine retention in lesions suspected to be squamous cell carcinoma or keratoacanthoma. *Aust J Dermatol*, 2019;60:in press (DOI https://doi.org/10.1111/ajd.12897).

19. Cameron A, Rosendahl C, Tschandl P, Riedl E, and Kittler H. Dermatoscopy of pigmented Bowen's disease. *J Am Acad Dermatol*, 2010;62:597.

20. Zalaudek I, Cota C, Ferrara G, *et al*. Flat pigmented macules on sun-damaged skin of the head/neck: junctional nevus, atypical lentiginous nevus, or melanoma in situ? *Clin Dermatol*, 2014;32:88.

21. Tschandl P, Rosendahl C, and Kittler H. Dermatoscopy of flat pigmented facial lesions. *J Eur Acad Dermatol Venereol*, 2015;29:120.

22. Akay BN, Kocyigit P, Heper AO, and Erdem C. Dermatoscopy of flat pigmented facial lesions: diagnostic challenge between pigmented actinic keratosis and lentigo maligna. *Br J Dermatol*, 2010;163:1212.

23. Lallas A, Tschandl P, Kyrgidis A, *et al*. Dermoscopic clues to differentiate facial lentigo maligna from pigmented actinic keratosis. *Br J Dermatol*, 2016;174:1079.

24. Rosendahl C, Cameron A, Argenziano G, Zalaudek I, Tschandl P, and Kittler H. Dermoscopy of squamous cell carcinoma and keratoacanthoma. *Arch Dermatol*, 2012;148:1386.

25. Rosendahl C, Cameron A, Bulinska A, and Weedon D. Cutaneous pigmented invasive squamous cell carcinoma: a case report with dermatoscopy and histology. *Dermatol Pract Concept*, 2011;1(1):14.

26. Lallas A, Pyne J, Kyrgidis A, *et al*. The clinical and dermoscopic features of invasive cutaneous squamous cell carcinoma depend on the histopathological grade of differentiation. *Br J Dermatol*, 2015;172:1308.

27. Bernard J, Poulalhon N, Argenziano G, Debarbieux S, Dalle S, and Thomas L. Dermoscopy of dermatofibrosarcoma protuberans: a study of 15 cases. *Br J Dermatol*, 2013;169:85.

28. Chamberlain AJ, Fritschi L, and Kelly JW. Nodular melanoma: patients' perceptions of presenting features and implications for earlier detection. *J Am Acad Dermatol*, 2003;48:694.

29. Rosendahl C, Cameron A, and Zalaudek I. Risk of ablative therapy for 'elevated firm growing' lesions: Merkel cell carcinoma diagnosed after laser surgical therapy. *Dermatologic Surg*, 2009;35:1005.

30. Jalilian C, Chamberlain AJ, Haskett M, *et al*. Clinical and dermoscopic characteristics of Merkel cell carcinoma. *Br J Dermatol*, 2013;169:294.

31. Bugatti L, and Filosa G. Dermatoscopic features of cutaneous atypical fibroxanthoma: three cases. *Clin Exp Dermatol*, 2009;34:e898.

32. Zaballos P, Ara M, Puig S, and Malvehy J. Dermoscopy of sebaceous hyperplasia. *Arch Dermatol*, 2005;141:808.

33. Khelifa E, Masouyé I, Kaya G, and Le Gal F-A. Dermoscopy of desmoplastic

trichoepithelioma reveals other criteria to distinguish it from basal cell carcinoma. *Dermatology,* 2013;226:101.

34. Horcajada-Reales C, Avilés-Izquierdo JA, Ciudad-Blanco C, *et al.* Dermoscopic pattern in facial trichilemmomas: Red iris-like structure. *J Am Acad Dermatol,* 2015;72(1 Suppl):S30.

35. Gencoglan G, Karaarslan IK, Akalin T, and Ozdemir F. Trichilemmal cyst with homogeneous blue pigmentation on dermoscopy. *Aust J Dermatol,* 2009;50:301.

36. Zaballos P, Llambrich A, Puig S, and Malvehy J. Dermoscopic findings of pilomatricomas. *Dermatology*, 2008;217:225.

37. Ferrari A, Buccini P, Silipo V, *et al.* Eccrine poroma: a clinical-dermoscopic study of seven cases. *Acta Derm Venereol*, 2009;89:160.

38. Marques-da-Costa J, Campos-do-Carmo G, Ormiga P, Ishida C, Cuzzi T, and Ramos-e-Silva M. Sebaceous adenoma: clinics, dermatoscopy, and histopathology. *Int J Dermatol,* 2015;54:e200.

39. Satomura H, Ogata D, Arai E, and Tsuchida T. Dermoscopic features of ocular and extraocular sebaceous carcinomas. *J Dermatol,* 2017;44:1313.

40. www.dermnetnz.org/cme/dermoscopy-course/dermoscopy-of-other-non-melanocytic-lesions/ [accessed 5 February 2018].

41. Lallas A, Apalla Z, Lefaki I, *et al.* Dermoscopy of early stage mycosis fungoides. *J Eur Acad Dermatol Venereol*, 2013;27:617.

42. Hu SC-S, Ke C-LK, Lee C-H, Wu C-S, Chen G-S, and Cheng S-T. Dermoscopy of Kaposi's sarcoma: areas exhibiting the multicoloured "rainbow pattern." *J Eur Acad Dermatol Venereol*, 2009;23:1128.

Index

f after a page number means the entry appears in a figure